L. G. KEMPE · OPERATIVE NEUROSURGERY

OPERATIVE NEUROSURGERY

Volume 2

Posterior Fossa, Spinal Cord, and Peripheral Nerve Disease

By

Ludwig G. Kempe

Col., M.C., U.S.A.

Fourth Printing

With 290 Partly Colored Figures

Springer-Verlag

Berlin · Heidelberg · NewYork · Tokyo

LUDWIG G. KEMPE, Col., M.C., U.S.A.

Chief, Neurosurgery Service
Walter Reed General Hospital
Washington, D.C.

Consultant in Neurosurgery to
The Surgeon General, U.S. Army

Associate Clin. Professor in Neurosurgery
George Washington University
Washington, D.C.

First printing 1970
Second printing 1975
Third printing 1981
Fourth printing 1986

ISBN 3-540-04890-1 Springer-Verlag Berlin Heidelberg New York
ISBN 0-387-04890-1 Springer-Verlag New York Heidelberg Berlin

Typesetting, printing, and bookbinding: Universitätsdruckerei H. Stürtz AG, Würzburg

2122/3130-54

Preface

Operative Neurosurgery, Volume II, presents the major neurosurgical procedures involving the posterior fossa, spinal cord and peripheral nerves. As in Volume I, the text describes and the figures illustrate the step-by-step surgical technique. Emphasis is placed on anatomical topographic views of the operative exposure as seen by the surgeon. The contents have been arranged on the basis of anatomical location rather than etiology.

Although this book is primarily based on the experience of the neurosurgical service at Walter Reed General Hospital, its content reflects only the views of the author and does not proport to reflect any official position of the Department of the Army or the Department of Defense.

Volume II is available at this time because of the tireless efforts of my associate, Major GARY D. VANDERARK, Assistant Chief of Neurosurgery Service, Walter Reed General Hospital. His critical review and support in every aspect of this work are gratefully acknowledged.

I also wish to thank Mr. HANS BRANDT of Heidelberg, Germany, who again has demonstrated his great talent in medical artistry. His enduring enthusiasm has also shortened the length of time necessary to prepare this volume.

Throughout my military surgical career and especially in the preparation of this work, I have received the unceasing support and encouragement of Lt. Gen. LEONARD D. HEATON, Surgeon General of the U.S. Army. My thanks are extended to this master teacher and surgeon.

I am most grateful for the patience and understanding of my wife, CZENTA, for toleration through the many years necessary to prepare this manuscript.

Dr. HEINZ GOETZE of Springer-Verlag has been a wise and helpful counsellor in the preparation and publication of this book.

Washington, January, 1970 L. G. KEMPE

Table of Contents — Volume 2

Table of Contents — Volume 1
Cranial, Cerebral, and Intracranial Vascular Disease

Chapter I

Suboccipital Craniectomy — Horseshoe Incision

Posterior Fossa Exploration

Except in infants, the sitting position is used most commonly in surgery of the posterior fossa. Certain precautions must be taken when using this position because of the danger of air embolism. The lower extremities must be wrapped with elastic bandages and elevated. An inflatable wrapping below the level of the diaphragm is an effective means of increasing the venous pressure thereby preventing air embolism. Bone wax must be used generously. Cut bone margins should be coated with wax even when not bleeding. Air emboli can be detected by an ultrasonic detector placed over the neck, blood gas analysis and/or by a stethoscope placed over the precordium. Treatment must be rapidly carried out. The patient's head must be lowered, and the embolus aspirated via a catheter previously placed in the right atrium.

Proper position of the head is also crucial in the sitting position. As illustrated in Fig. 1a and b, the head should not be flexed to the degree that venous drainage is obstructed. After positioning the head properly, the entire table is then tilted forward as shown in Fig. 1c.

The height of the table is very important. A common mistake is made in keeping the table too low with the result that the surgeon goes through back-breaking contortions especially in exposure of the cerebropontile angle and tentorial incisura. The author has observed that the most comfortable height is achieved when the posterior rim of the foramen magnum is at the level of the surgeon's eyes. The arms will not tire at this level because the elbows can be rested on the back support of the operating table.

Controlled respiration with a negative pressure phase is contraindicated. In any posterior fossa surgery the patient should trigger his own respiration. The form, frequency and volume of respiration is the most sensitive indicator of brain stem function while working in the posterior fossa with the patient under general anesthesia.

The patient's head must be draped in such a way that the occipital region as well as the suboccipital and cervical areas are exposed. It is wise to place a right occipital burr hole 4 cm. lateral to the midline 6-8 cm. above the external occipital protuberance (Fig. 2) so that the lateral ventricle can be tapped at any time during the procedure. When the suboccipital dura is tense, the lateral ventricle should be vented before proceeding any further.

The horseshoe incision is not used as frequently as it once was, but there are still indications for this approach. It is especially useful in patients who have been previously irradiated in this area. In these patients a midline incision may heal slowly or even lead to a postoperative false meningocele.

The incision is made from mastoid tip to mastoid tip in an arch which curves upward 2 cm. above the external occipital protuberance (Fig. 2). The skin incision is carried down to the pericranium which is not incised at this level. Hemostasis is attained using Rainey clips. The skin flap is retracted downward (Fig. 2) to expose the superior nuchal line. The trapezius, splenius capitis and semispinalis capitis muscles are then incised transversely a short distance below their insertion so that a good closure of this muscle layer can be obtained later. These muscles are stripped from the occipital squama with a periosteal elevator down to the posterior rim of the foramen magnum and laterally to the level of the mastoid processes. The mastoid emissary veins will be encountered laterally and generous amounts of bone wax should be used to plug any bony venous channels. The arch of the atlas is palpated with an index finger to ascertain the level of the foramen magnum. In stripping the muscles from the suboccipital region, pressure in this area must be avoided. The rectus capitis posterior major and minor muscles are stripped from their insertion at the inferior nuchal line. The origin of the rectus capitis posterior minor muscle from the arch of the atlas should be removed by sharp dissection. The periosteum of the arch of the atlas is incised in the midline and then stripped laterally (Figs. 3 and 18). The dense fibrous tissue in the deep suboccipital triangle can best be stripped laterally by grasping the muscle fibers and fibrous tissue with a pair of forceps and using a slightly opened straight scissors (Fig. 17). The position of the vertebral artery laterally must be kept in mind during this maneuver. Spring retractors are inserted to maintain the exposure thus gained.

The arch of the atlas is removed in all midline exposures using a sharp Kerrison rongeur. Multiple burr holes are placed in the exposed suboccipital bone and the intervening bone is removed by rongeurs. The bone must be removed superiorly until the transverse sinus comes into view for maximal exposure and so that the bridging cerebellar veins can be dealt with if necessary. If the dura remains tense even after cannulating a lateral ventricle and draining off the cerebrospinal fluid, an exploring needle should be passed into each cerebellar hemisphere in search of a cyst which can be aspirated.

The dura is opened with a *Y*-shaped incision (Figs. 4 and 20) which crosses the marginal sinus and not the occipital sinus. Because the occipital sinus is located immediately over the falx cerebelli it is not as easily clipped as the marginal sinus. The dura is reflected superiorly and laterally. The cerebellar hemispheres, vermis and tonsils can be inspected through the intact arachnoid. Any deviation from the midline, discoloration or asymmetry is noted. Almost invariably the tonsil will be lowest on the side of the cerebellar hemisphere containing a mass lesion. Symmetry, folial pattern and vascularity of the hemispheres are observed. The arachnoid over the cisterna magna is opened and cerebrospinal fluid escapes. This usually makes the pulsation of the intracranial structures much more obvious. The anesthetist is informed of the change in intracranial dynamics and reminded that from this point any change in the patient's vital signs must be reported immediately.

The cerebellar hemispheres are then gently palpated. An underlying cyst will give a boggy feeling; whereas, a solid tumor may make the cerebellum feel firmer than the other hemisphere.

If no abnormality is apparent at this point, the tonsils should be carefully separated to visualize the posterior end of the fourth ventricle.

A word is in order at this point with regard to the use of retraction in the posterior fossa. This area, even more than other intracranial compartments, does not tolerate faulty insertion or application of instruments without disastrous sequelae. As in the above mentioned exposure of the foramen of Magendie, the surgeon guides and holds the retractors on each side of the vallecula. When a retractor is held by an assistant he must be able to see what he is retracting. The position of a retractor is the responsibility of the surgeon even when he is not holding it; and, if it is incorrectly positioned, he must replace it. Tilting of a retractor is particularly hazardous. Even when retracting a cerebellar hemisphere, tilting can cause bleeding deep between the folia which can be difficult to localize and disastrous for the patient.

Having explored the distal fourth ventricle and still not discovering the pathology, the next step in a posterior fossa exploration is to split the vermis in the midline posteriorly (Fig. 6). Gentle retraction laterally then allows complete inspection of the remainder of the fourth ventricle up to the anterior medullary velum and distal aqueduct. Hemispheric tumors usually cause a deformity of the ventricular wall on the side of the lesion.

If a deep hemispheric tumor is suspected, an exploring needle is inserted (Figs. 8 and 9) into the center of the inferior surface of each cerebellar hemisphere. The needle must be directed superior to the brain stem and lateral to the dentate nucleus (Fig. 9).

Attention is finally turned to the extra axial subarachnoid space. The lateral recess of the medullary cistern and the posterior portion of the cerebellopontine angle are inspected. The ease of this exposure is directly related to the width of the craniectomy exposure at the posterior rim of foramen magnum. Once again the position of the brain spatula and direction of retraction are important. Compare these two essential elements in Fig. 10, where the posterior portion of the cerebellopontine angle is exposed, and Fig. 11 in which the anterior portion of the cerebellopontine angle is seen.

At the termination of any posterior fossa craniectomy in the sitting position, the anesthetist should be asked to compress the jugular veins so that hemostasis can be checked. If a tumor is totally removed and no swelling is present, the dura is closed. If only an incomplete excision is accomplished and decompression is required, the dura is not re-approximated; but a thin absorbable gelatin sponge is tucked inside the dural opening. When the lateral ventricle has been cannulated, the need for continued ventricular drainage must be considered. Usually the catheter is kept in place for at least 24 to 48 hours.

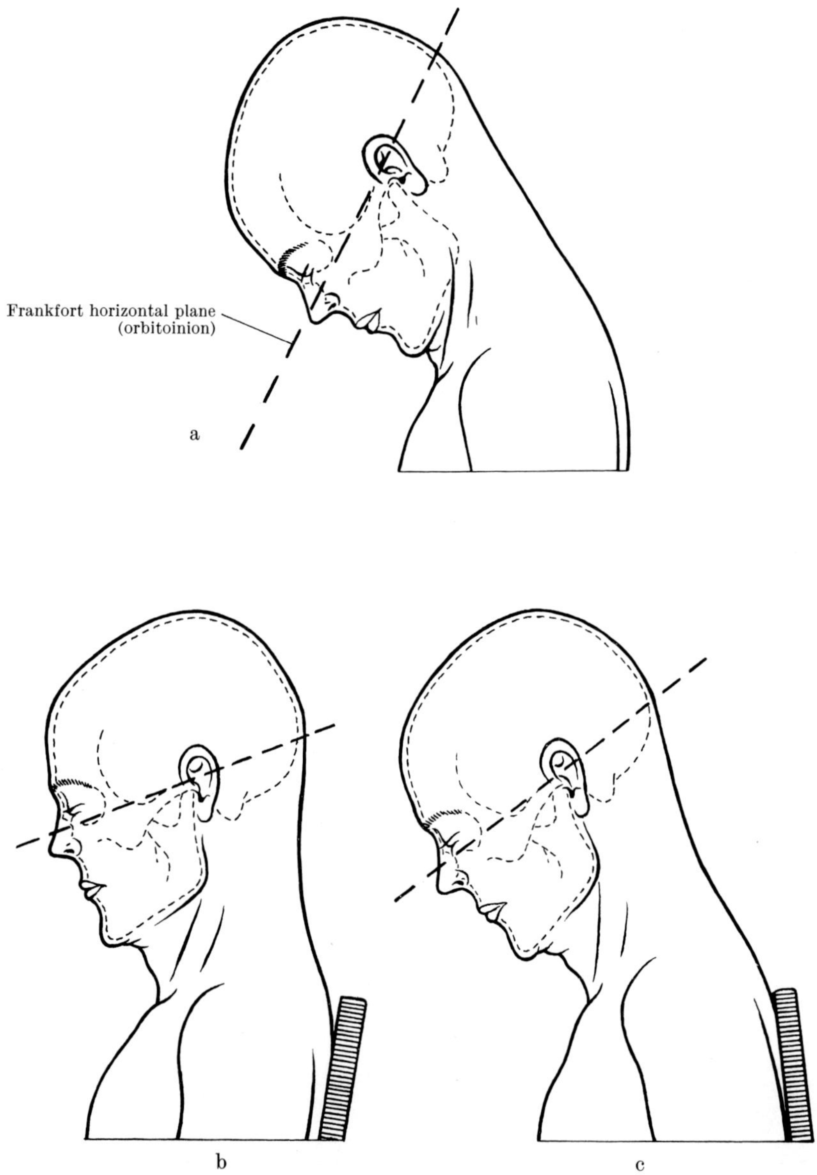

Fig. 1. Suboccipital craniectomy: Sitting position for posterior fossa surgery.
Observe: a The head is flexed too far forward causing venous obstruction. b Correct position. c The degree of flexion is the same as in b but the entire operating table has been tilted forward giving the final optimal position.

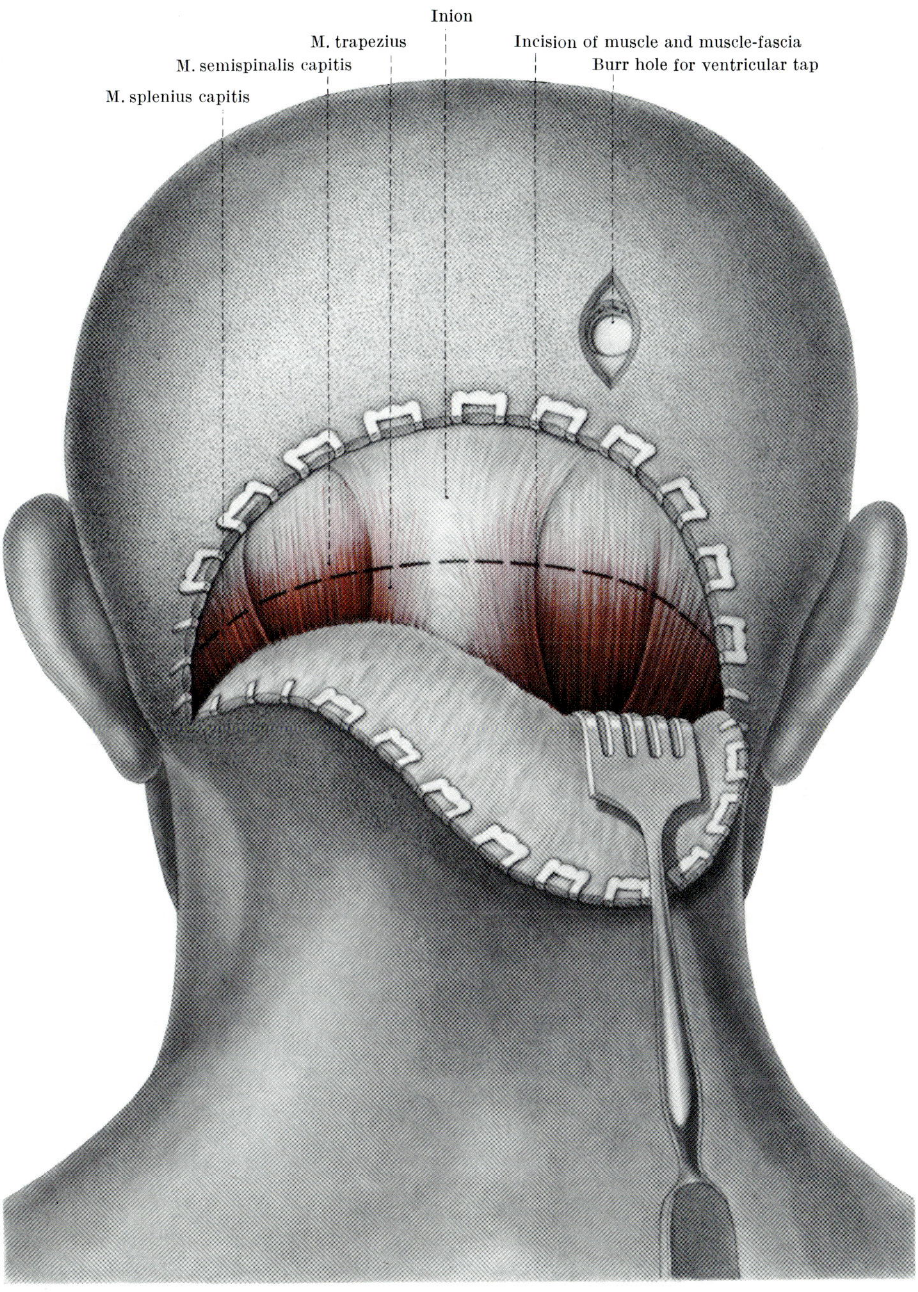

Fig. 2. Suboccipital craniectomy: Horseshoe incision for posterior fossa surgery.

Observe: 1. Occipital burr hole for possible ventricular drainage. 2. Line of incision of muscle and fascia below their insertion to facilitate closure.

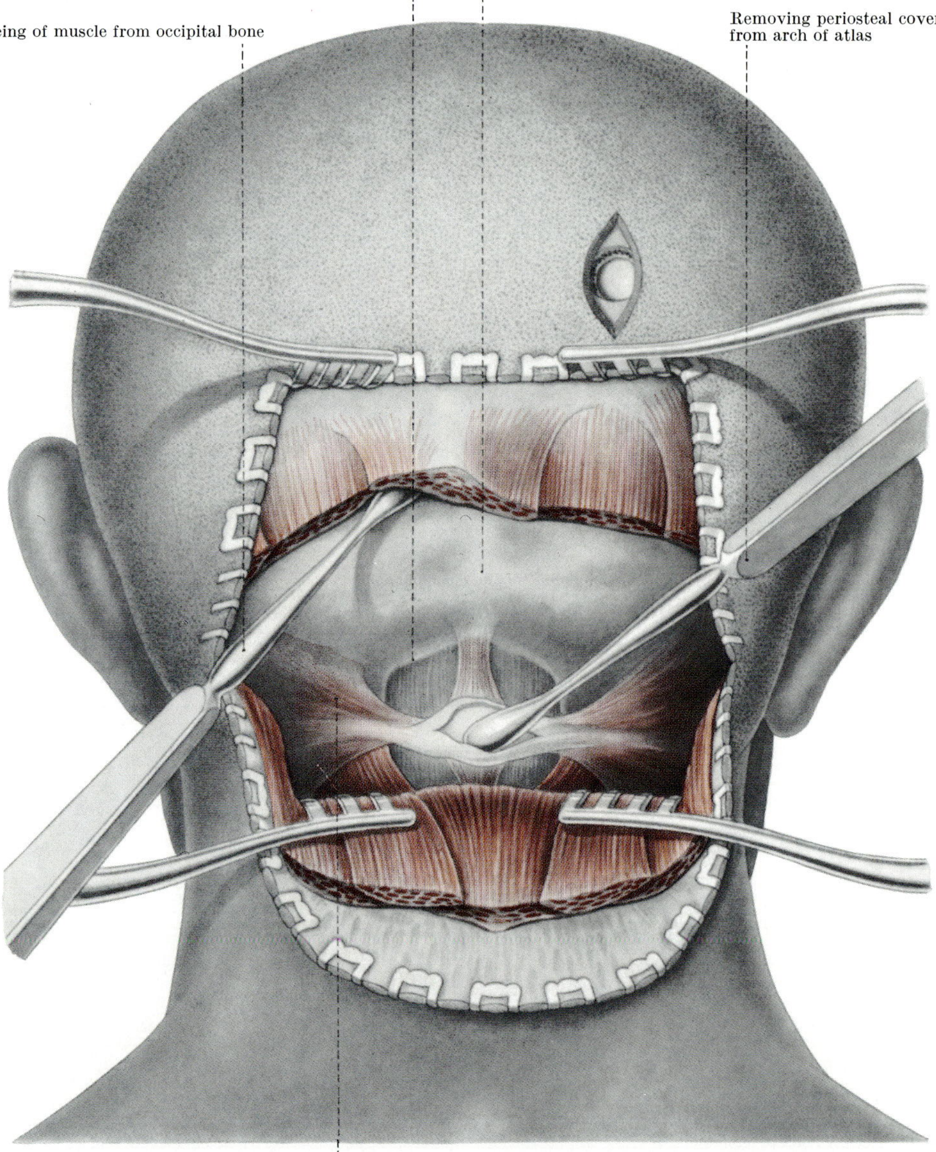

Fig. 3. Suboccipital craniectomy: Exposure of suboccipital squama and arch of atlas.

Observe: 1. Subperiosteal dissection of arch of atlas prior to removal of the arch. 2. Subperiosteal stripping to the superior nuchal line.

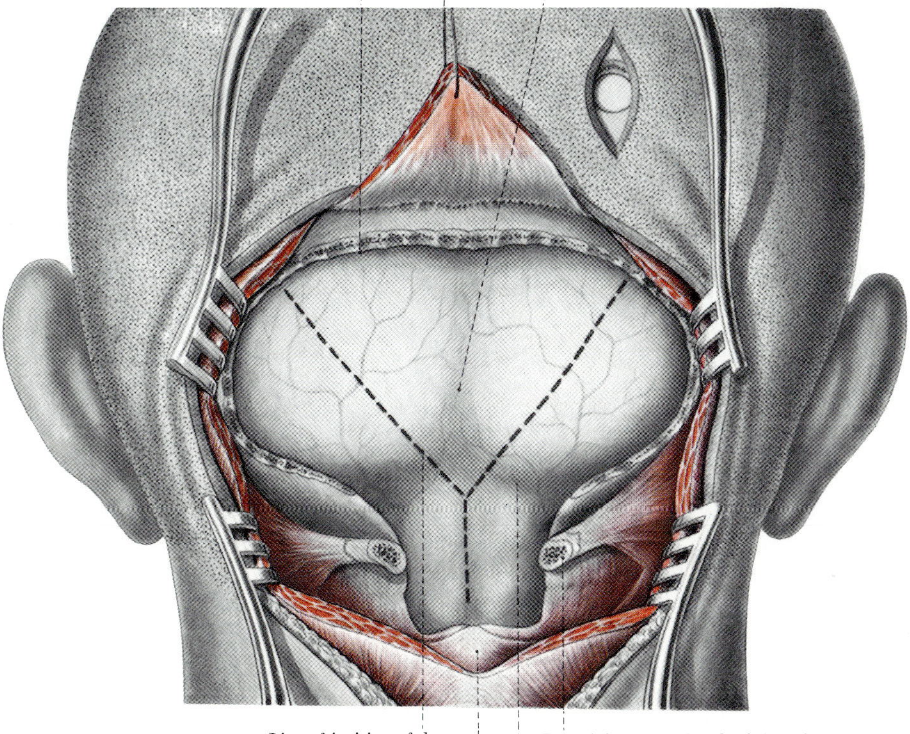

Fig. 4. Suboccipital craniectomy: Dural incision.

Observe: 1. Extent of craniectomy to level of transverse sinus for control of bridging veins. 2. *Y*-shaped dural incision avoids opening of occipital sinus: only the marginal sinus at the level of the foramen magnum will be transversed.

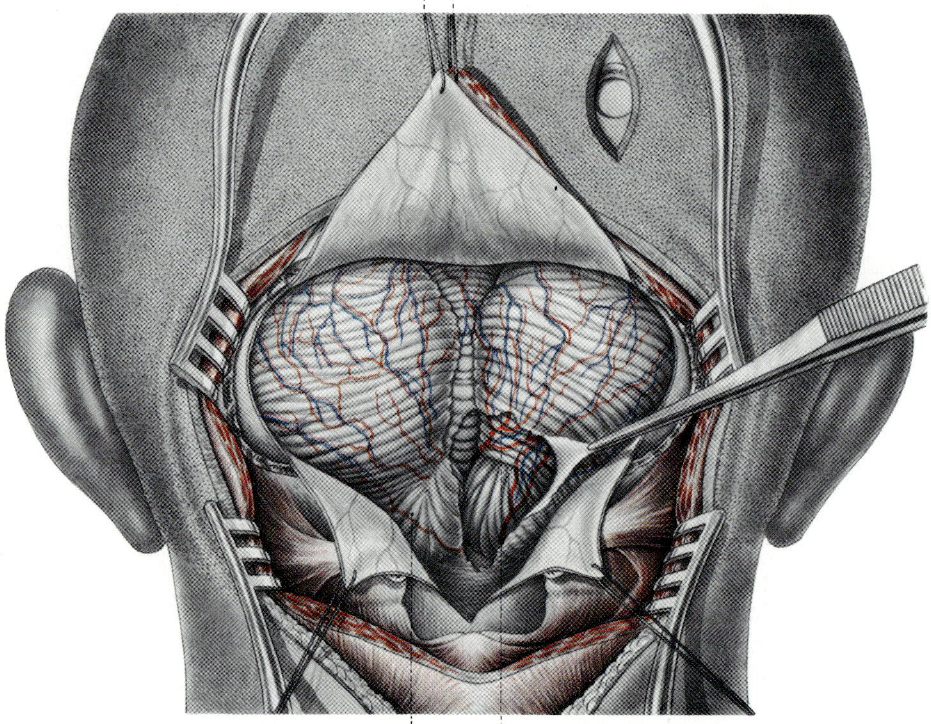

Fig. 5. Suboccipital craniectomy: Operative exposure of cerebellum.
Observe: 1. Retraction of dura by sutures. 2. Opening of arachnoid over cisterna magna.

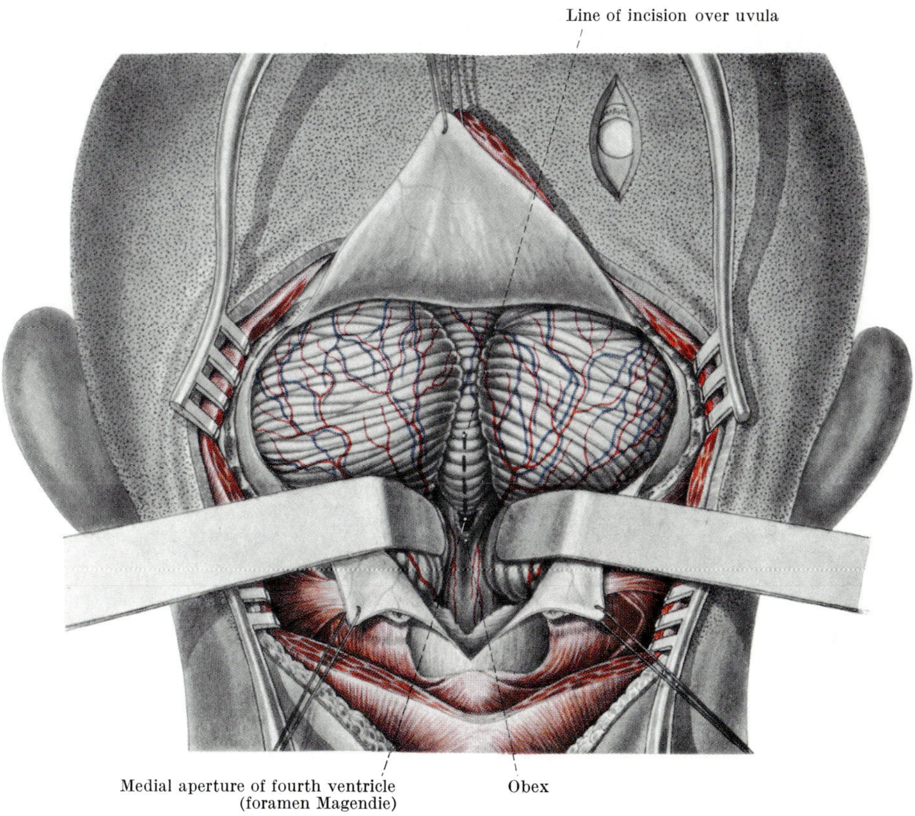

Fig. 6. Suboccipital craniectomy: Posterior fossa exploration.

Observe: 1. Cerebellar tonsils retracted laterally to expose the obex and the foramen Magendie.
2. Extent of vermal incision necessary to inspect the fourth ventricle.

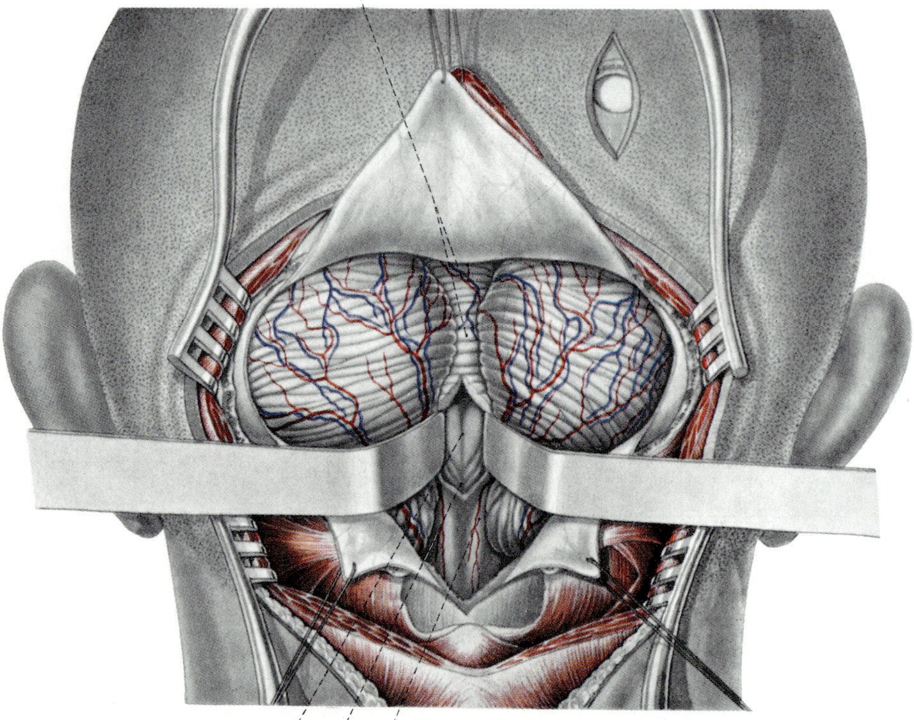

Fig. 7. Posterior fossa exploration: The floor of fourth ventricle as seen through a vermis splitting incision.

Observe: Normal anatomy of fourth ventricular floor.

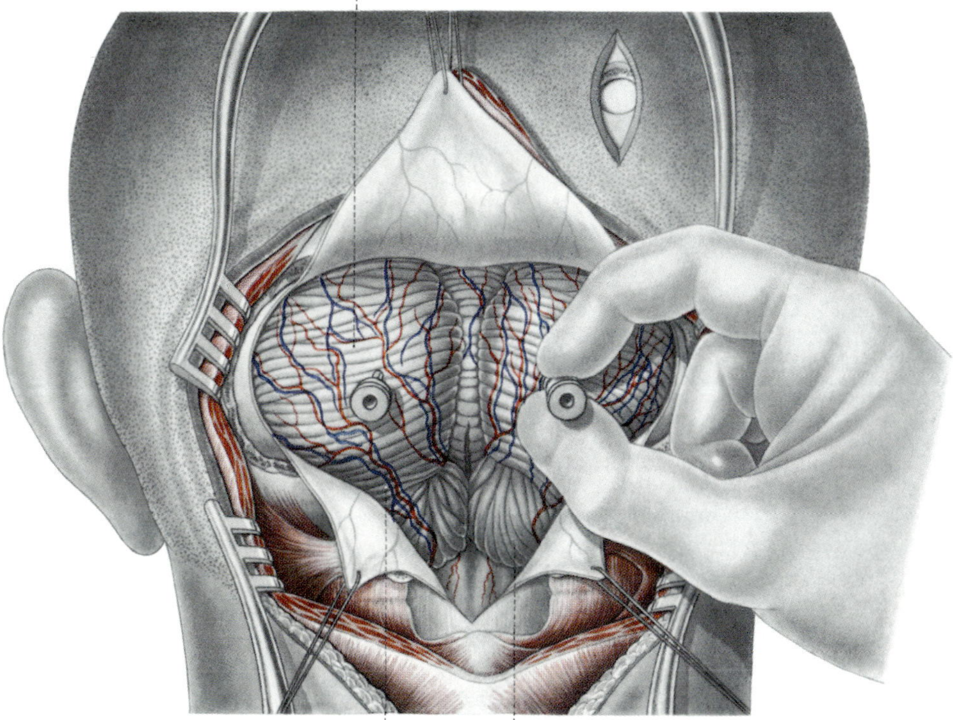

Fig. 8. Posterior fossa exploration: Insertion of ventricular needle into each cerebellar hemisphere in search of possible deep seated tumor.

Observe: Compare position of needle with Fig. 9.

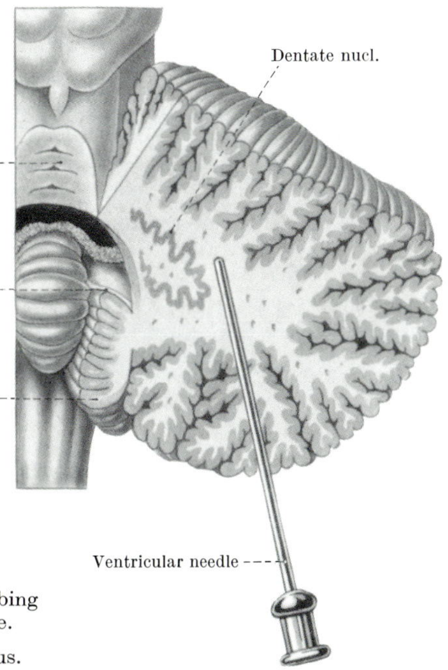

Fig. 9. Posterior fossa exploration: Position of probing ventricular needle in right cerebellar hemisphere.

Observe: Direction of needle avoids dentate nucleus.

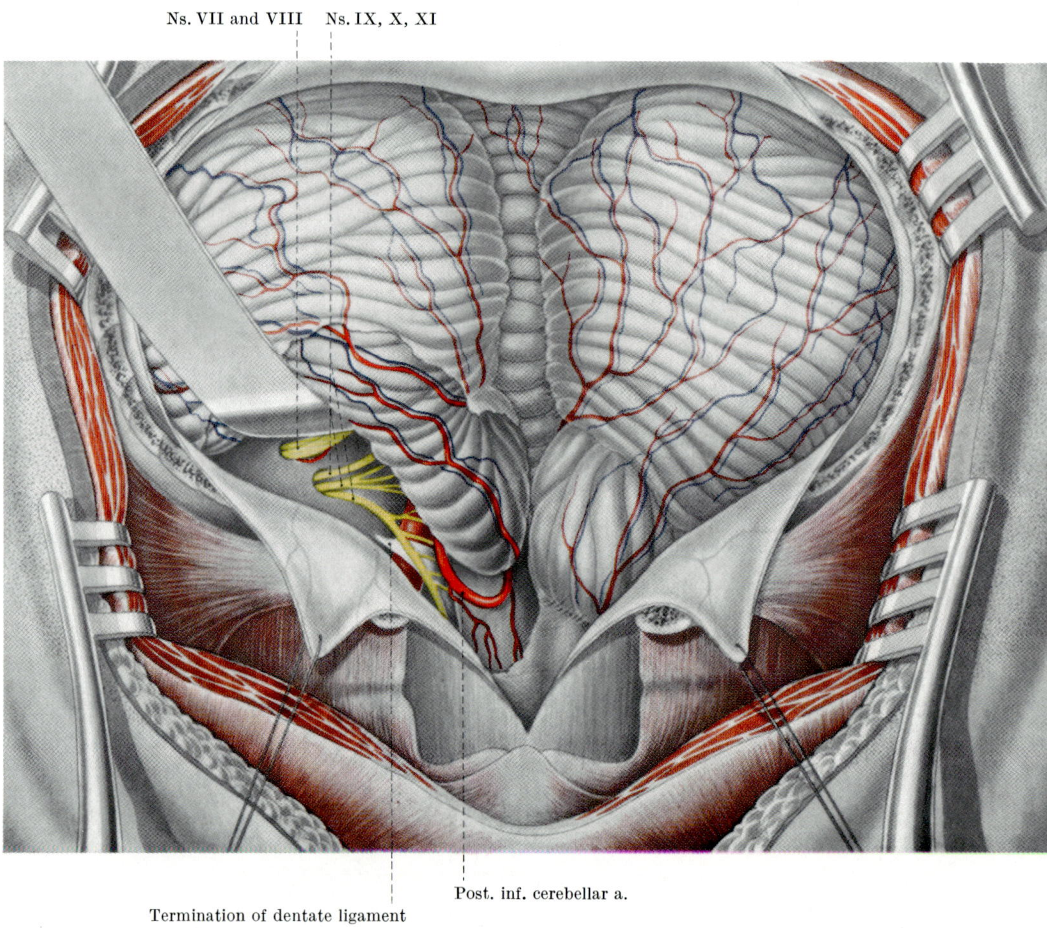

Fig. 10. Posterior fossa exploration: Inspection of lateral recess of medullary cistern and posterior portion of left cerebellopontine angle.

Observe: 1. Retraction is upward, away from the brain stem. 2. Exposure of Ns. VII, VIII, IX, X, XI.

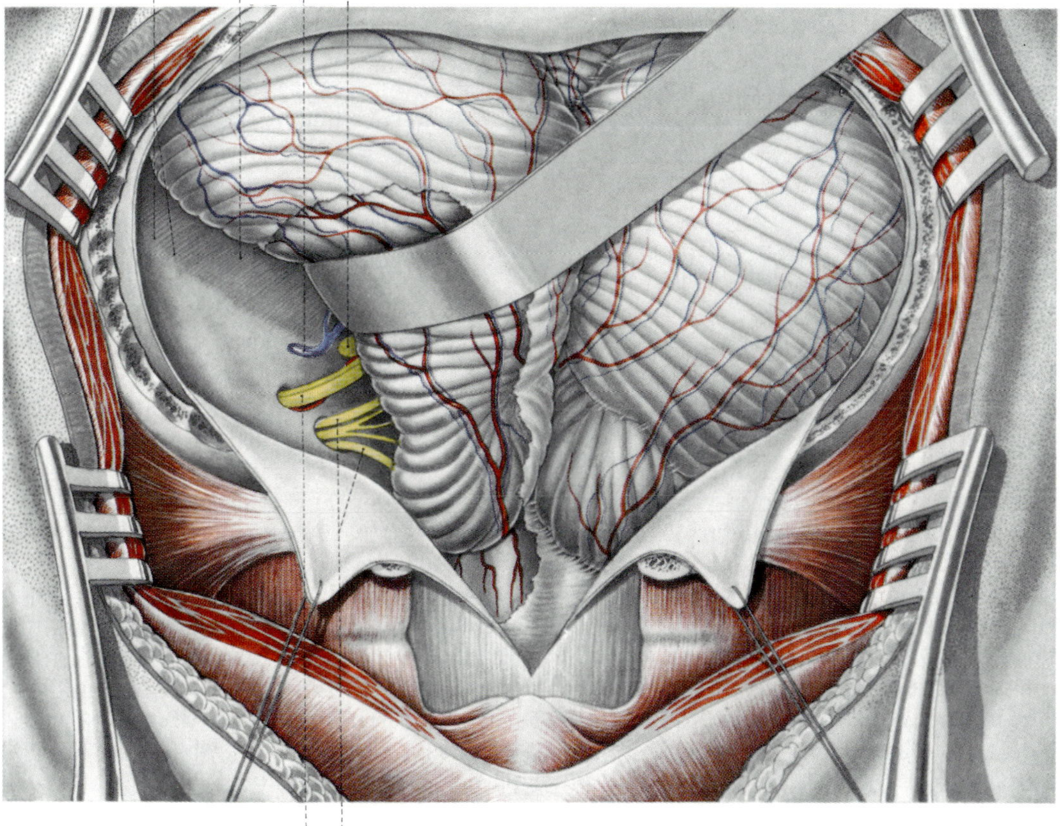

Fig. 11. Posterior fossa exploration: Inspection of entire cerebellopontine angle.

Observe: 1. Retraction is medially and superiorly. 2. Compare position of brain spatula with Fig. 10. 3. Ns. V VII, VIII, IX, X, XI are exposed.

Chapter II

Suboccipital Craniectomy — Median Incision

A. Metastatic Tumor of the Cerebellar Vermis

To illustrate the midline incision in a suboccipital craniotomy, a metastatic tumor of the vermis and right cerebellar hemisphere has been chosen (Figs. 13 and 14). Solitary metastases within the central nervous system should be removed. Many years of functional activity have been added to patients lives even when repeated operations are necessary to remove "solitary" lesions. One patient especially comes to mind. She had three posterior fossa operations over a 12-year period for a metastatic breast lesion. The patient finally died 15 years after her first neurosurgical procedure, and at autopsy the only tumor found was within the cerebellar vermis. Another patient returned to our hospital yearly for seven years to have the current senior resident remove his "solitary" metastatic melanoma.

The most common incision used in suboccipital craniectomies for intracerebellar pathology is in the midline (Fig. 15). The proper position of the sitting patient has been described in Chapter I. The skin incision is made from four cm. above the external occipital protuberance (inion) to over the spinous process of C_5. This length of incision is necessary for lateral exposure to the mastoid air cells on each side. The skin margins are freed from the deep fascia and retracted. A *Y*-shaped incision is made into the deep fascia (Fig. 16). The midline can easily be determined by intermittently palpating the inion and the spinous process of C_2. The *V* portion of the fascial incision is elevated and suspended by a silk suture. The importance of this type of fascial opening will be very apparent when it is time to close the wound. The incision is then continued in the midline down to the occipital bone and to the spinous process of C_2. The median raphe is most easily split by using a straight scissors. By staying precisely in the midline, bleeding is kept at a minimum. The insertion of the muscles to the occipital squama are stripped laterally by subperiosteal elevation. The spinous process of C_2 is exposed using a sharp knife which can be kept against the bony contours of this bifid spinous process. The origins of the obliquus inferior and rectus capitus major muscles are transected, and the muscles are retracted laterally by a self-retaining retractor. The dorsal surface of the arch of the atlas is exposed by cutting the origin of the rectus capitus minor muscle and then stripping the fibrous tissue from the arch subperiosteally using a straight scissors as described in Chapter I (Figs. 17, 18, 19). The bone in the suboccipital region and the arch of the atlas is removed as previously described (Fig. 20). A right occipital burr hole is also made at this point as illustrated.

After opening the dura, inspection of the cerebellum reveals an asymmetry of the cerebellar tonsils and hemispheres. The right cerebellar hemisphere is bulging across the midline and the right tonsil is larger and lower than the opposite one (Fig. 21). The arachnoid over the foramen magnum is opened and the cerebrospinal fluid is allowed to drain out. The vermis can be visualized only after the hemispheres are retracted laterally (Figs. 22 and 23). Flattening of the vermis indicates that the lesion extends across the midline. This means that the tumor should be approached by beginning in the midline and retracting laterally that is, away from the brain stem. A midline pial incision into the vermis is made using electrocautery and a fine neurosurgical scissors (compare p. 78, Vol. I). Because metastatic tumors are surrounded by edematous brain, a cleavage plane is easily developed around the tumor using suction and cotton pledgets. A spoon-shaped

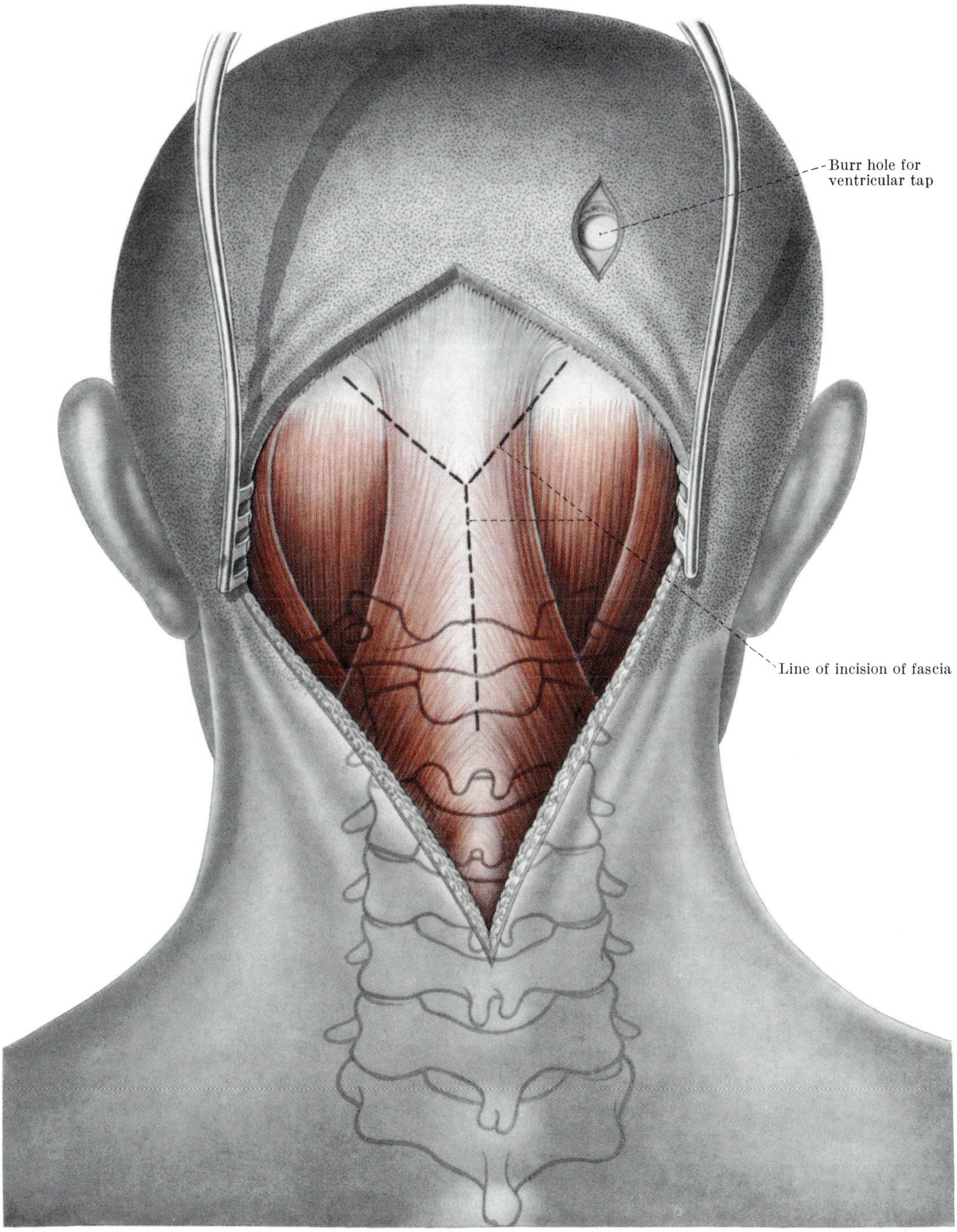

Fig. 16. Suboccipital craniectomy: Midline incision.

Observe: 1. *Y*-shaped incision of fascia will give supportive strength to closure. 2. Right occipital burr hole for possible ventricular drainage.

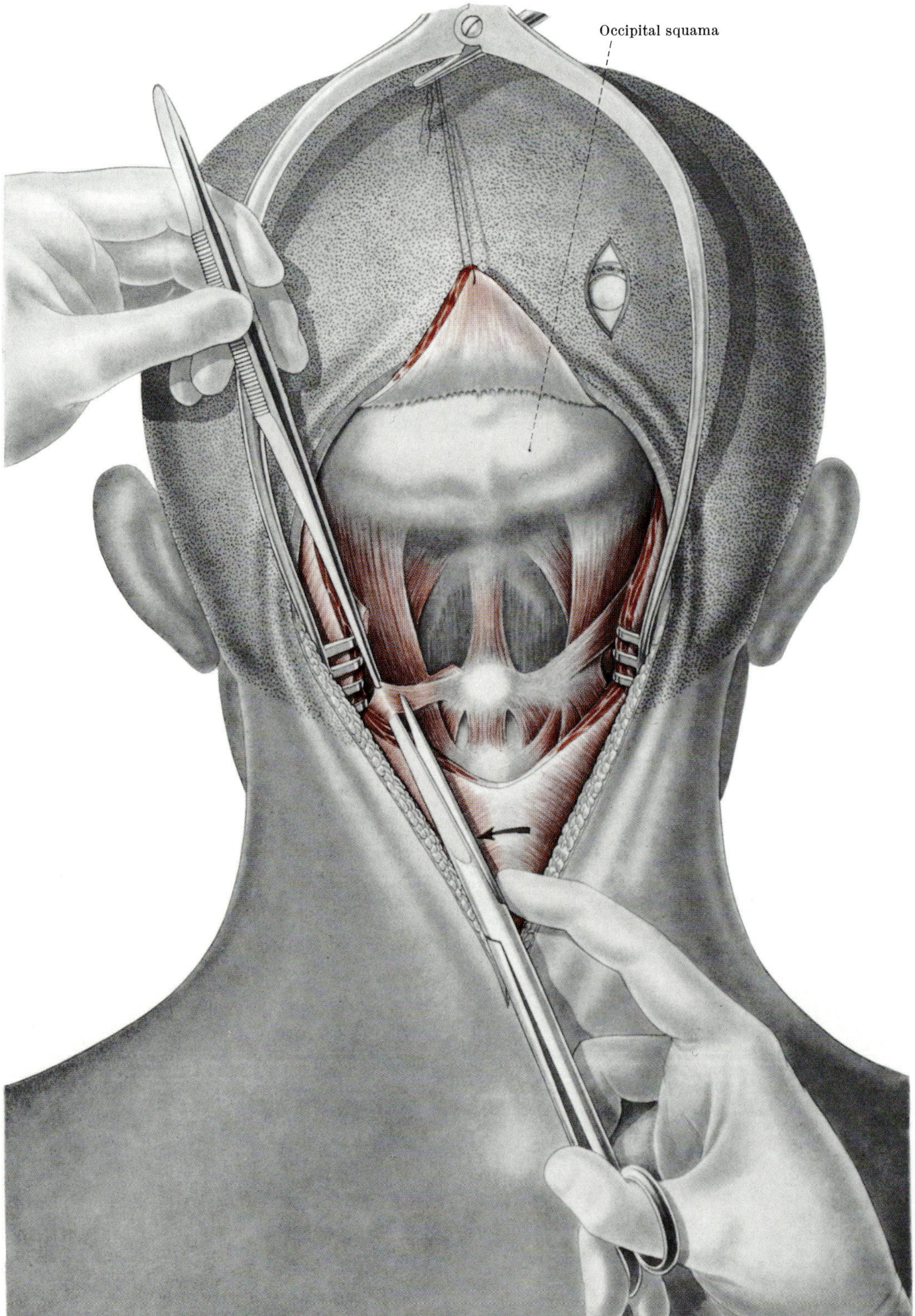

Fig. 17. Suboccipital craniectomy: Subperiosteal exposure of occipital squama.
Observe: Dissection of the deep suboccipital triangle using straight scissors.

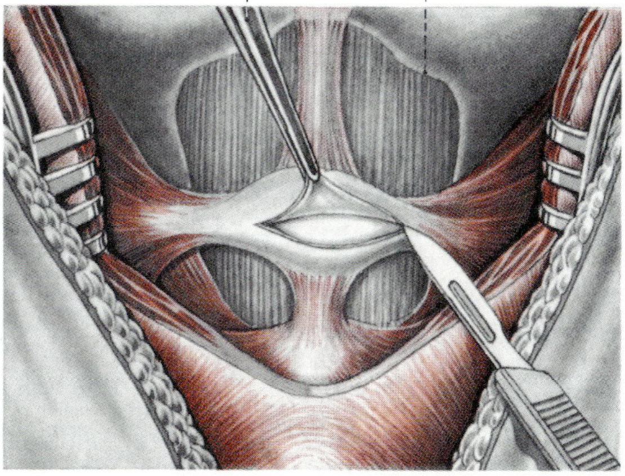

Fig. 18. Suboccipital craniectomy: Subperiosteal exposure of arch of atlas.

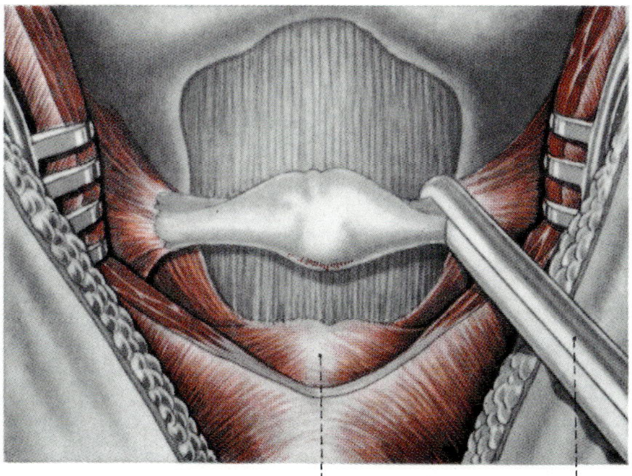

Fig. 19. Suboccipital craniectomy: Removal of the arch of the atlas.

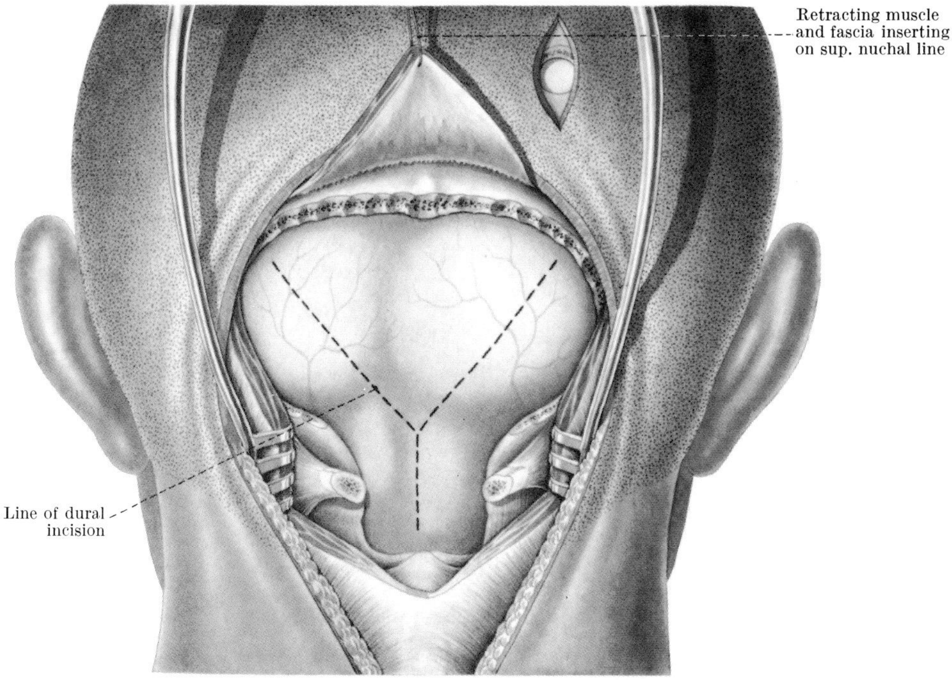

Fig. 20. Suboccipital craniectomy with posterior arch of the atlas removed.

Observe: 1. *Y*-shaped dural incision (compare Fig. 4). 2. Asymmetrical contour of the posteroinferior surface of the cerebellum visible through the unopened dura.

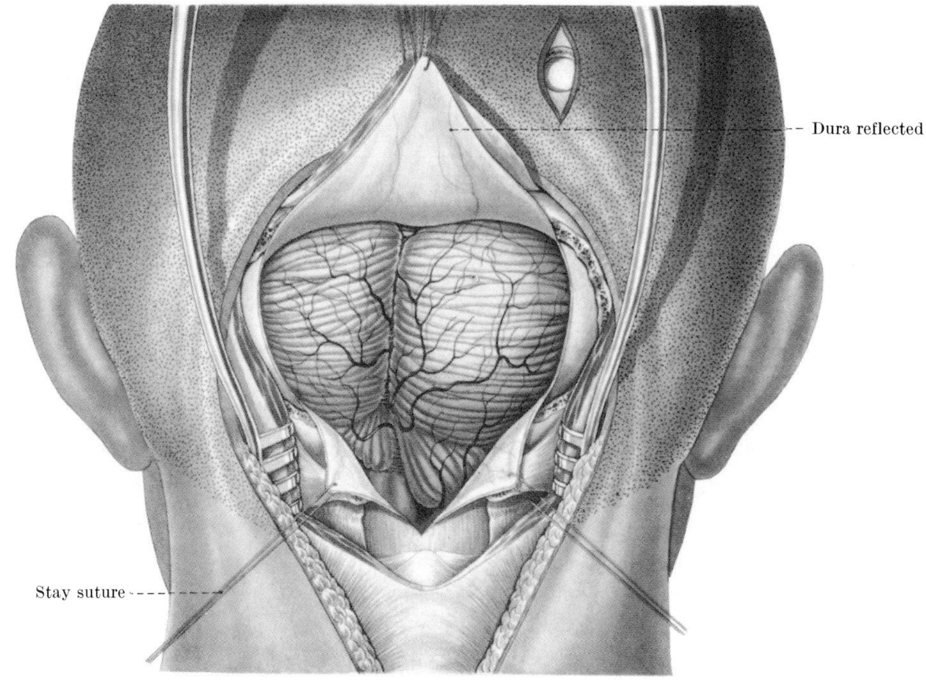

Fig. 21. Suboccipital craniectomy for cerebellar tumor: Inferior surface of cerebellum exposed.

Observe: 1. Difference in size of cerebellar hemisphere and particularly of cerebellar tonsil on the side of the lesion. 2. Retraction of dura by stay sutures.

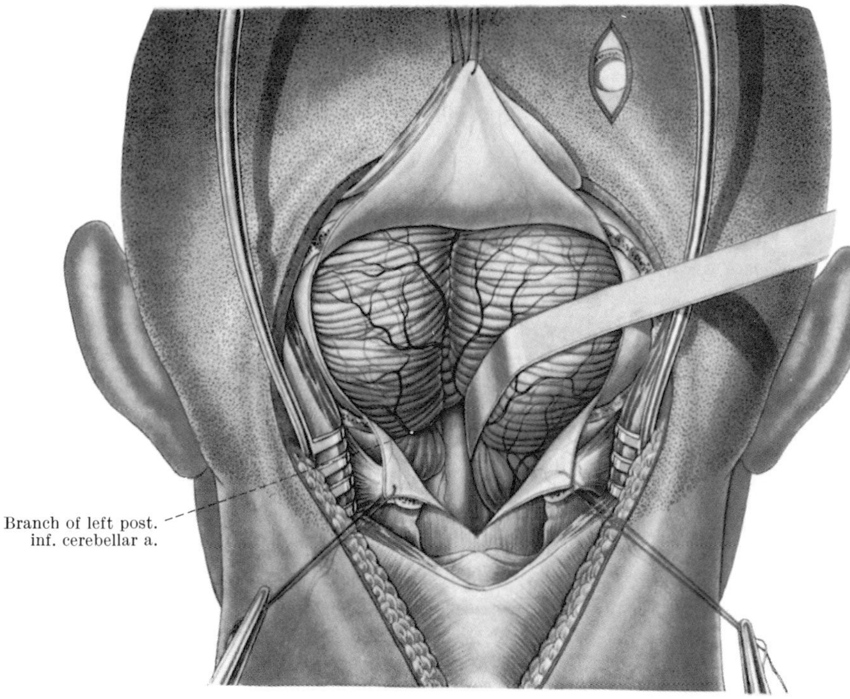

Fig. 22. Suboccipital craniectomy for cerebellar tumor: Exposure of the inferior part of the vermis.

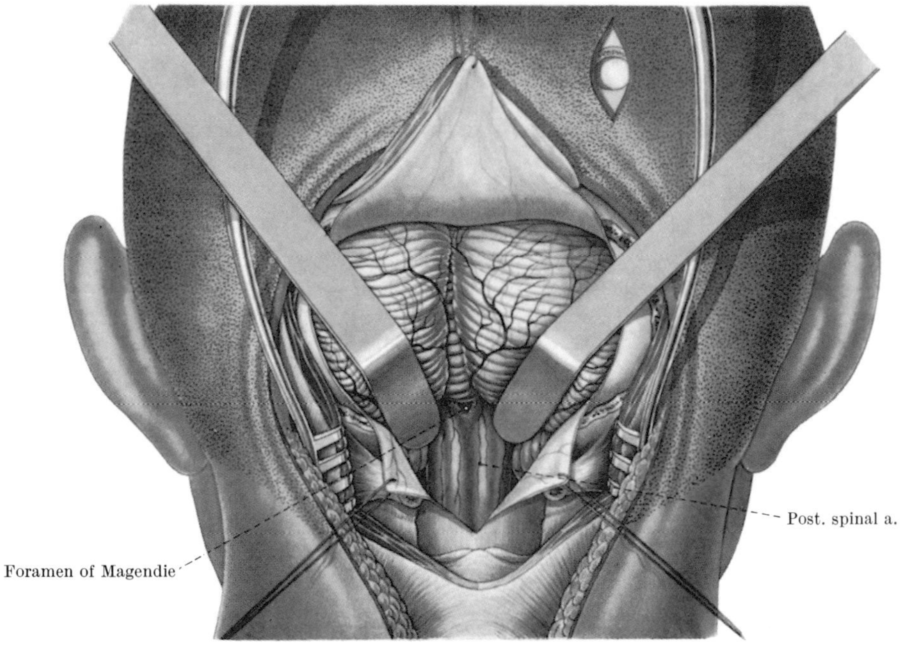

Fig. 23. Suboccipital craniectomy for cerebellar tumor: Exposure of the obex and the foramen of Magendie.

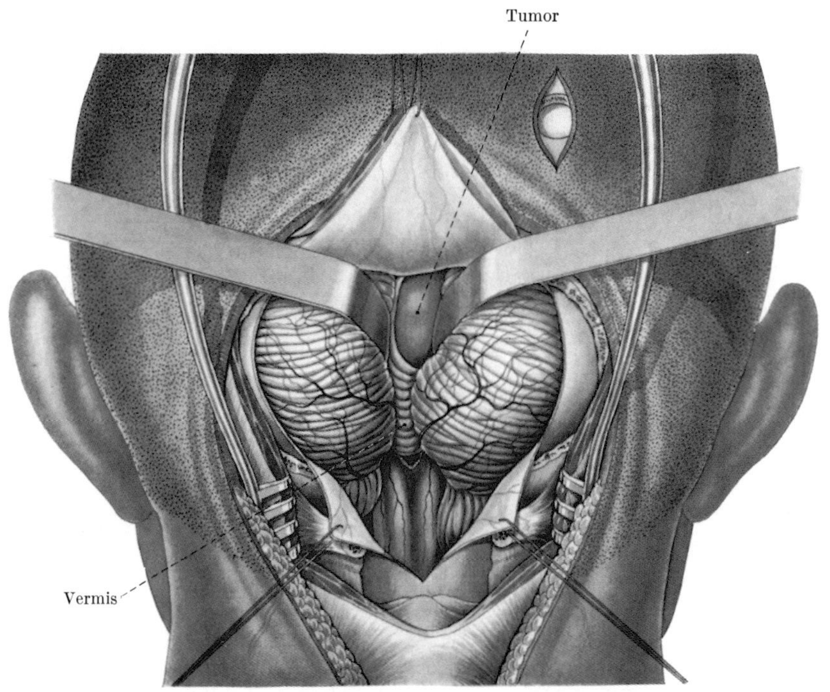

Fig. 24. Suboccipital craniectomy for cerebellar tumor: Retracting the cerebellar hemispheres to expose vermal tumor.

Observe: Paravermal incision has been made through edematous cortex to expose the tumor.

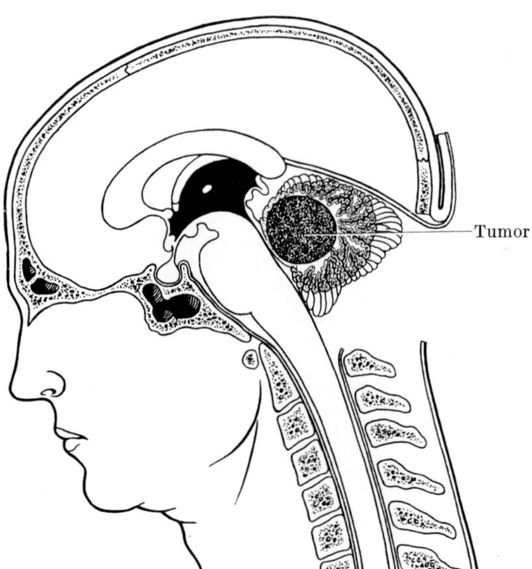

Fig. 25. Suboccipital craniectomy for cerebellar tumor: Midline sagittal section of head showing position of tumor.

Observe: The bone has been removed and the dura is reflected.

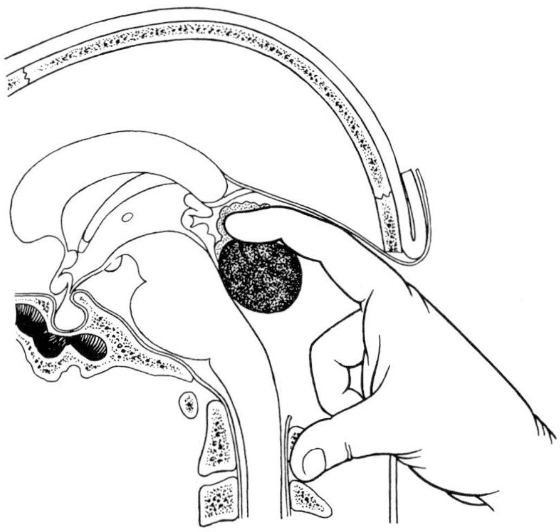

Fig. 26.

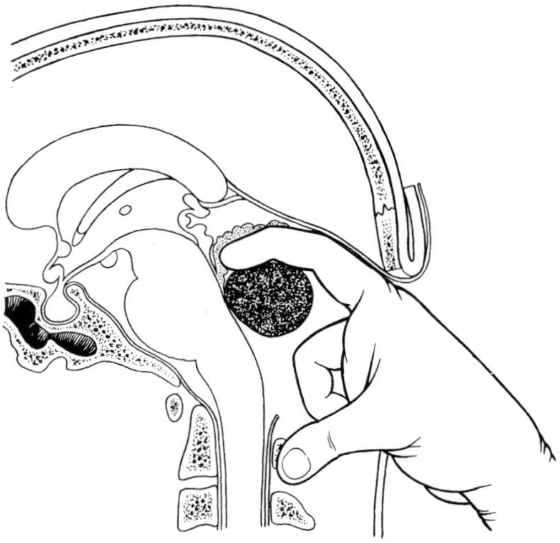

Fig. 27.

Fig. 26. Use of index finger in dissection and delivery of the tumor (metastatic nodule). *Observe:* The finger is moved up over the tumor without ever pressing the lesion anteriorly.

Fig. 27. Use of index finger in dissection and delivery of the tumor. *Observe:* The finger has passed over superior extent of the tumor.

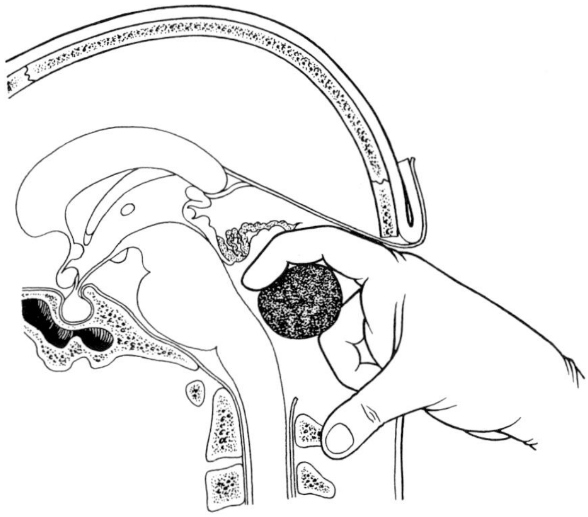

Fig. 28.

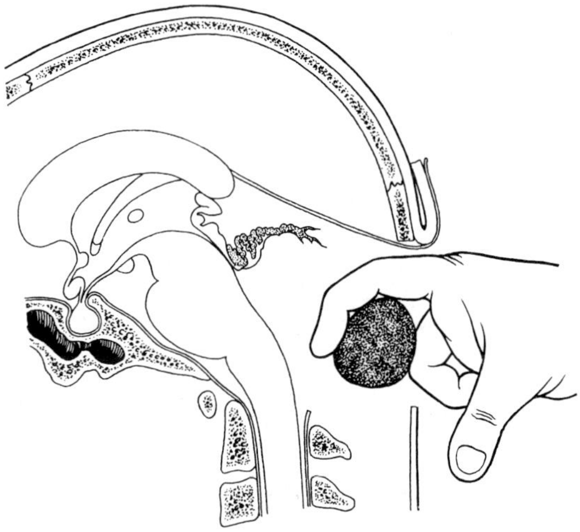

Fig. 29.

Fig. 28. Use of index finger in dissection and delivery of the tumor (metastatic nodule). *Observe:* Direction of movement is inferiorly and posteriorly.

Fig. 29. Use of index finger in dissection and delivery of the tumor (metastatic nodule).

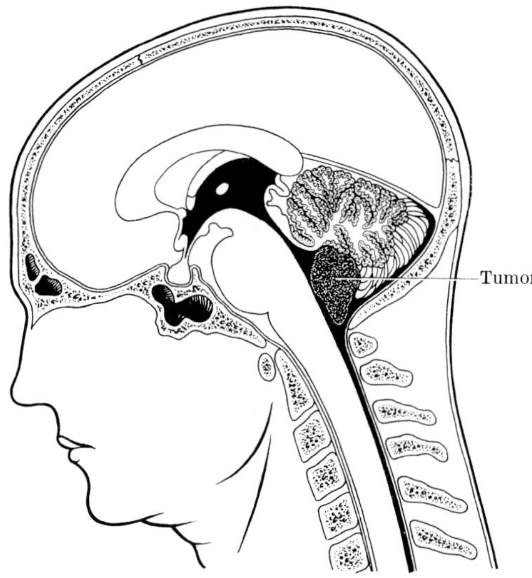

Fig. 30. Median sagittal section of lower fourth ventricular tumor (cerebellar medulloblastoma).

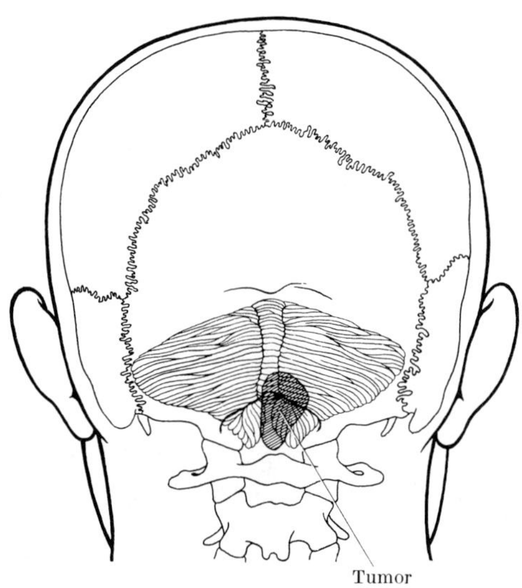

Fig. 31. Lower fourth ventricular tumor (cerebellar astrocytoma) projected on an outline of the head and spine in position for surgery.

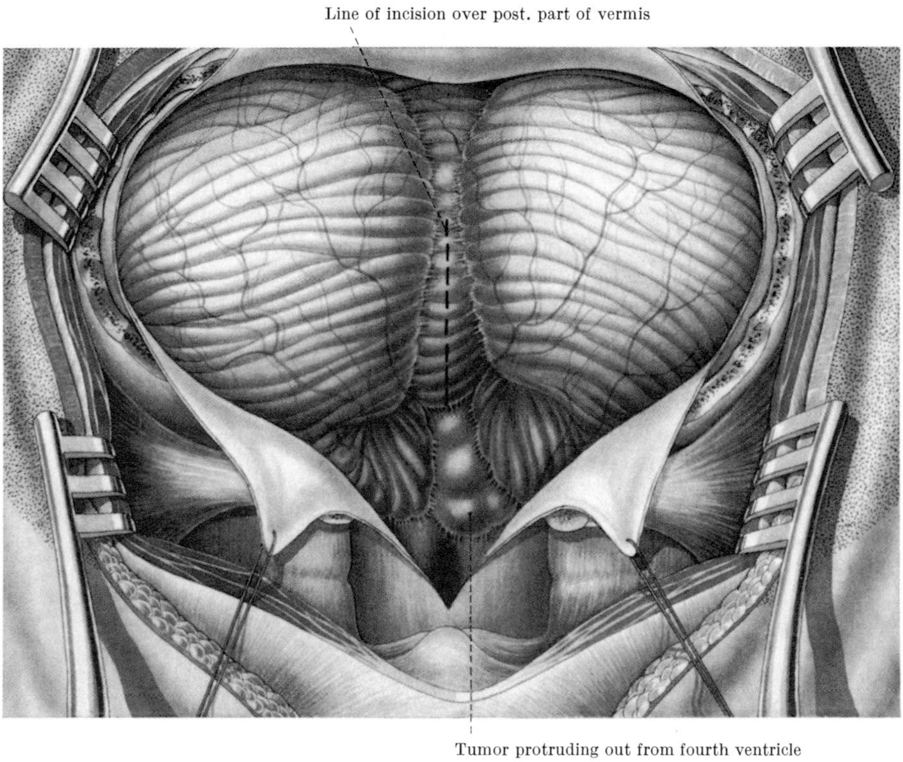

Fig. 32. Medulloblastoma of the lower part of the fourth ventricle.
Observe: 1. Arachnoid remains intact. 2. Tumor protruding from beneath the vermis and between the tonsils. 3. Dotted line indicates extent of incision of the vermis.

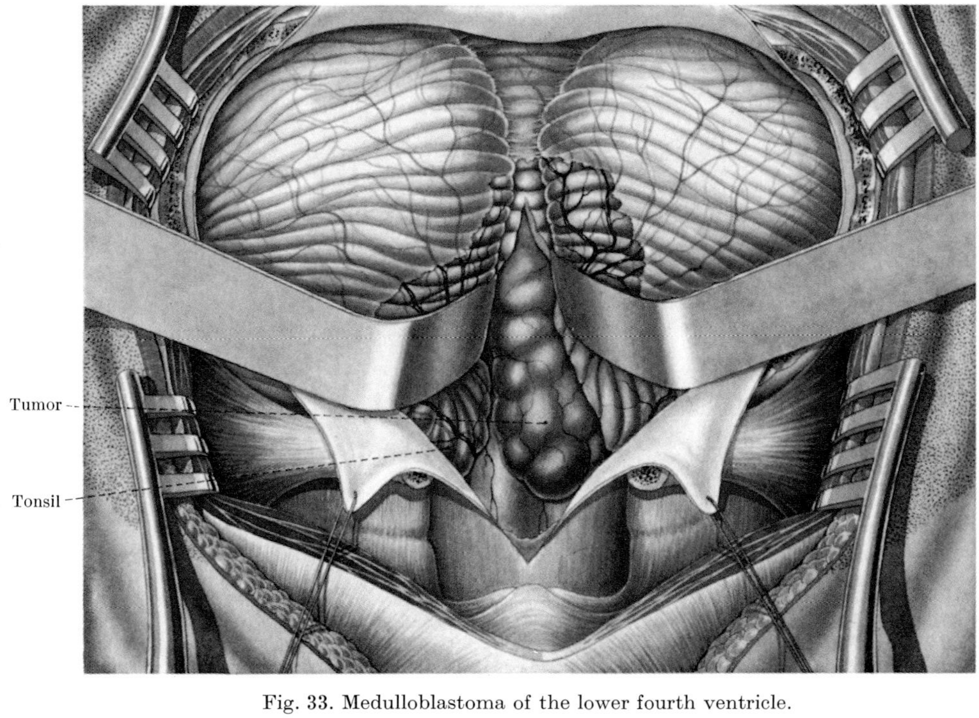

Fig. 33. Medulloblastoma of the lower fourth ventricle.
Observe: Tumor presenting through the vermal incision.

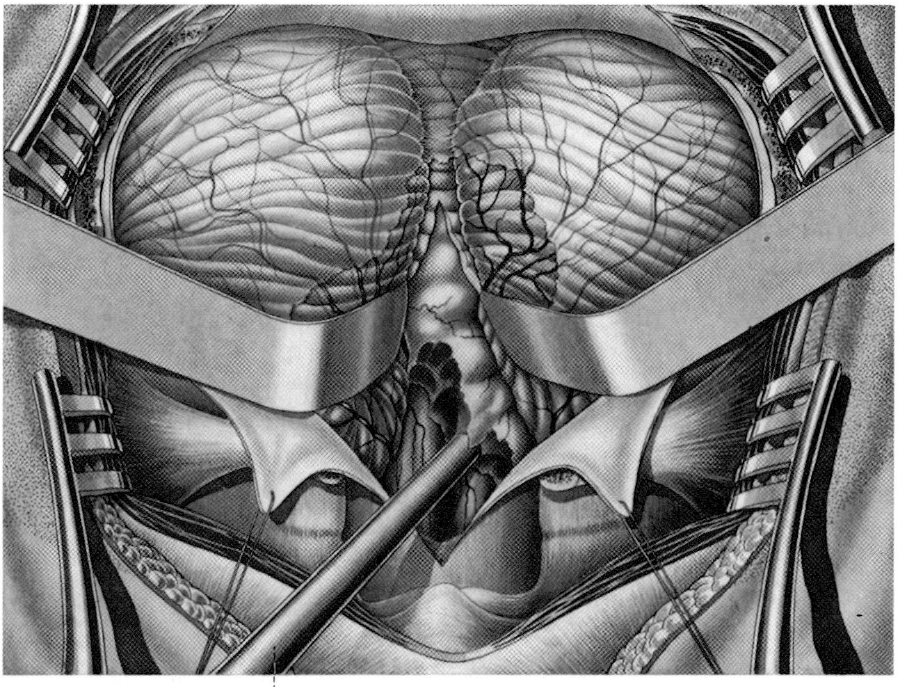

Fig. 34. Medulloblastoma of the lower fourth ventricle being removed by suction.

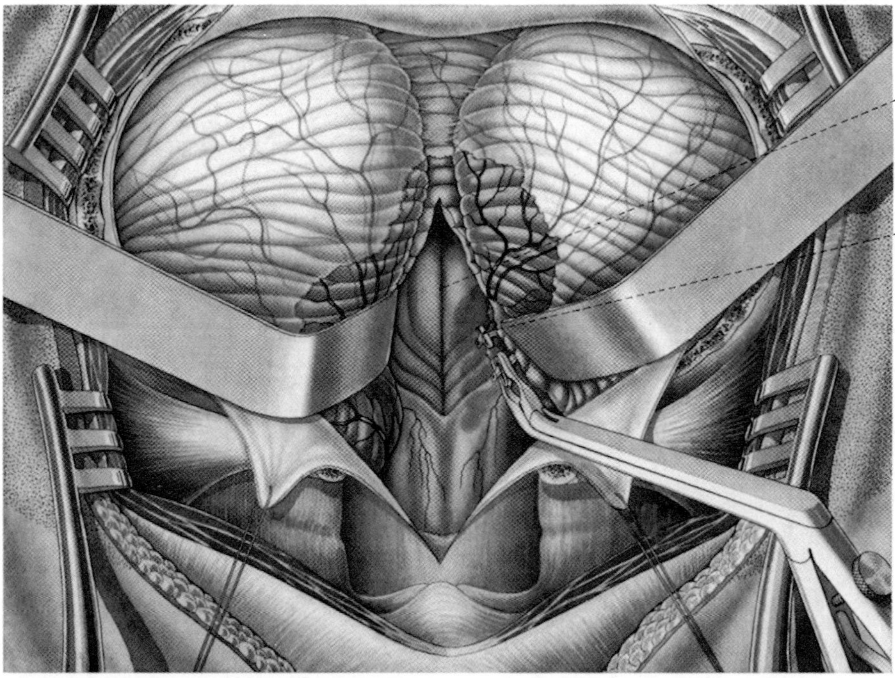

Fig. 35. Medulloblastoma of the lower fourth ventricle: Control of feeding vessels, which are branches of the choroidal arteries, by silver clips.

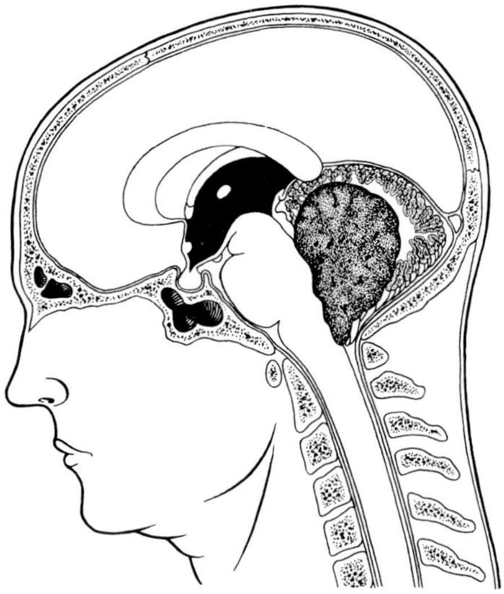

Fig. 36.

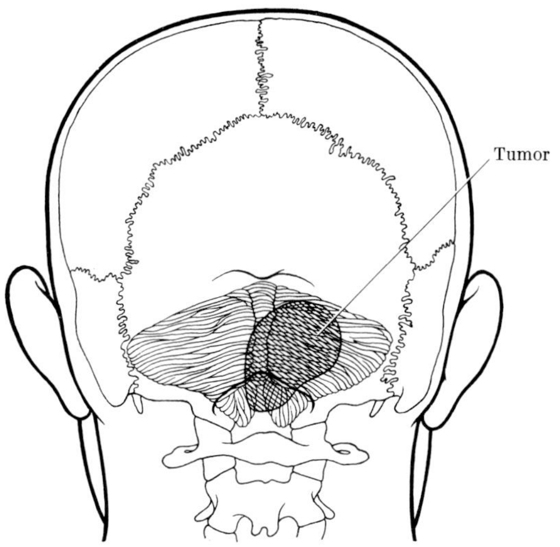

Fig. 37.

Fig. 36. Fourth ventricular tumor (Ependymoma): midline sagittal section.

Observe: Attachment to the floor of the fourth ventricle.

Fig. 37. Intraventricular tumor (Ependymoma) projected on an outline of the head and spine in position for surgery.

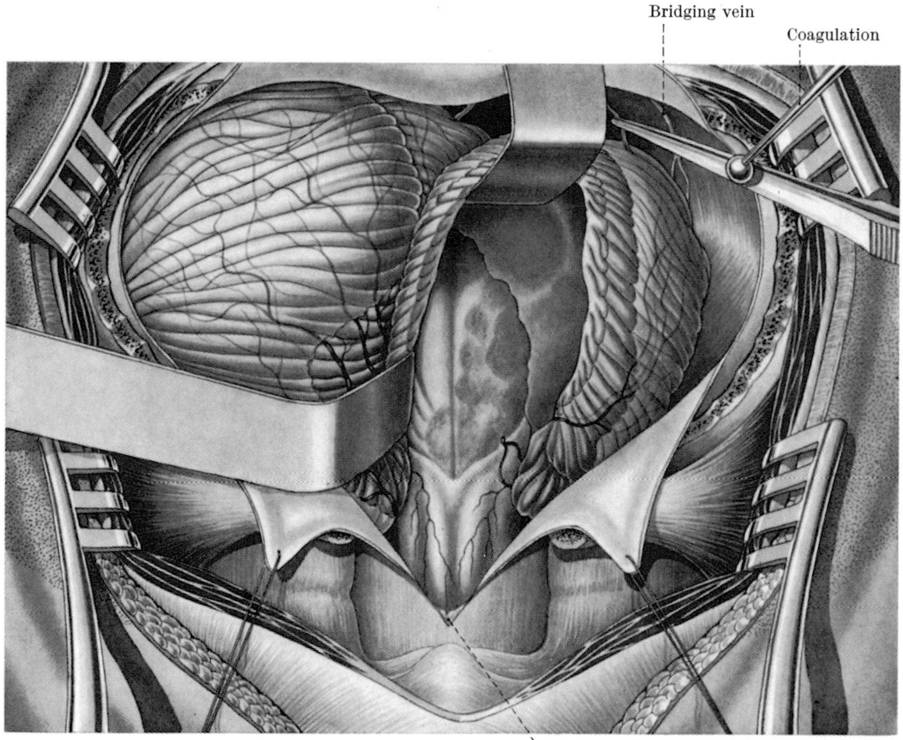

Fig. 38. Fourth ventricular tumor (Ependymoma): Subtotal removal of tumor leaving that part which is adherent to the floor of the IV. ventricle.

Observe: Following removal of this large tumor, the right cerebellar hemisphere has collapsed. As a result the bridging veins must be electrocoagulated.

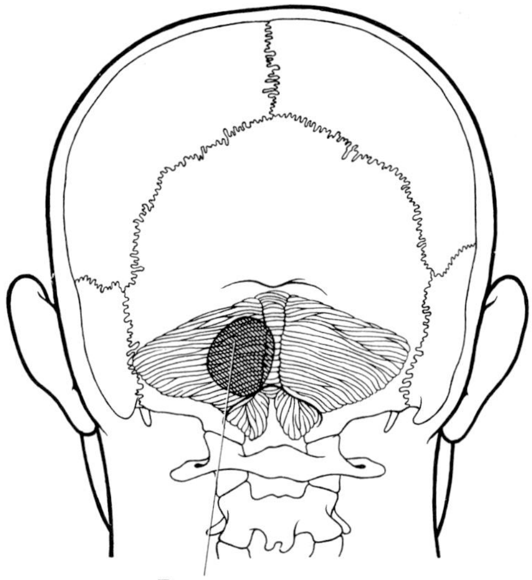

Fig. 39. Left lateral cerebellar intrahemispheric glioma (juvenile astrocytoma) projected on an outline of the head and spine in position for surgery.

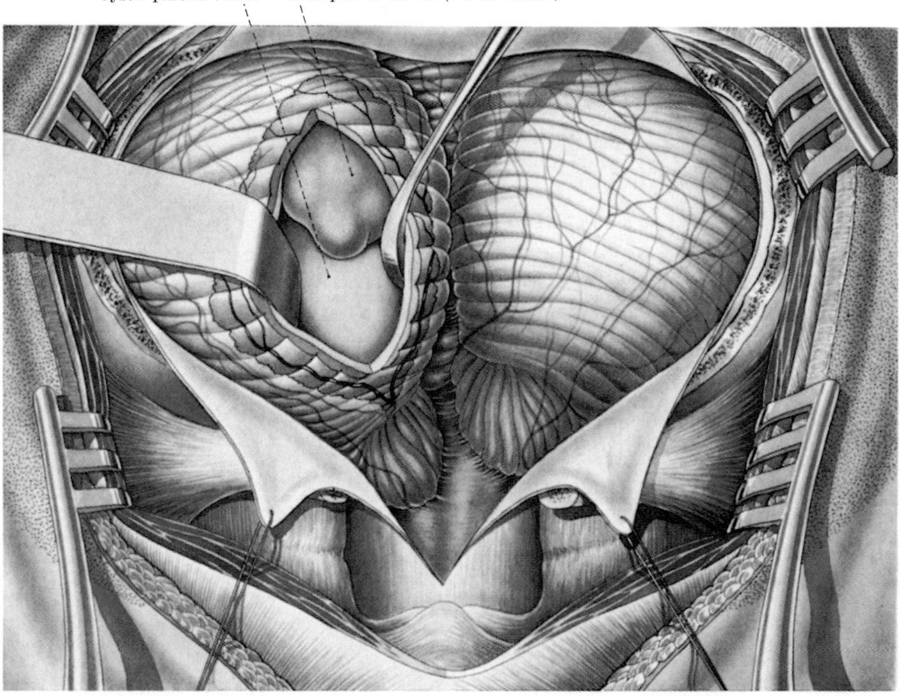

Fig. 40. Cerebellar astrocytoma.

Observe: 1. Cyst has been entered to reveal mural nodule projecting into the cyst cavity.
2. Cyst wall is white and smooth.

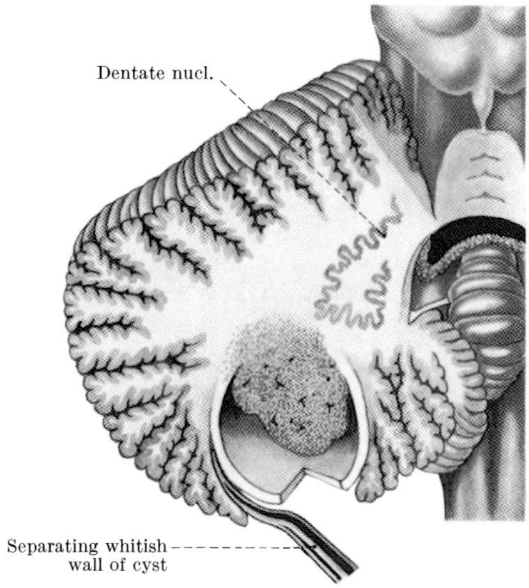

Fig. 41. Cerebellar astrocytoma: Oblique section through the cerebellar hemisphere with the tumor reveals indefinite border between solid tumor and normal brain tissue.

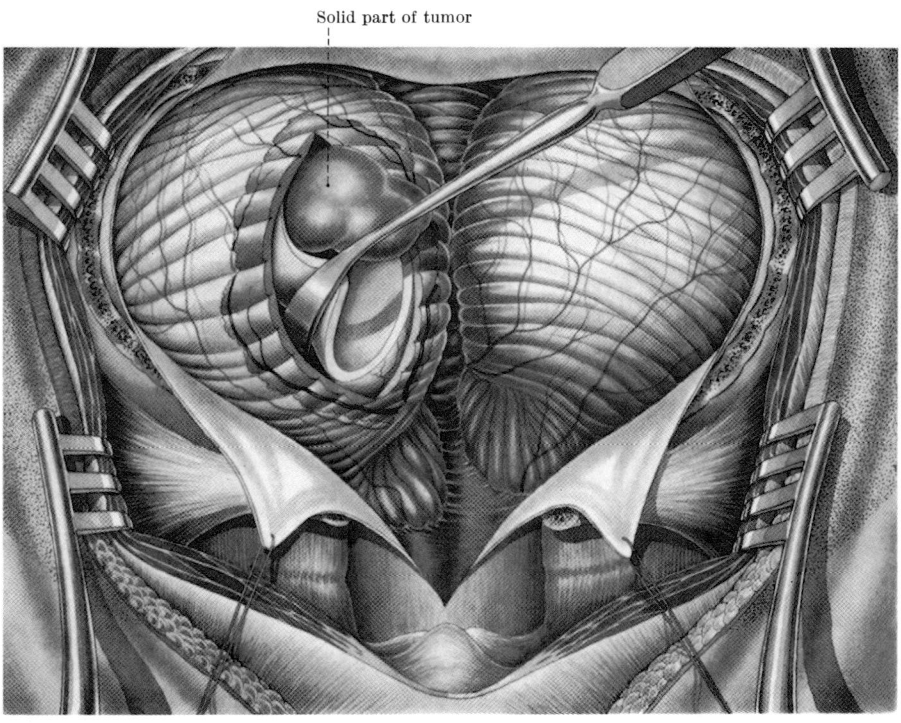

Fig. 42. Removal of cystic cerebellar astrocytoma.

Observe: The capsule of the cyst, as well as the solid tumor, is removed.

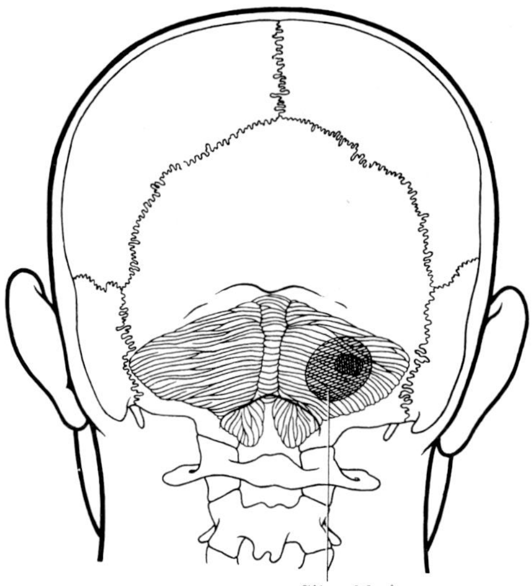

Fig. 43. Hemangioblastoma of the right cerebellar hemisphere projected on an outline of the head and spine in position for surgery.

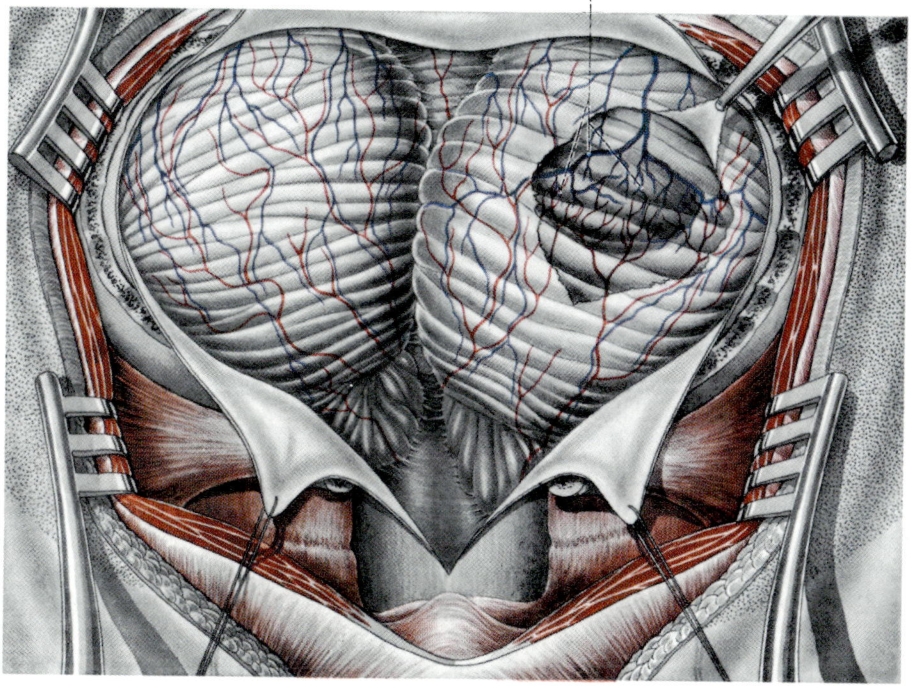

Fig. 44. Hemangioblastoma right cerebellar hemisphere: Surface exposure.
Observe: Increased vascularity and discoloration over the site of the lesion.

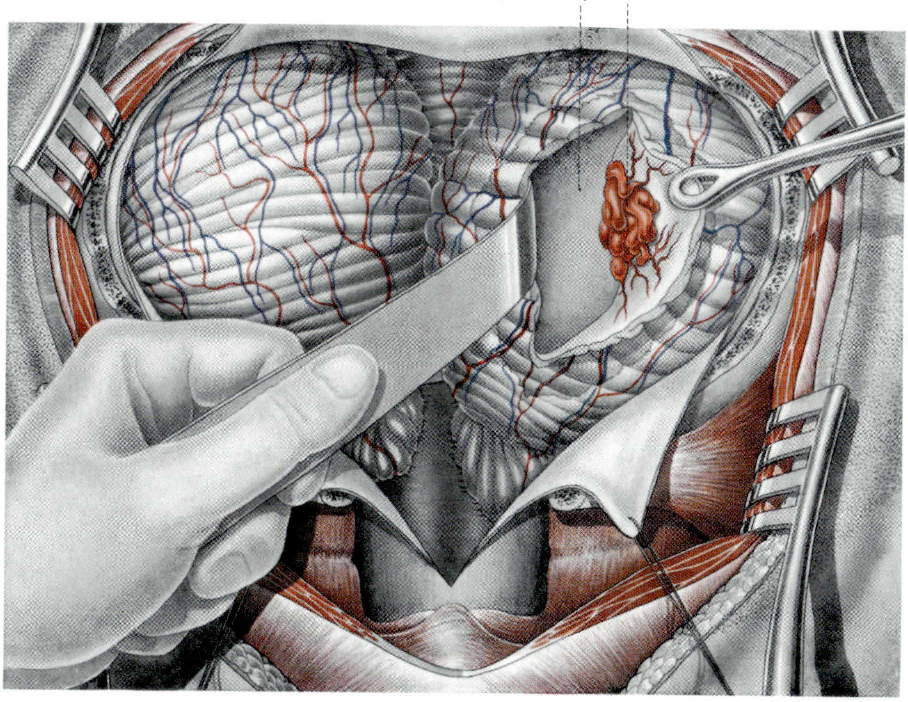

Fig. 45. Hemangioblastoma right cerebellar hemisphere: Cystic tumor with mural nodule.
Observe: 1. The tumor is located close to the surface of the cerebellum.

Chapter III

Suboccipital Craniectomy — Paramedian Incision

Acoustic Neurinoma

Acoustic neurinomas usually arise from the vestibular portion of the eighth cranial nerve within the internal auditory meatus (porus acousticus). Increasingly sensitive tests (Bekesy audiometry, Short Increment Sensitivity Index, Alternate Binaural Loudness Balance, caloric vestibular response, positive contrast studies, etc.) allow earlier diagnosis; and, as a result, smaller tumors are now being removed. However, even today, many tumors still come to our attention only after they have produced pressure on the pons, medulla and cranial nerves or have caused increased intracranial pressure.

The anatomical relationships of this tumor are illustrated in Figs. 46 and 47. The facial nerve, more or less adherent to the tumor capsule, is pushed toward the ventral surface of the tumor. It then passes anteriorly toward the roots of the trigeminal nerve. The facial nerve enters the internal auditory meatus at its anterior extent either in the upper or lower quadrant (see Figs. 53—59).

The main vascular supply to this tumor is from the posterior inferior and anterior inferior cerebellar arteries as shown in Figs. 46 and 47. Venous drainage is from the dorsal aspect of the tumor to the petrosal sinus.

The goal in the surgical treatment of this lesion is total removal of the tumor with preservation of the facial nerve. This goal is not always attainable. The tumor capsule may be so adherent to the pons and medulla that total removal would result in contusion or infarction of the brain stem. Pathological specimen often demonstrate many fine branches passing directly from the basilar artery into the tumor. Obviously, a radical intracapsular excision will occasionally have to be the treatment of choice.

It is not always possible to preserve the seventh nerve. Even though it is carefully identified proximally, close to the brain stem, and distally, as it leaves through the porus acousticus, the facial nerve is most easily injured in the area inbetween. The nerve often is thin and spread out over the capsule of the tumor. The larger the tumor the more difficult it will be to preserve the facial nerve.

The patient is placed in the sitting position with the head turned toward the side of the lesion. The ideal position will place the petrous ridge on the side of the tumor in a straight antero-posterior direction (Fig. 48). This rotation of the head is most advantageous in exposing the cerebellopontine angle since it requires less retraction on the cerebellum and permits easier illumination of the operative field.

A 12 cm. vertical incision is made beginning four cm. above the superior nuchal line half way between the inion and the mastoid process (Fig. 49). A unilateral suboccipital craniectomy is performed using multiple burr holes and then rongeuring between them. Fig. 49 illustrates the limits of the craniectomy. There is no need to extend the craniectomy into the foramen magnum nor to remove the arch of the atlas. It is important to remove the bone up to the transverse sinus and laterally to the mastoid air cells of the temporal bone (Fig. 50). A cruciate dural incision will allow maximal exposure (Fig. 50).

The cerebellum is gently elevated to expose the tumor. A majority of acoustic neurinomas have a cystic component and there is often a cyst over the postero-inferior portion of the tumor. On aspirating the cyst an amber highly proteinatious fluid is obtained. With collapse of the cyst and opening of the arachnoid, the limits and size of the lesion can now be established. If, at this point, it is apparent that the tumor is so large that a great deal of retraction of the cerebellum is necessary to gain exposure, the lateral one-third of the hemisphere should be removed.

In referring to the illustrations, remember that for the sake of clarity cotton pledgets have not been included. In Fig. 51, for example, the cerebellar hemisphere would not be retracted without a protecting cottonoid strip. The importance of wet cotton pledgets in protecting the cerebellum cannot be overemphasized.

The IX, X and XI cranial nerves are identified at the lower pole of the tumor (Fig. 51). The tumor capsule is entered in an avascular area. The tumor is gutted using a fairly large curette (Fig. 52). In intracapsular removal, two points must be kept in mind: 1. Since the medial extention of the tumor has not been defined, extreme caution must be taken to avoid injury to the brain stem. 2. Since the facial nerve is usually anterior or ventral to the tumor, the capsule must not be violated in these areas. Hemostasis within the capsule is attained using absorbable gelatin sponges soaked in thrombin, and attention is once again directed outside the capsule.

The IX, X and XI nerves are now freed from the capsule of the tumor and covered with a protecting, wet cotton pledget. In the dissection of the inferior capsule, large feeding branches from the posterior inferior cerebellar artery or directly from the vertebral artery must be clipped and divided. Monopolar coagulation should be avoided in this area.

The tumor capsule is then gently elevated and the facial nerve is identified on its ventral aspect (Fig. 53). Electrical stimulation will aid in identifying the nerve. It may be possible to isolate the facial nerve for only a few millimeters at this point since the nerve passes anteriorly toward the roots of the trigeminal nerve on its way toward the porus acousticus, and this portion of the course of the nerve is still obscured by the tumor.

Having identified the facial nerve proximally (Fig. 53), it must now be exposed distally at the internal auditory meatus. As the seventh nerve is protected the tumor is then divided at the meatus (Fig. 54).

Attention is now directed to the antero-superior extension. As the tumor is most gently retracted inferiorly, the veins draining from the tumor into the superior petrosal Sinus can be identified. These vessels are clipped or coagulated with bipolar current and divided. Moving medially, arterial branches to the tumor from the anterior inferior cerebellar artery are visualized, clipped and divided (Fig. 55). If the tumor extends upward through the tentorial incisura, it may even be supplied by branches from the superior cerebellar artery. The fifth nerve is almost always very easily dissected free of the tumor capsule, but it is at this point anteriorly that the facial nerve is most difficult to preserve. As the tumor is gradually retracted inferiorly the facial nerve may be identified as many thinned out single fascicles. Magnification, in this situation, may provide the only possible way to preserve the continuity of the facial nerve.

The angle of retraction is changed from inferiorly to laterally, and the crucial medial dissection is now carried out. As previously mentioned, at times it will be best for the patient if a small portion of the capsule which is adherent to the brain stem is left behind. After removing the remaining capsule, bleeding veins on the surface of the pons and medulla can be controlled by applying a wet cotton fluff and temporarily leaving that area.

Having removed the bulk of the tumor, attention is turned to the remaining nubbin in the porus acousticus. Under magnification the dura is incised at the posterior aspect of the porus and elevated (Figs. 56 and 57). A high speed drill, cooled by irrigation, can be used to remove the posterior wall of the porus and expose the remaining tumor.

It is important to coat this bony margin with bone wax since post operative cerebrospinal fluid fistulae have been reported. The tumor is teased out of the canal while the facial nerve is protected (Fig. 58). The small artery accompanying the facial nerve is protected and preserved in the same manner. Any bleeding from within the canal can be controlled with bipolar coagulation.

The tumor bed is checked for meticulous hemostasis. All cotton fluffs and strips are freed using irrigation and removed. A water-tight dural closure is attained and the remainder of the wound closed in layers.

Fig. 46. Acoustic neurinoma: Ventral view of the cerebellopontine angle demonstrating the relationship of an acoustic neurinoma to adjacent structures.

Observe: 1. Deformation of brain stem. 2. Elongation and displacement of N. V. 3. Cut surface of part of tumor entering internal acoustic meatus. 4. Vascular supply to the tumor capsule. 5. Thinned out N. VII running over the tumor capsule.

Fig. 47. Acoustic neurinoma: Ventral view of cerebellopontine angle following removal of acoustic neurinoma.

Observe: Vein draining into the superior petrosal sinus.

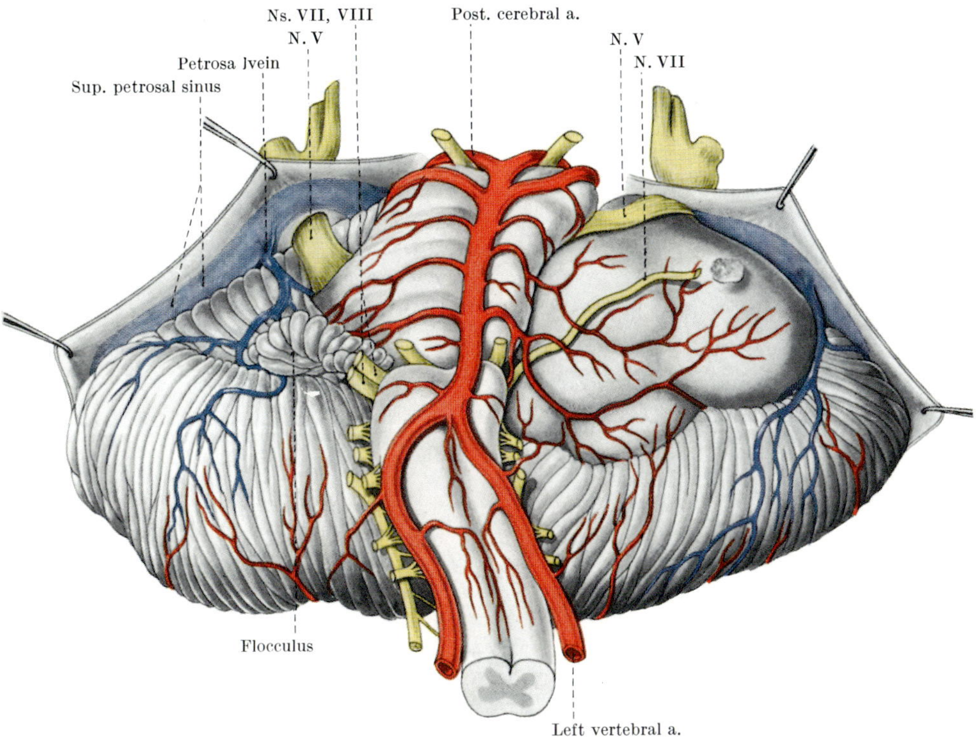
Ns. VII, VIII
N. V
Petrosa }vein
Sup. petrosal sinus
Post. cerebral a.
N. V
N. VII
Flocculus
Left vertebral a.

Fig. 46.

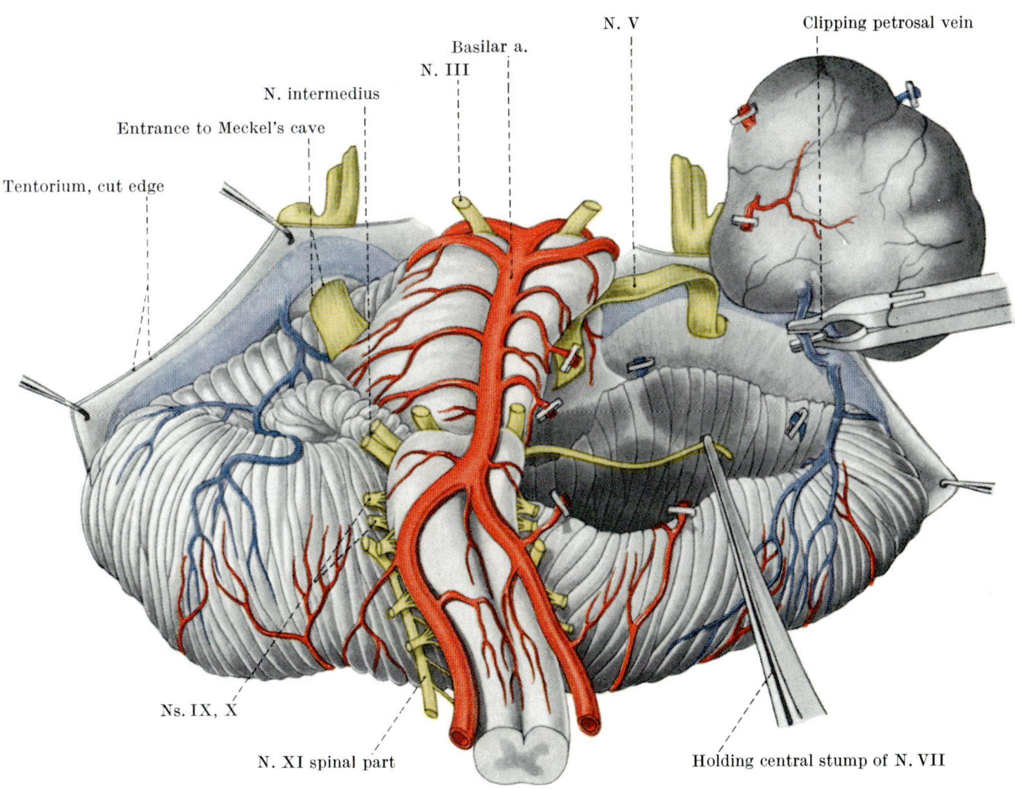
N. V
Clipping petrosal vein
Basilar a.
N. III
N. intermedius
Entrance to Meckel's cave
Tentorium, cut edge
Ns. IX, X
N. XI spinal part
Holding central stump of N. VII

Fig. 47.

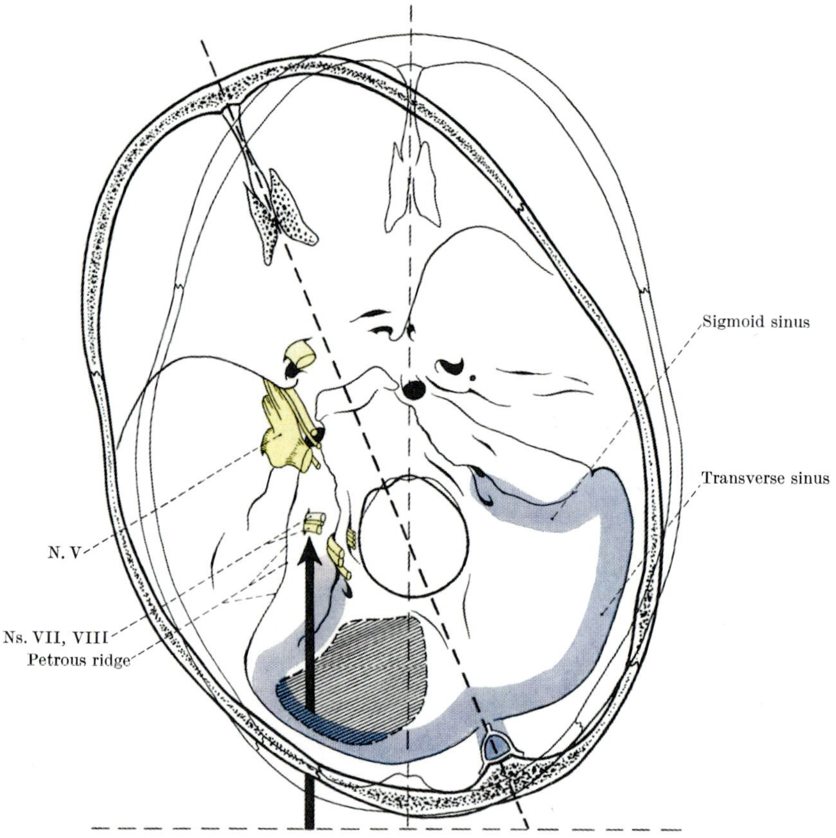

Fig. 48. Acoustic neurinoma: Schematic drawing of the base of the skull to demonstrate optimal rotation around vertical axis of the head for unilateral suboccipital craniectomy for a left sided acoustic neurinoma.

Observe: 1. The left petrous ridge runs nearly in a straight a-p direction. 2. Shaded area outlines craniectomy.

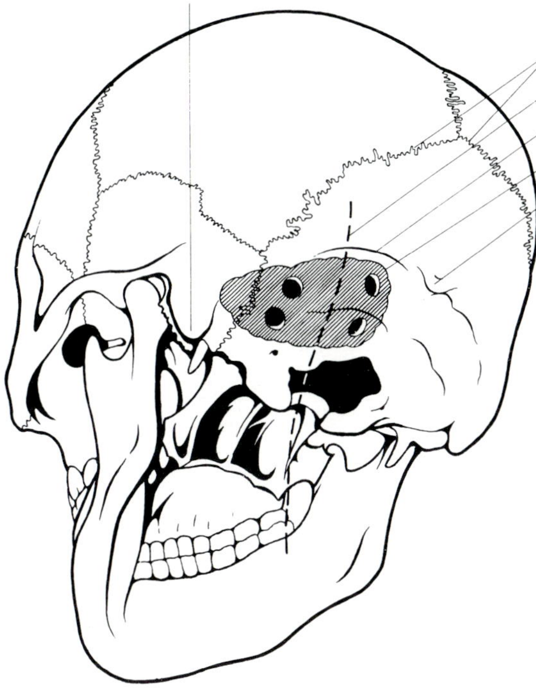

Fig. 49. Acoustic neurinoma: Outline of skin incision and craniectomy for unilateral approach to the left cerebellopontine area.

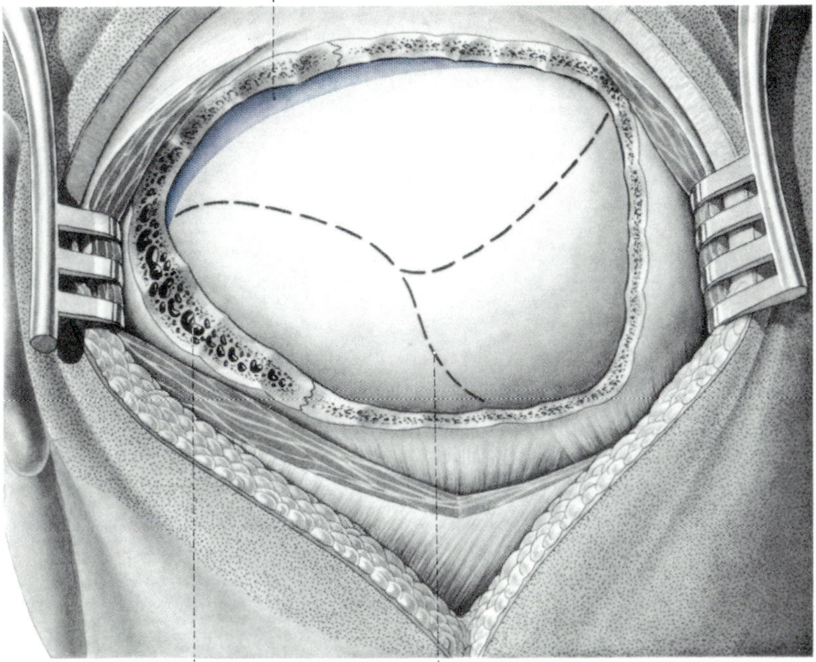

Fig. 50. Acoustic neurinoma: Dural exposure after left suboccipital craniectomy for exposure to the cerebellopontine angle.

Observe: 1. The craniectomy extends far enough superiorly to bring the transverse sinus into view. 2. The dural incision is shown by the dotted line.

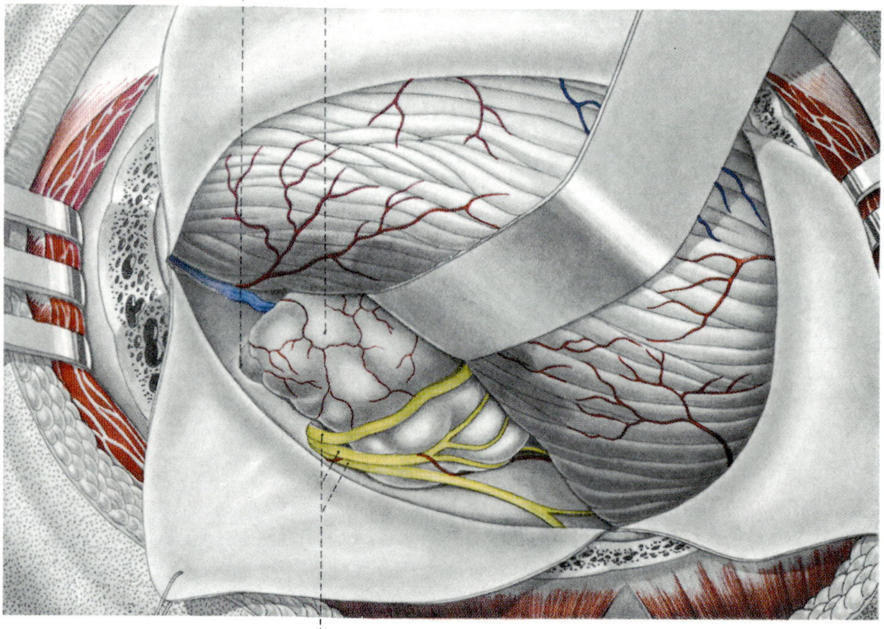

Fig. 51. Acoustic neurinoma: Exposure of cerebellopontine angle. The lower pole and lateral extent of tumor are visible.

Observe: 1. Relationship of Ns. IX, X and XI to lower pole of tumor. 2. Extention of tumor out the internal acoustic meatus.

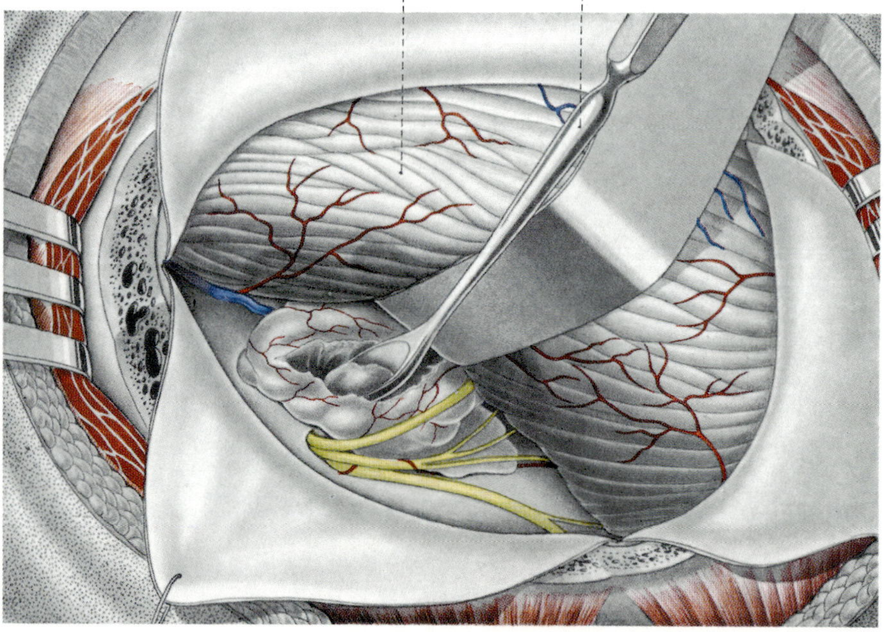

Fig. 52. Acoustic neurinoma: Incision of tumor capsule permits intracapsular removal.

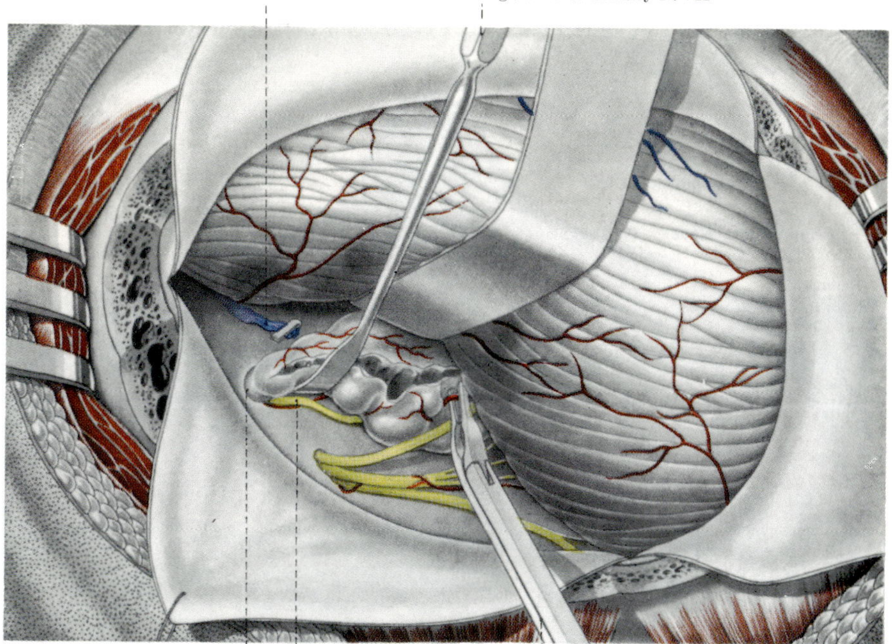

Fig. 53. Acoustic neurinoma: Dissection of the capsule and remaining tumor from surrounding structures.

Observe: 1. Identification of N. VII at the internal acoustic meatus. 2. Clipping and sectioning of the vascular supply to the tumor.

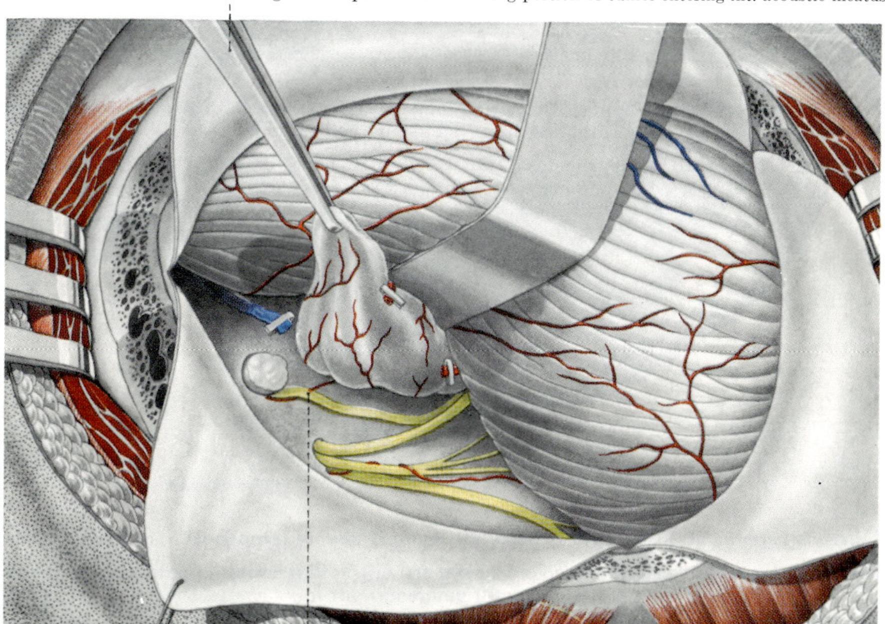

Fig. 54. Acoustic neurinoma: Removal.

Observe: 1. After identifying N. VII at the internal acoustic meatus, the extention of the tumor into the meatus is sectioned permitting further dissection of the tumor capsule.

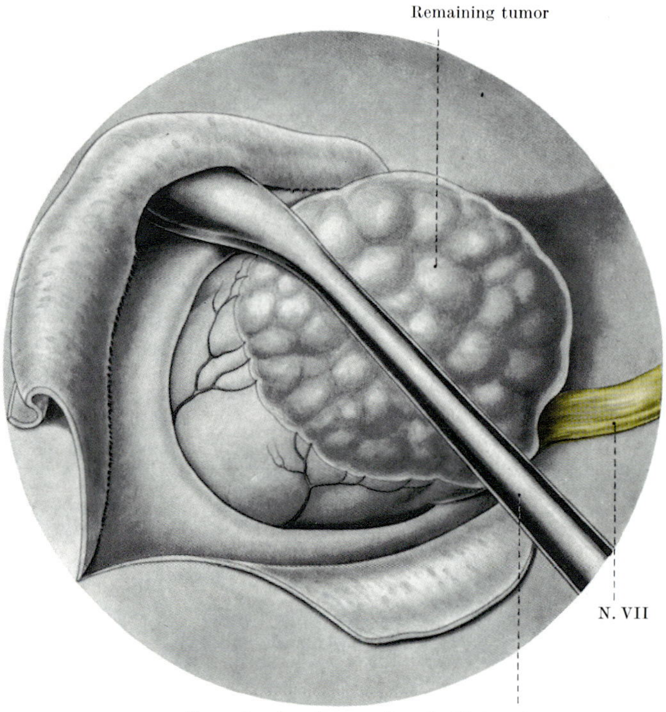

Fig. 57. Acoustic neurinoma: View of remaining tumor in the internal acoustic meatus as seen through the surgical operating microscope.

Fig. 58. Acoustic neurinoma: The posterior wall of the internal acoustic meatus is removed by a high speed drill. *Observe:* 1. Location of N. VII in fundus of the internal acoustic meatus. 2. Dissection of the tumor from N. VII.

Fig. 59. Acoustic neurinoma: Fundus of the internal acoustic meatus after removal of acoustic neurinoma with preservation of N. VII as seen through the surgical operating microscope.

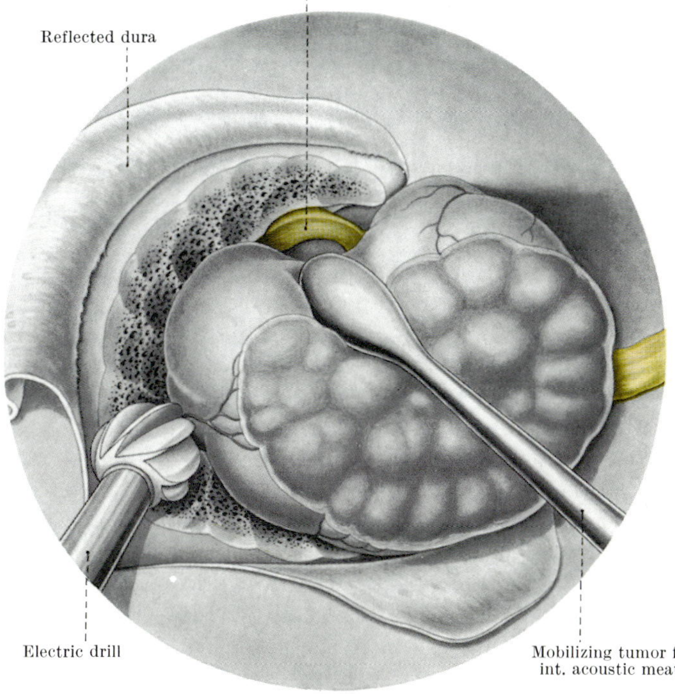
N. VII
Reflected dura
Electric drill
Mobilizing tumor from
int. acoustic meatus

Fig. 58.

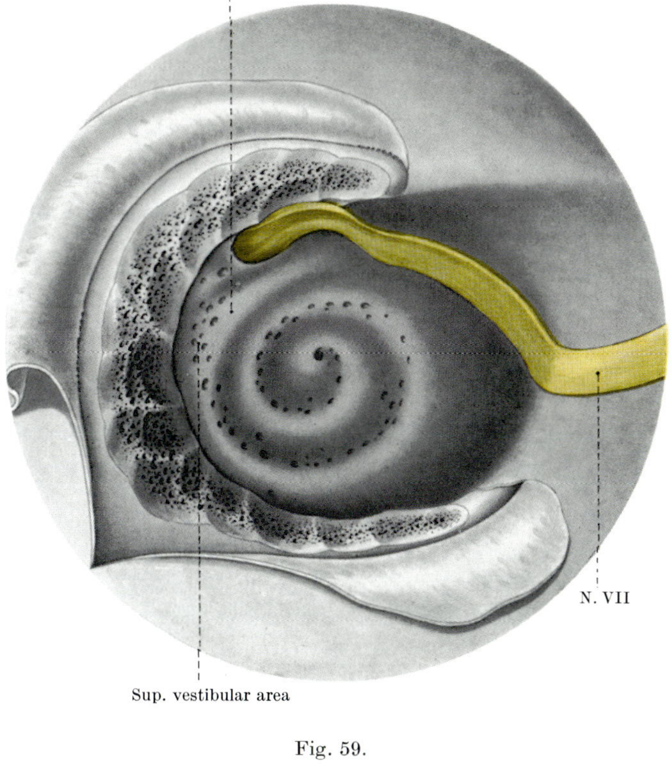
Transverse crest
N. VII
Sup. vestibular area

Fig. 59.

Chapter IV

Suboccipital Craniectomy — Occipital Craniotomy

Meningioma of the Posterior Surface of the Petrous Bone

The most frequent location for meningiomas of the posterior fossa, in our experience, is on the posterior surface of the petrous bone (see Fig. 60; compare Chapter XXI, Vol. I, p. 215). The major blood supply to these very vascular tumors arises from short branches of the internal carotid artery as it passes through the carotid canal within the petrous bone. Additional vessels from the posterior branches of the middle meningeal artery feed the tumor. In medially placed tumors near the clivus, the blood supply may be identical to that for a clivus meningioma, as described in Chapter XXII, Vol. I, p. 223 and Fig. 291. These tumors are attached to the dura over the posterior surface of the petrous bone anterior and superior to the internal auditory meatus and to the undersurface of the tentorium. The tentorium may be perforated by the tumor just as the falx is often penetrated by meningiomas in that location.

Meningiomas in this location are most readily removed by a combined supra- and infra-tentorial approach. This operation is also done with the patient sitting. All of the precautions against a sudden fall in blood pressure and air embolism, as described in Chapter I, must be taken.

A 20 cm. curvilinear scalp incision is made beginning 5 cm. above the lambdoidal suture, bisecting the superior nuchal line half way between the inion and the mastoid process, and then turning straight down the neck (Fig. 61). Subgaleal and subperiosteal dissection then allows the bony exposure shown in Fig. 61. Burr holes are placed both above and below the transverse sinus. A small free bone flap is elevated above the sinus and a suboccipital craniectomy is completed below the sinus.

The occipital dura is opened so that the base of the dura flap is at the sinus (Fig. 62). A few occipital bridging veins are coagulated and the occipital lobe is elevated to expose the tentorium. The superior surface of the tentorium is inspected for supratentorial extension of the tumor. If the tumor has perforated the tentorium, it should be incised so that the tentorial flap will be based at the superior petrosal sinus. At times it is better to expose the incisura from above and begin the tentorial incision at that point. In the case illustrated, the tumor did not perforate the tentorium; and, therefore, the small tentorial incision is based posteriorly (Figs. 63 and 64). Cerebellar veins may be draped over the tumor as they pass to the superior petrosal sinus. These veins must be coagulated and divided. The tumor capsule is coagulated and a window is made into the tumor. The tumor is then gutted using a sharp curette or occasionally, in very vascular tumors, the electrocautery loop (Fig. 65). Depending on the size of the tumor, the tentorium may be opened up to the transverse sinus which gives a beautiful view of the cerebellopontine angle from above.

The dura over the posterior fossa is then opened as shown in Fig. 62. Depending on the size of the tumor, it may be covered by only a shell of cerebellum or it may be so large that it is necessary to resect a lateral portion of the hemisphere. As the cerebellum is retracted, it must be covered by wet cotton pledgets; and when the cerebellum is dissected from the tumor capsule, cotton pledgets should be advanced into the line of cleavage. The cranial nerves, which are stretched by the tumor (Fig. 66), are also protected with a wet cottonoid as the tumor is now morselized from below (Fig. 67). Feeding vessels from the superior and anterior inferior cerebellar arteries will become visible as the tumor is reduced in size and must be clipped and cut. It is often necessary to alternate back and forth between the supra- and infra-tentorial exposure as the tumor is gradually reduced in size. The facial nerve may be found displaced ventrally or it may be pushed superiorly toward the root of the trigeminal nerve. This means that the seventh nerve must always be kept in mind since it can be found at any site around the tumor.

The outstanding hazard of this operation is the relationship of the tumor to surrounding vascular structures. The basilar artery may be adherent to, or even enveloped by, the tumor. This means that occasionally a small portion of this tumor will have to be left behind. The superior petrosal sinus is usually obliterated by the tumor. After reducing the size of the tumor so that its dura attachments can be seen from above and below, it is excised. Perforating channels from the internal carotid artery in the carotid canal are plugged with bone wax. The tumor bed is thoroughly coagulated under continuous irrigation (Fig. 68).

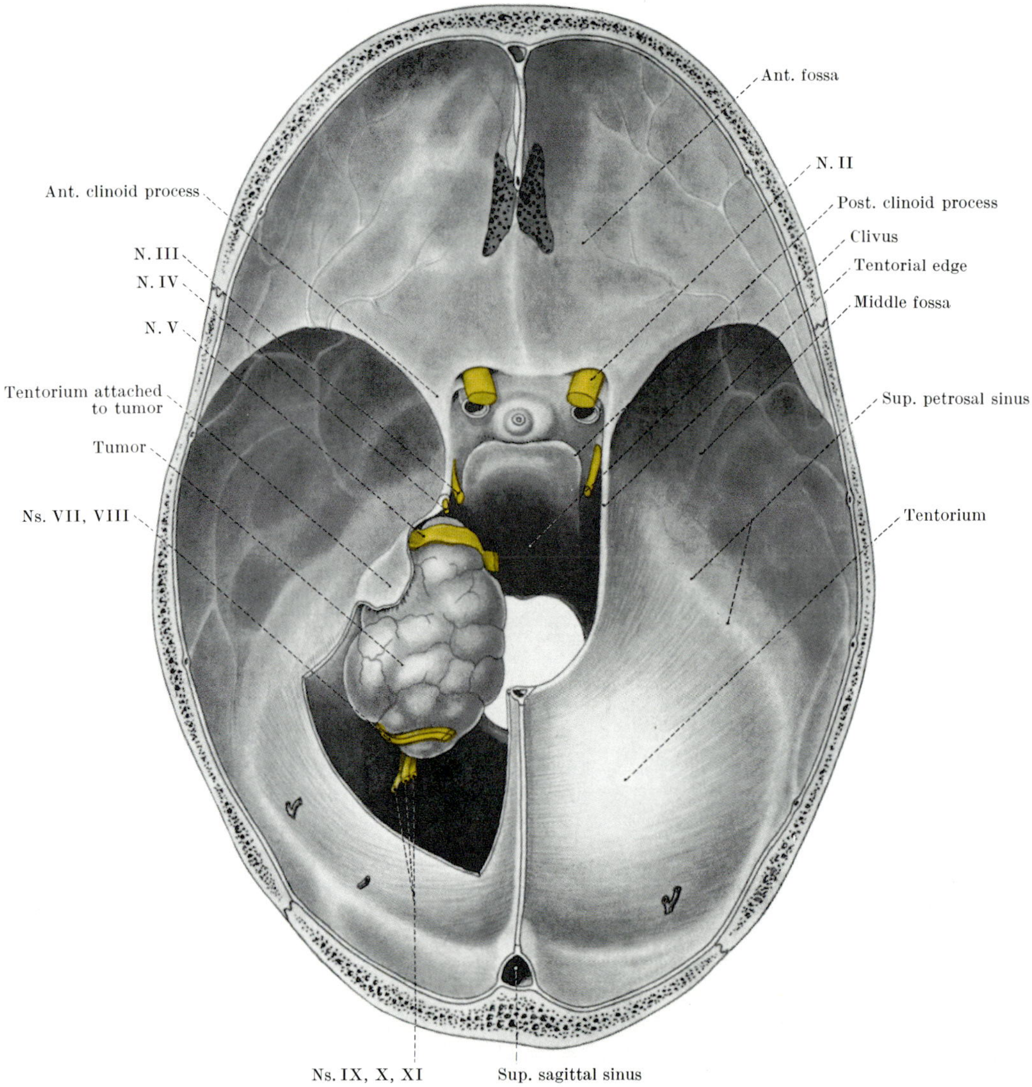

Fig. 60. Anatomico-topographical demonstration of a meningioma over posterior surface of right petrous bone. *Observe:* 1. Displacement and stretching of cranial nerves. 2. The tumor is also adherent to undersurface of the tentorium. 3. Compare with Figs. 46 and 47 to visualize the displacement of the brain stem and cerebellum.

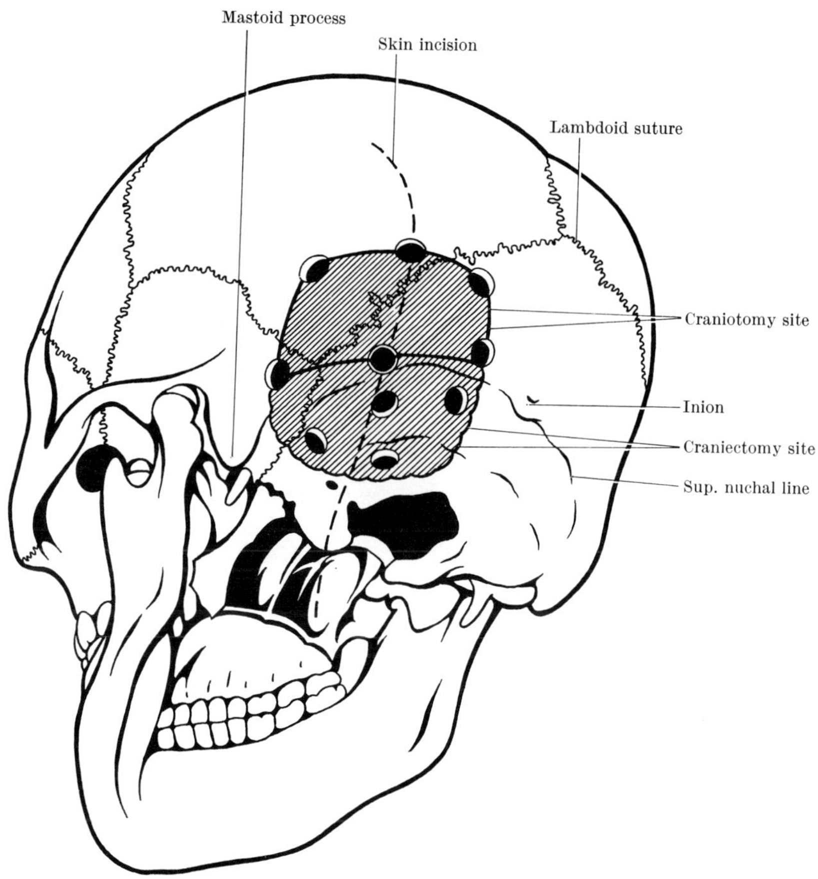

Fig. 61. Unilateral occipital craniotomy and suboccipital craniectomy for meningioma of the posterior surface of the petrous bone.

Observe: Interrupted line indicates the skin incision.

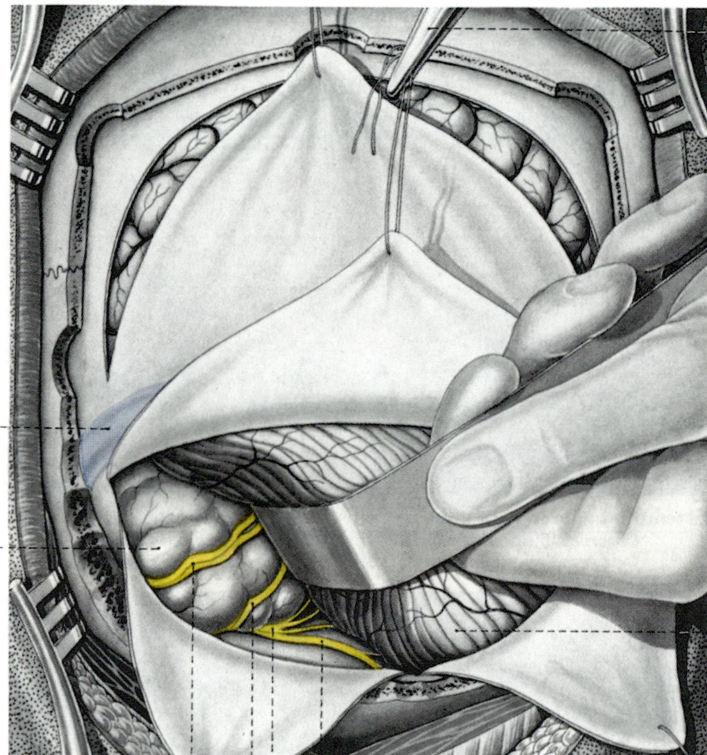

Fig. 66. Exposure of inferior aspect of a meningioma of the posterior surface of the petrous bone. *Observe:* Ns. VII and VIII coursing over the capsule of the tumor.

Fig. 67. Meningioma of the posterior surface of the petrous bone: Reduction of tumor bulk using a sharp spoon curette.

Fig. 68. Meningioma of the posterior surface of the left petrous bone: Operative field after total removal. *Observe:* Use of bipolar coagulation for hemostasis.

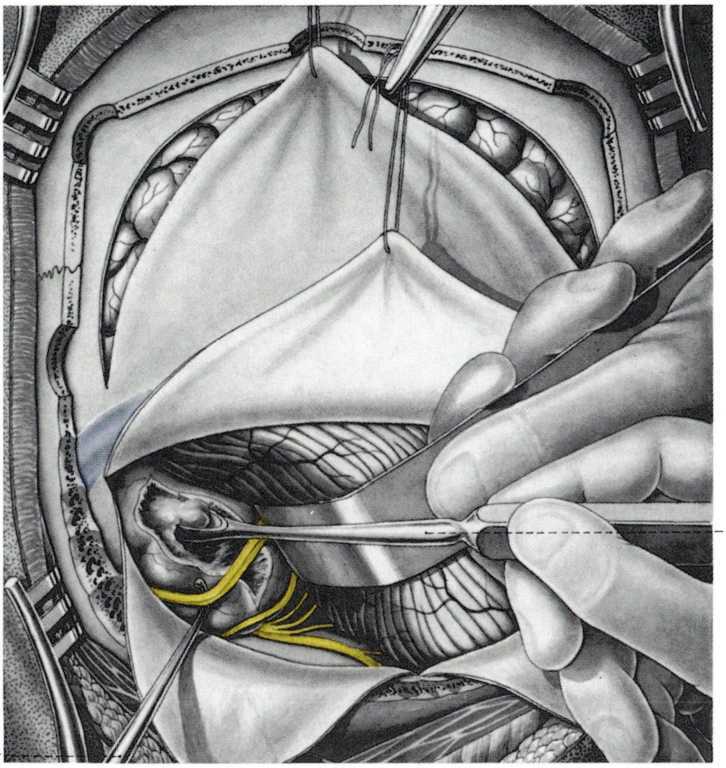
Sharp spoon curette
Retracting Ns. VII, VIII

Fig. 67.

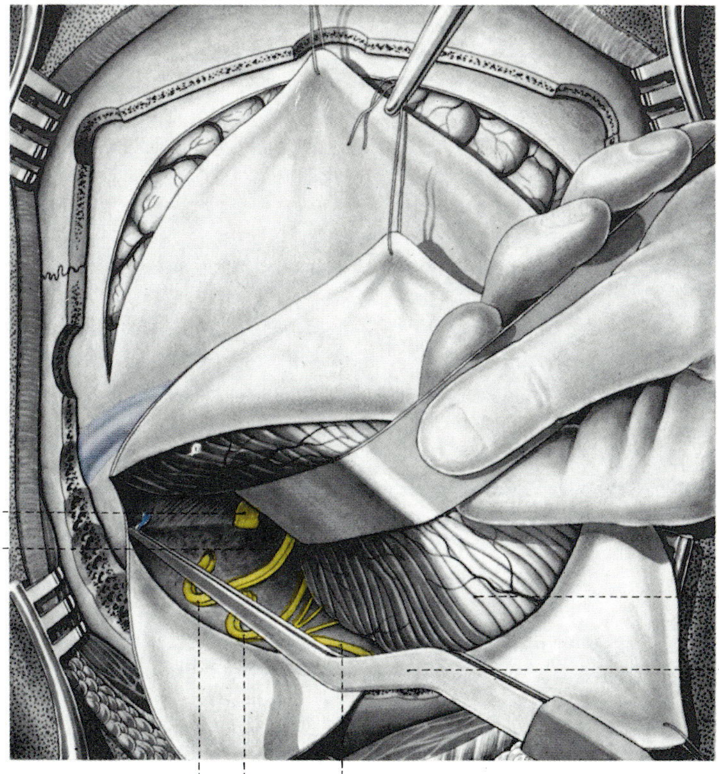
N. V
Posterior surface of petrous bone
Left cerebellar hemisphere
Bipolar coagulation
N. XI
Ns. VII, VIII
Ns. IX, X

Fig. 68.

Chapter V

Posterior Fossa Rhizotomies

A. Trigeminal Rhizotomy

Since 1955 we have used the posterior fossa approach exclusively in the surgical treatment of tic douloureux. This exposure is preferable because, as DANDY [1] pointed out many years ago, light touch is preserved in all three divisions. This means that the corneal reflex is not disturbed. It would also seem that this is a less hazardous approach as far as injury to the motor root is concerned. Because tic douloureux may result from compression of the nerve roots by various causes, this route also offers the advantage, in these cases, of exposing the pathology.

The patient is operated on in the sitting position. The head is turned slightly toward the side of the facial pain. This position is identical to that illustrated in Fig. 48 for acoustic neurinomas. This position allows the easiest exposure of the cerebellopontine angle and optimizes the angle of retraction on the cerebellum.

A 12 cm. vertical scalp incision is made beginning four cm. above the superior nuchal line and bisecting this line midway between the inion and the mastoid process. The muscles and pericranium are incised in the same line and elevated. A self-retaining retractor is used to maintain the bone exposure. The unilateral suboccipital craniectomy is identical to that which is used for an acoustic tumor (Fig. 49). The laterosuperior extent of the craniectomy should expose the lower margin of the transverse sinus. By removing the bone this far laterally (Figs. 49 and 50) the mastoid air cells will be opened and they must be obliterated using bone wax. The lateral limits of the craniectomy are absolutely critical for gaining the optimal exposure of the cerebellopontine angle (Fig. 70).

The dura is opened as illustrated in Fig. 50. A retractor is placed over the lateral extent of the cerebellar hemisphere and the cerebellum is retracted medially. The cerebellum is not elevated but merely retracted medially. If this brain spatula is correctly inserted and retracted, the seventh and eighth cranial nerves and the petrosal vein covered by the bulging arachnoid of the cerebellopontine cystern will be seen. Note that to this point the arachnoid has not been entered. The arachnoid is torn between the seventh nerve and the petrosal vein. Cerebrospinal fluid is evacuated. At the inferior portion of the exposure, the IX, X, and XI nerves are also visible. The cranial nerves from VII to XI in the lateral gutter are covered with a moist cottonoid for protection. The petrosal vein must be coagulated or clipped and divided (Fig. 70). The cerebellar retractor is now advanced a few millimeters by removing it and reapplying it. The nerve roots of the trigeminus may be covered by webs of arachnoid which must be carefully removed. The nerve roots are inspected for any vessels which may be adherent or close to the nerve. These vessels must be separated from the nerve roots so that they will not be inadvertantly torn in sectioning the nerve root. A sharp-angled Dandy nerve hook is introduced from below (see arrow in Fig. 69) to separate the caudal one-third to one-half of the rootlets (Fig. 71). The portion of the nerve within the hook is coagulated and divided.

[1] DANDY, W.: An operation for the cure of Tic Douloureux. Arch. Surg. 18, 687—734 (1929).

B. Nervus Intermedius Rhizotomy

Rhizotomy of the nervus intermedius may be done for geniculate neuralgia or intractable pain secondary to a malignancy. In recent years this operation has been recommended in the treatment of Horton's cephalgia (histamine headaches). In our experience the most common indication is intractable pain about the ear in patients with a malignancy who have been treated with irradiation.

The position of the patient, scalp incision, craniectomy and operative exposure are identical to that already described and illustrated for the trigeminal rhizotomy. The retraction of the cerebellum, however, is different. In this operation the cerebellum is gently elevated rather than retracted medially (Fig. 72; compare with Figs. 70 and 71). Having exposed the seventh and eighth cranial nerves in the cerebellopontine angle, magnification becomes essential to the successful completion of this rhizotomy. Magnification is not only helpful in preventing injury to the facial and auditory nerves and accompanying vessels but is also of aid in identifying the nerve of Wrisberg (nervus intermedius). This nerve may consist of only two to four tiny fascicles. The nerve is usually, at least over part of its intracranial course, closely adherent to the vestibular nerve. A very fine blunt nerve hook or a mastoid seeker is used to gently separate the seventh and eighth nerve roots on their dorsal surface. When a plane has been developed so that the nerve hook "falls" between the nerves, the nerve hook is gently turned around and the nervus intermedius is "fished" out from this interval (Fig. 72). After ascertaining that no vessels are with this fine strand of nerve, it is coagulated and divided with a fine scissors. If cautery is used, extreme care must be taken to avoid injuring the seventh and eighth nerves.

C. Glossopharyngeal Rhizotomy

Glossopharyngeal neuralgia and intractable pain secondary to malignancy constitute the indications for glossopharyngeal neuralgia.

The surgical exposure is identical to that used in trigeminal rhizotomy. The angle of retraction in this case is different. As in exposing the seventh and eighth cranial nerves, the brain spatula should elevate the cerebellum. The position of this retractor is emphasized in this chapter because it should not be moved repeatedly since the cerebellum can be very easily injured. The surgeon must have sufficient knowledge of the anatomical relationships within the posterior fossa so that the retractor can be placed definitively in one motion.

The glossopharyngeal nerve is easily identified as the most rostral nerve in the IX, X and XI group. Magnification will aid in demonstrating that this nerve passes through a separate opening in the dura. The two rostralmost strands of the vagus nerve are included with the glossopharyngeal nerve in a blunt nerve hook or mastoid seeker. These fibers are elevated and separated from any vascular structure. Before the nerves are divided, the anesthetist is advised that the blood pressure may dramatically increase. This carotid sinus reflex is most striking in older individuals and in patients having bilateral rhizotomies. The nerves are divided using coagulation and a fine scissors (Fig. 73).

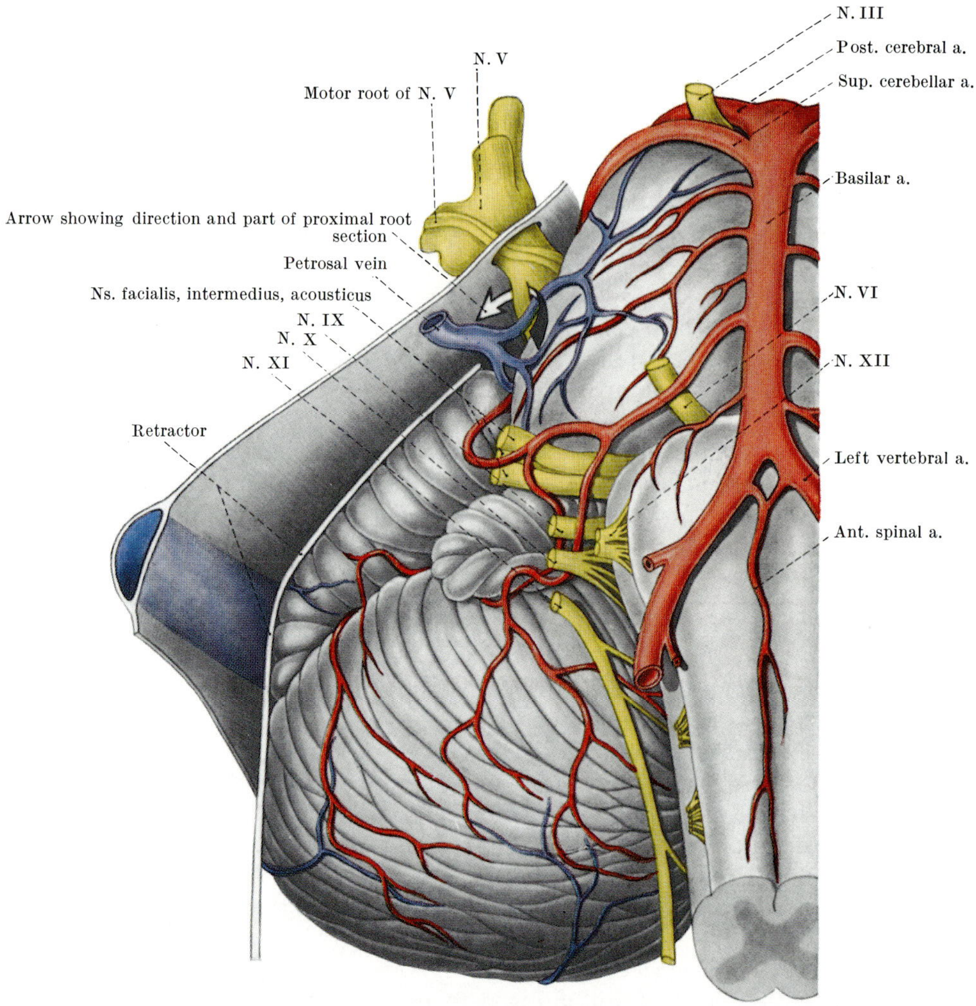

Fig. 69. Anatomico-topographical demonstration of the operative approach to the Vth nerve root via the posterior fossa.

Observe: The arrow indicates the approach and the direction of the Dandy nerve hook for partial division of the nerve root.

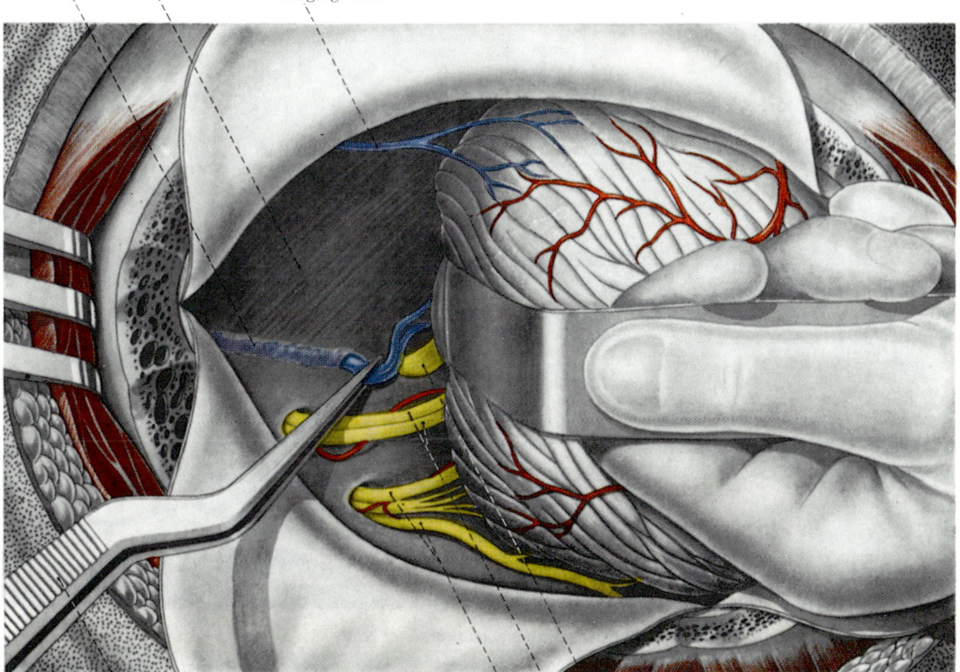

Fig. 70. Exposure of the left cerebellopontine angle for rhizotomy of N. V.

Observe: 1. Typical position of petrosal vein. 2. The exposed cranial nerves Ns. VII to XI will be covered by cottonoid after identification to prevent accidental injury while coagulating the petrosal vein.

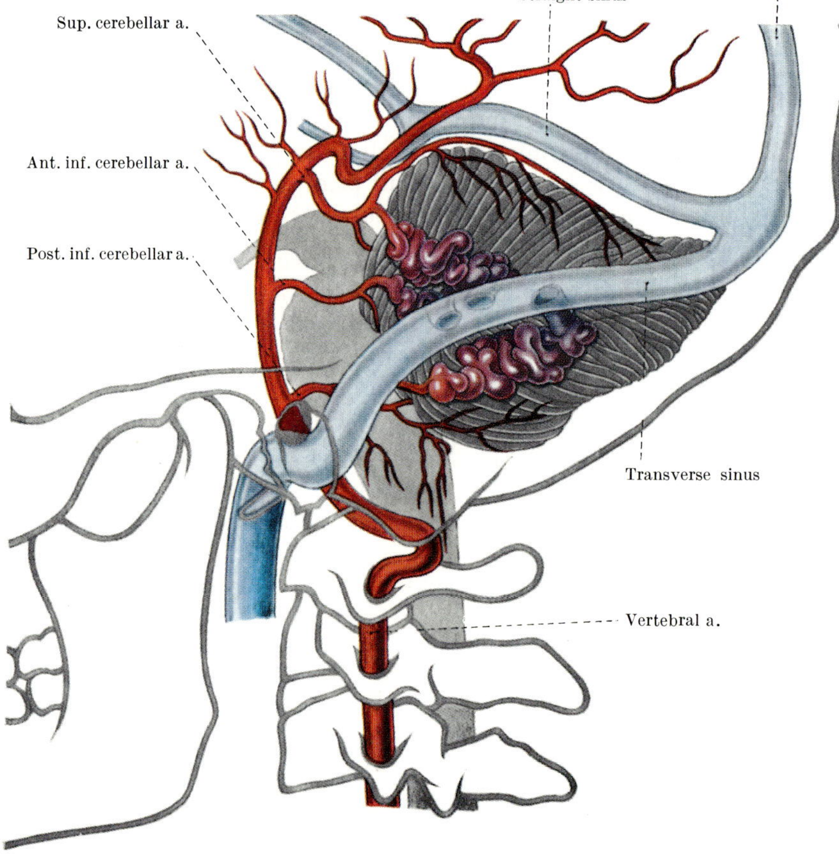

Fig. 74. Schematic presentation of an arterio-venous malformation over the left cerebellar hemisphere. *Observe:* Feeding arteries come from the major intracranial branches of the basilar and vertebral arteries.

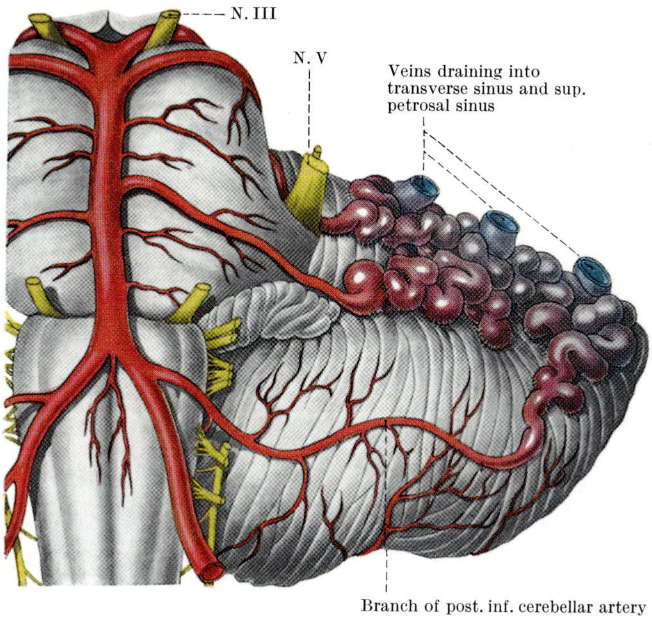

Fig. 75. Ventral view of an arterio-venous malformation over the left cerebellar hemisphere.

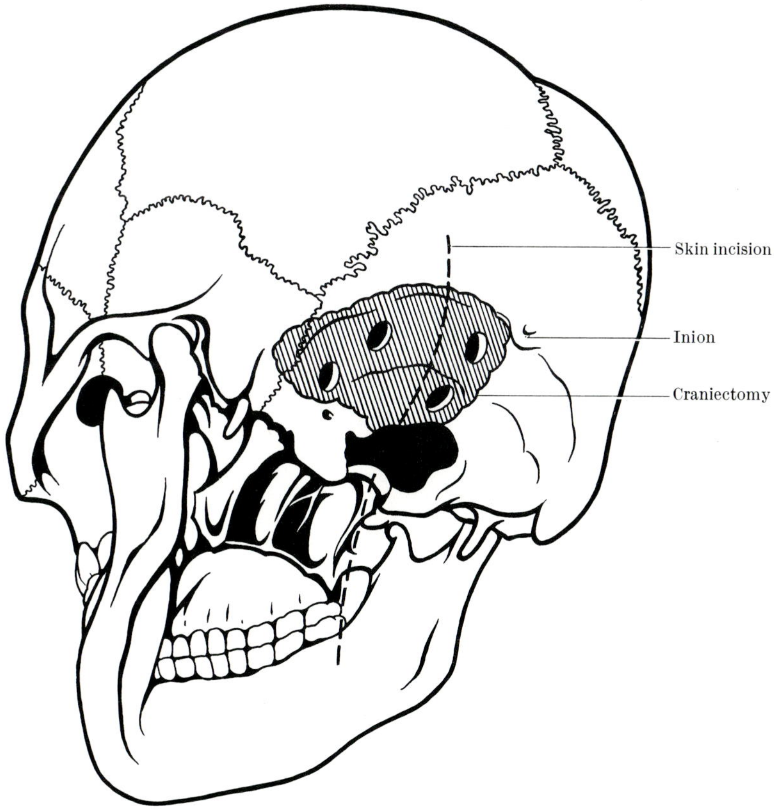

Fig. 76. Skin incision and craniectomy for an arterio-venous malformation over the left cerebellar hemisphere.

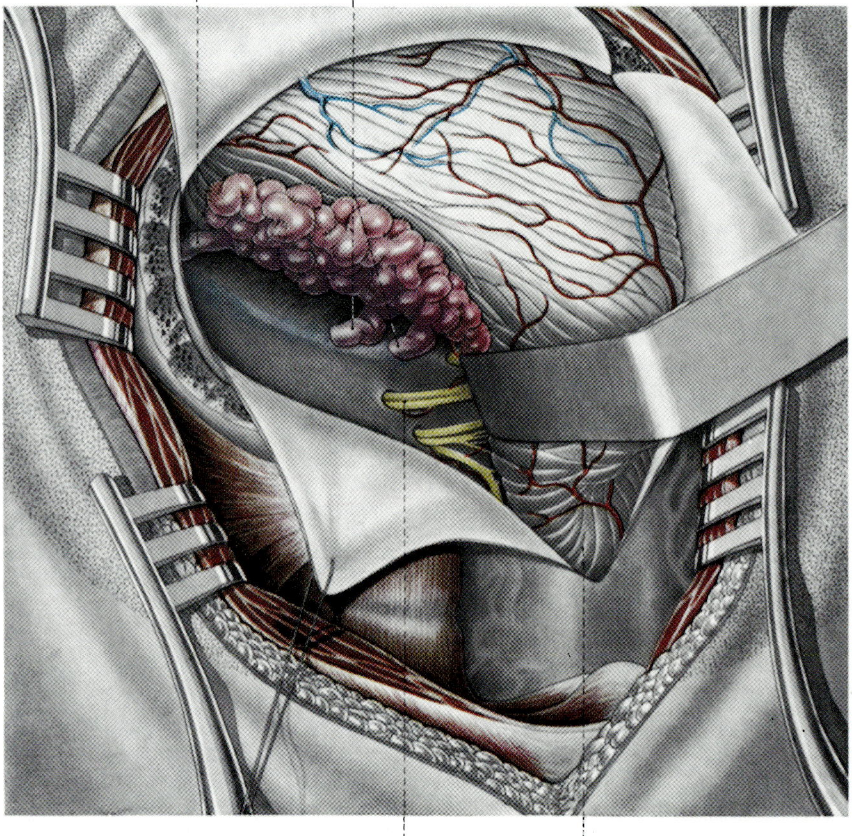

Fig. 77. Operative exposure of an arterio-venous malformation over the left lateral cerebellar hemisphere.

Observe: Venous drainage into superior petrosal and sigmoid sinuses.

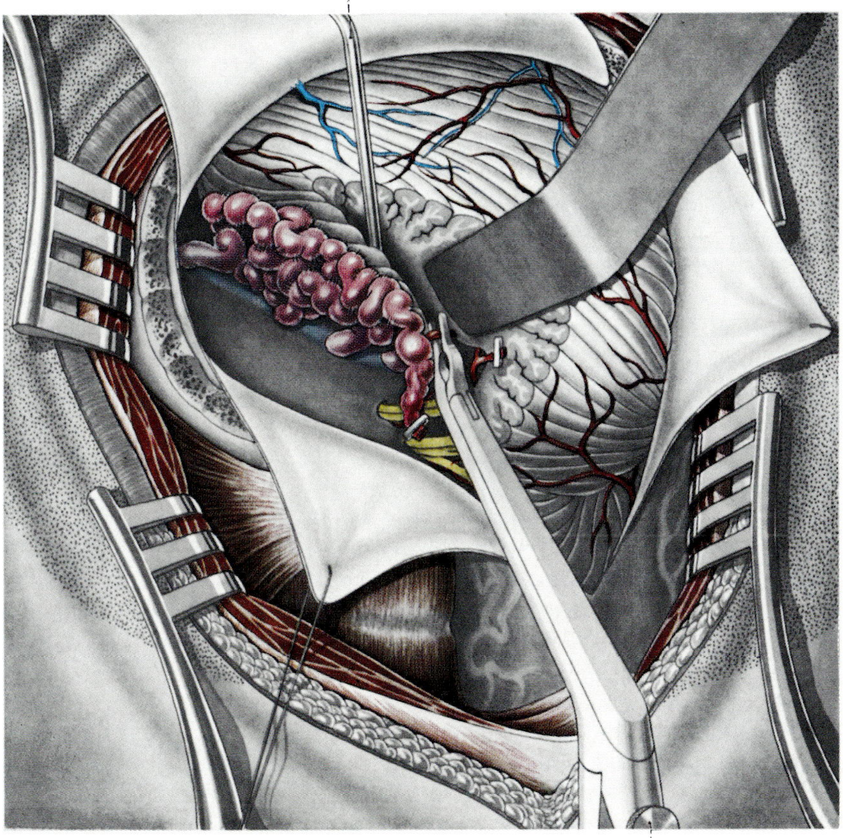

Fig. 78. Removal of an arterio-venous malformation of the left lateral cerebellar hemisphere.
Observe: 1. Feeding arteries are clipped. 2. Draining veins are taken last.

Chapter VII

Aneurysms of the Vertebral Artery

The first aneurysm in the posterior fossa successfully operated upon at Walter Reed General Hospital was in 1947 [1]. This aneurysm arose from the posterior inferior cerebellar artery. Since that time there have been four intracranial vertebral artery aneurysms. The origin of these aneurysms is often near the site where the vertebral artery passes through the dura. In fact, in two of our patients the aneurysms arose precisely as the vertebral artery passes intrathecally. This necessitates opening the dura to the base of the aneurysm so that the neck can be isolated. These aneurysms sometimes lie beneath the highest denticulate ligament which has to be transected to expose the lesion. These lesions do not have to rupture to cause symptoms. Aneurysms pointing rostrally along the lateral medullary cistern may cause irritative symptoms in the glossopharyngeal nerve (Fig. 79).

Aneurysms of the posterior fossa are diagnosed by vertebral angiography. The subtraction technique is often essential (Fig. 80a and b). In addition to routine half axial and lateral series, a base view (submental-vertex) is often of value.

The posterior fossa is exposed with the patient sitting by using a median incision and a bilateral suboccipital craniectomy (Fig. 81). It is important to remove the arch of the atlas so that the exposure will be low enough. The dura is opened in the shape of a *Y* (Fig. 4). The arachnoid is opened over the foramen magnum. The cerebellar hemisphere is gently elevated at its junction with the tonsil. Fig. 82 illustrates the area of aneurysm with the arachnoid still intact over most of the exposure. The arachnoidal opening is enlarged toward the lateral gutter. The highest denticulate ligament is identified, transected and reflected (Fig. 83). This permits exposure of the vertebral artery as it enters the dura. The vertebral artery is followed rostrally. The IX, X and XI cranial nerves are encountered as they lie stretched over the aneurysm (Fig. 82). These nerves as well as the posterior inferior cerebellar artery are separated from the aneurysm using a fine nerve hook, mastoid seeker or a variety of aneurysm needles. These instruments are also used to probe and define the size of the neck of the aneurysm. If the neck is broad we prefer to use a 00 oiled silk suture to ligate the aneurysm. In small-necked aneurysms a metallic clip is sometimes easier to apply.

The reader is referred to Vol. I, Chapter II for a more complete description and illustration of the technique of dissection and isolation of berry aneurysms.

---

[1] Rizzoli, H. V., Hayes, G. J.: Congenital berry aneurysm of the posterior fossa. J. Neurosurg. **10**, 550—551 (1953).

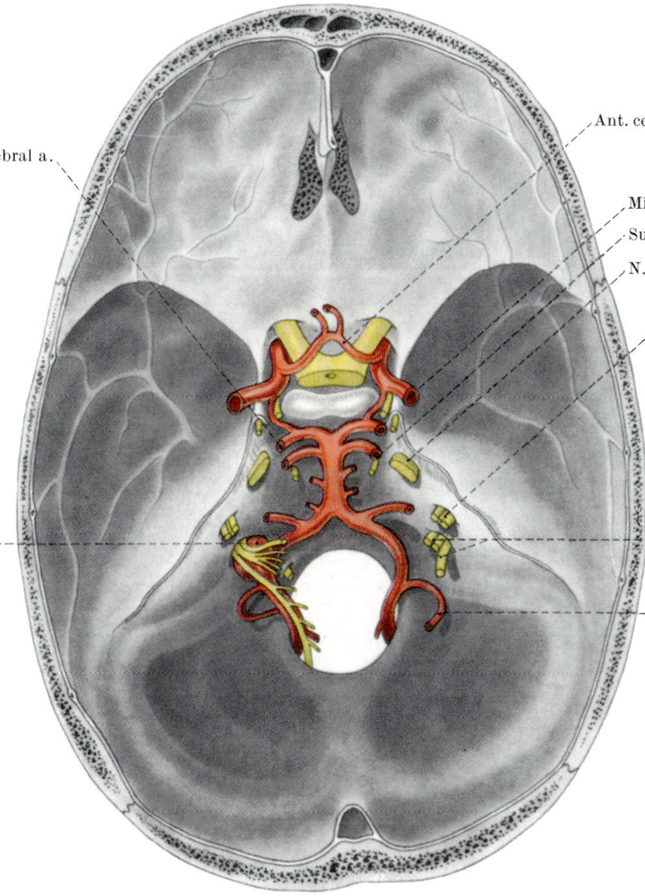

Fig. 79. Anatomico-topographical demonstration of an aneurysm of the left vertebral artery at the origin of the posterior inferior cerebellar artery.

Observe: Relationship of aneurysm to Ns. IX, X, XI.

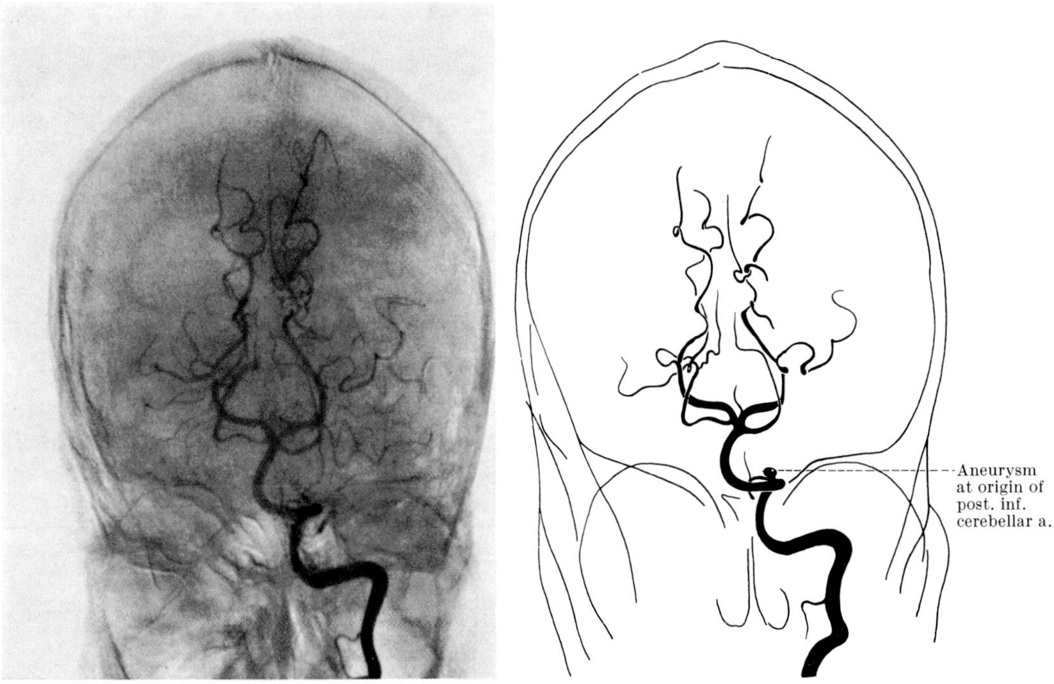

a b

Fig. 80a. Angiography: Aneurysm of the left vertebral artery at the origin of the posterior inferior cerebellar artery (subtraction film).

Fig. 80b. Line drawing elucidating X-ray of Fig. 80a.

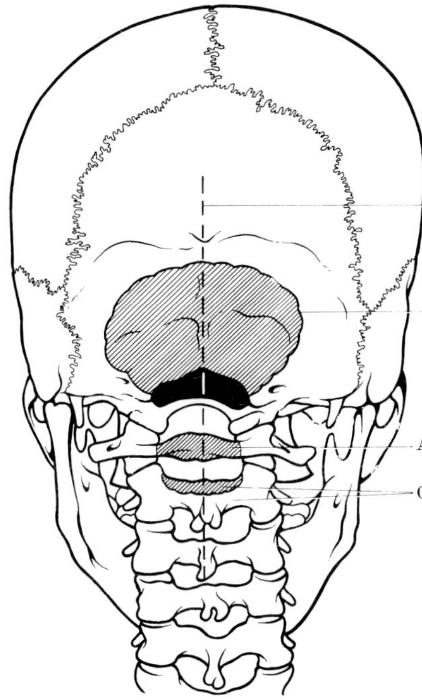

Fig. 81. Skin incision and craniectomy for an aneurysm of the vertebral artery. *Observe:* Posterior arch of atlas and part of C_2 are also removed.

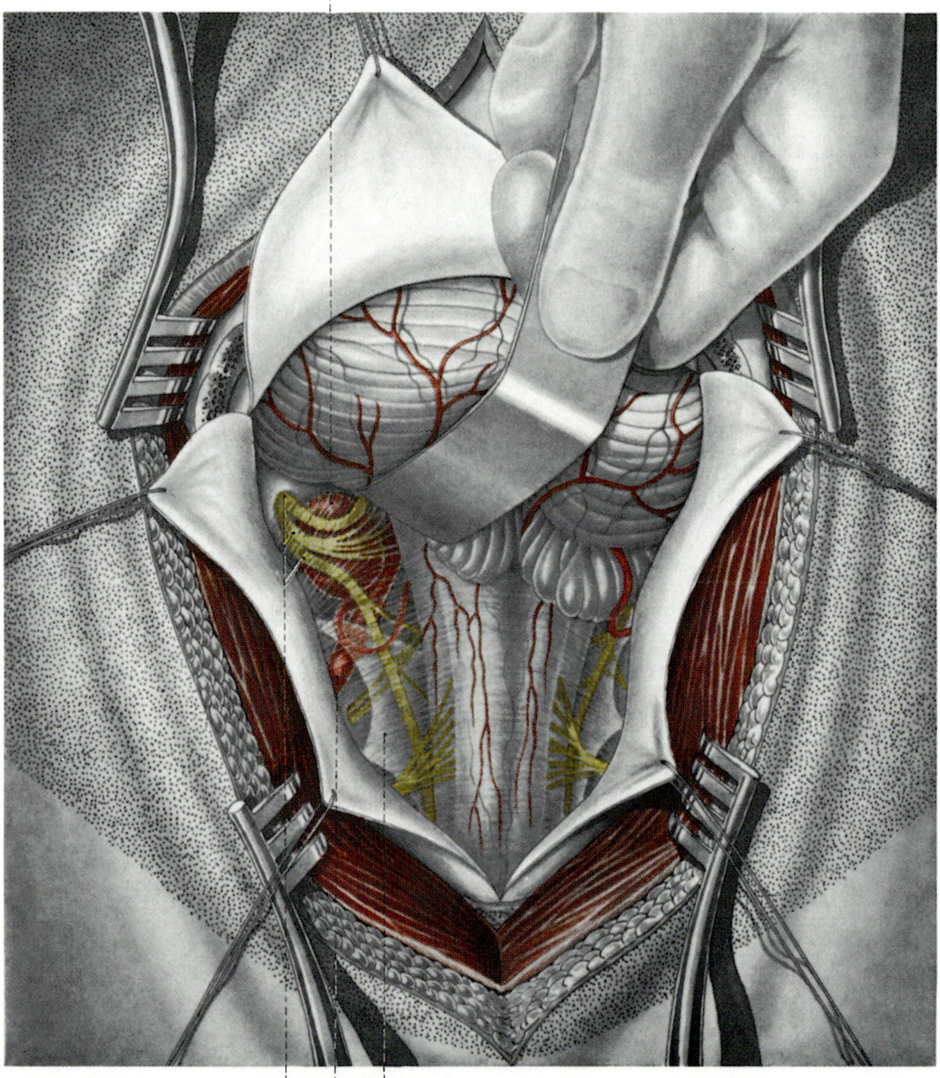

Fig. 82. Operative exposure of an aneurysm of the left vertebral artery at the origin of the posterior-inferior cerebellar artery.

Observe: 1. Arachnoid remains intact. 2. Cranial nerves Ns. IX, X, XI are partly displaced by aneurysm.

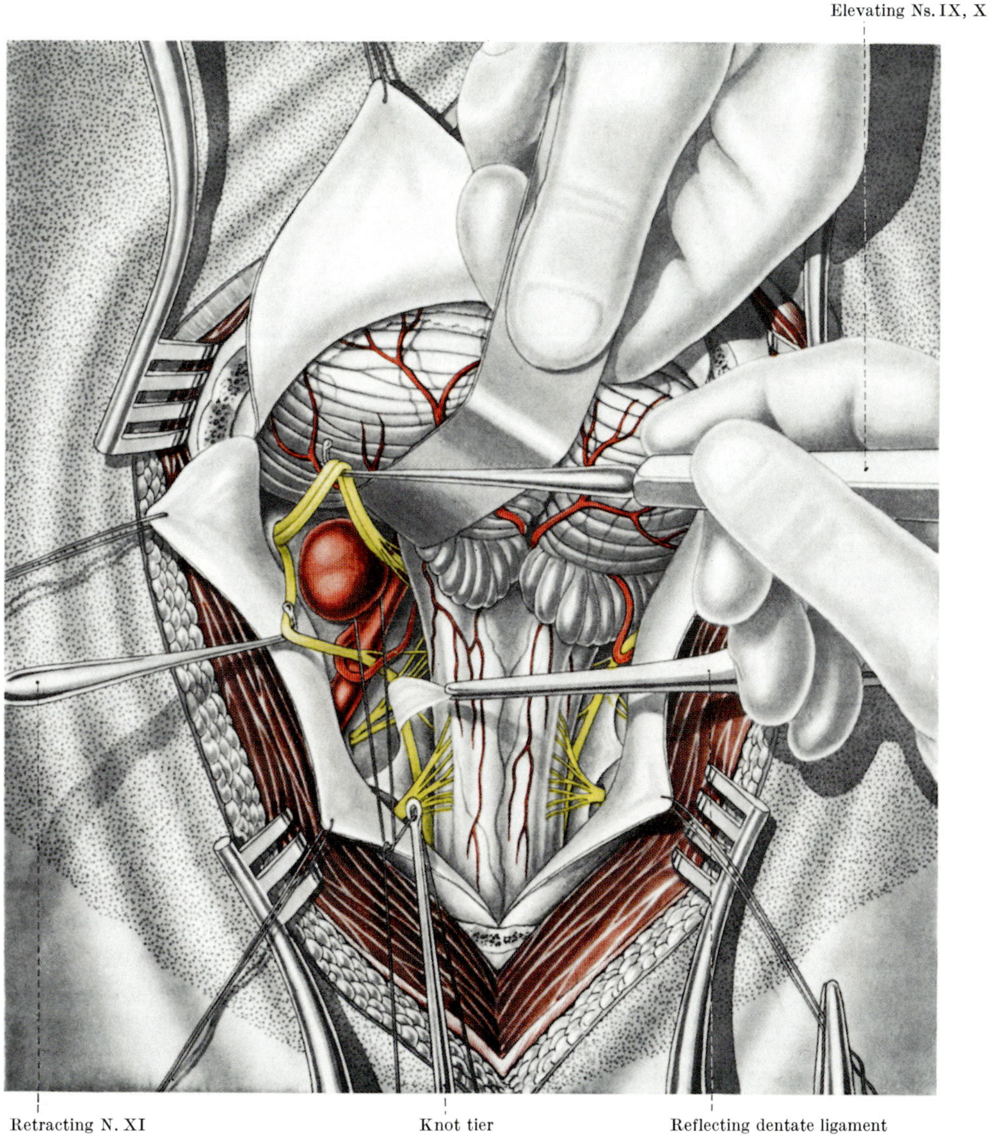

Fig. 83. Aneurysm of the left vertebral artery.

Observe: 1. Uppermost insertion of dentate ligament sectioned and reflected. 2. Cranial nerves Ns. IX, X, XI separated from the aneurysm. 3. Ligature around the neck of the aneurysm preserves the posterior inferior cerebellar artery.

Chapter VIII

Glomus Jugulare Tumor (Chemodectoma)

Glomus jugulare tumors have their origin from a small (0.25—0.5 mm.) group of cells in the adventitia of the jugular bulb. These paraganglia have recently been identified in different places in the petrous bone such as in the tympanic branch of the glossopharyngeal nerve, in the canaliculus tympanicus and in the submucosa of the promentory [1]. Glomus jugulare tumors receive their blood supply from the ascending pharyngeal artery. This observation is important in the surgical removal of these vascular tumors. It is often wise to ligate not only the external carotid artery but the ascending pharyngeal artery as well.

These lesions tend to be locally invasive. They erode the petrous portion of the temporal bone. Glomus jugulare tumors often enter the internal jugular vein as well as the dural sinuses. The tumor may penetrate the dura to compress the posterior fossa structures. Characteristically, this lesion presents as a reddish-blue mass penetrating the tympanic membrane. When the otologist biopsies the tumor it usually bleeds profusely.

Our experience with 12 of these tumors has convinced us that surgical excision is the treatment of choice. Irradiation is of absolutely no value in glomus jugulare tumors[2]. We have seen a relatively small tumor which was treated by irradiation present seven months later with massive destruction of the petrous bone. This made a formidable surgical task out of a much simpler operation.

Preoperatively these patients are evaluated with tomography of the temporo-occipital bone and angiography. Using arteriography or venography, the patency of the lateral and sigmoid sinuses and internal jugular vein should be ascertained. The development of the subtraction technique has greatly aided the quality of positive contrast studies in this area. In larger tumors a good sized ascending pharyngeal artery may be visualized.

To illustrate the surgical technique for removing chemodectomas of this area, a relatively small tumor is presented. The lesion depicted in Fig. 84 is filling the jugular bulb and could be expected to cause symptoms relative to the IX, X and XI nerves.

The operative procedure begins by ligating the external carotid artery and, when indicated, the ascending pharyngeal artery in the neck. The patient is then placed in the prone or lateral decubitus position and the head turned so that the mastoid process and asterion on the side of the lesion are uppermost. The surgeon's view of the skull appropriately positioned for surgery is shown in Fig. 85. The head and trunk are elevated slightly.

A skin incision is made beginning three cm. above the lambdoidal suture midway between the inion and the mastoid process and carried downward 12 cm. (Fig. 87). In larger lesions, greater exposure is necessary. In this situation, a skin incision is made beginning in front of the ear and then passing posteriorly in the shape of a question mark. The incision for ligating the external carotid artery in the neck can be included in this incision by prolonging the inferior extent anteriorly across the sternocleidomastoid muscle. The incision is carried down to the bone which is then stripped subperiosteally to expose the temporo-occipital junction.

---

[1] Kleinsasser, O.: Handbuch der Neurochirurgie, vol. IV, pt. I, p. 466—472. Berlin-Göttingen-Heidelberg: Springer 1966.

[2] McMeeken, R. R., Hardman, S. M., Kempe, L. G.: Multiple sclerosis after X-radiation. Activation by treatment of metastatic glomus tumor. Arch. Otolaryng. **90**, 617—621 (1969).

Multiple burr holes are placed above and below the level of the lateral sinus. The craniectomy is then completed using a rongeur. The extent of the craniectomy is shown in Figs. 85 and 87. It is important to expose the area of the entrance of the superior petrosal sinus into the lateral sinus to form the sigmoid sinus. Whenever possible the sigmoid sinus proximal to this point is ligated rather than ligating both the superior petrosal and lateral sinuses. Fig. 86 shows the anatomical relationship of the sinuses and mastoid emissary vein. The craniectomy is continued antero-inferiorly into the petrous bone until the tumor is recognized (Fig. 87). A high speed drill is then used and additional bone is removed following the tumor and sigmoid sinus inferiorly (Fig. 88). Great care is necessary to avoid injurying the facial nerve. In Fig. 89 the facial nerve is seen partially unroofed.

Small dural flaps are elevated anteriorly and posteriorly to the sinus just above the tumor (Fig. 88). Since these dural incisions flank the sigmoid sinus, rather than the transverse sinus, they will both be below the tentorium. The sinus is ligated with 00 silk and opened longitudinally below the ligature. A tongue of tumor will be seen in the lumen of the sinus. The soft tumor is removed by suction and curettage (Fig. 90). Additional bone is removed as necessary. No tumor should be left within the mastoid air cells. The internal jugular vein is followed inferiorly through the skull. The vein then passes just in front of the transverse process of C_1. This transverse process is exposed subperiosteally and removed. The jugular vein and its tributaries are ligated at this level. In doing this, care must be taken to avoid injurying the VII, IX, X and XI nerves (Fig. 91). The vein is opened longitudinally above the level of the ligature and the tumor removal is completed.

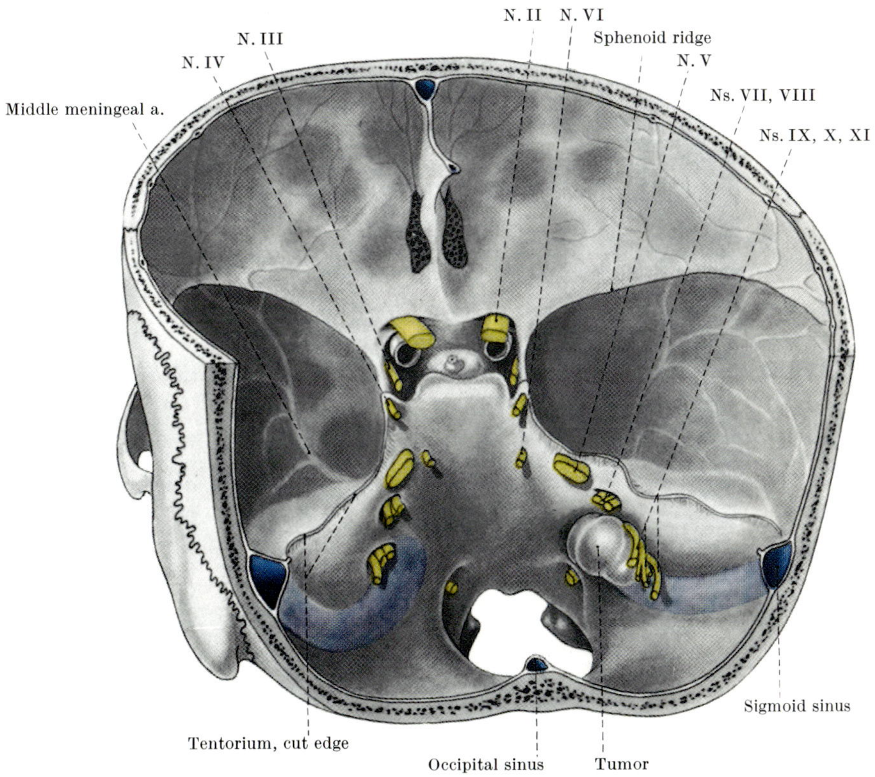

Fig. 84. Anatomico-topographical demonstration of a right glomus jugulare tumor.
Observe: Dura remains intact over the tumor.

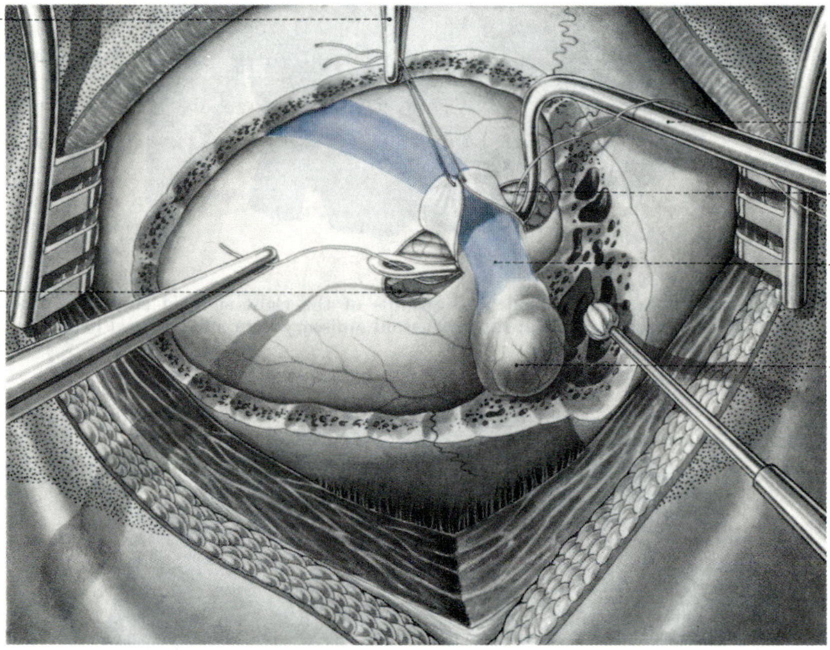

Fig. 88. Glomus jugulare tumor. Ligation of the sigmoid sinus and further removal of petrous bone.

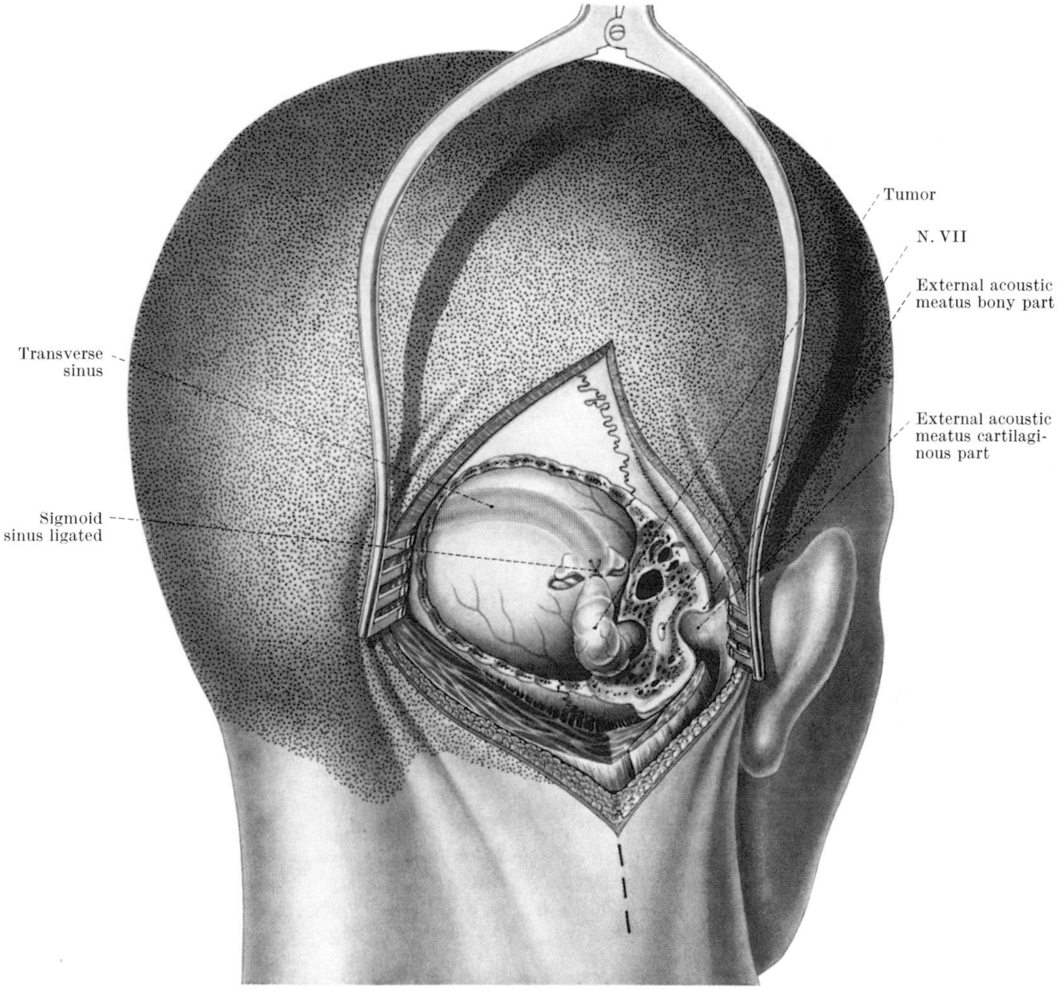

Fig. 89. Glomus jugulare tumor.

Observe: Extent of petrous bone removed.

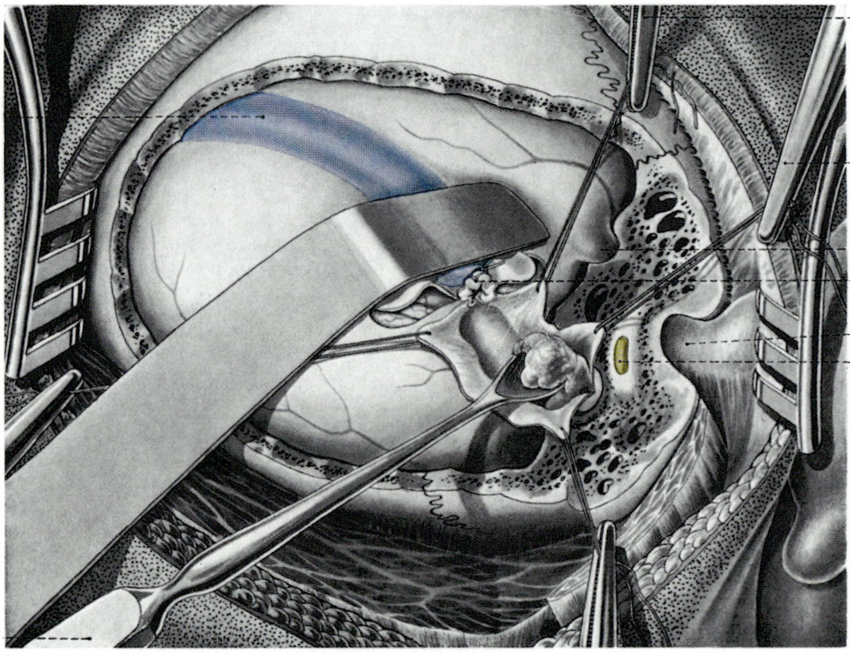

Fig. 90. Glomus jugulare tumor.

Observe: Ligated sigmoid sinus is opened to remove tumor which has grown within the lumen of the sinus.

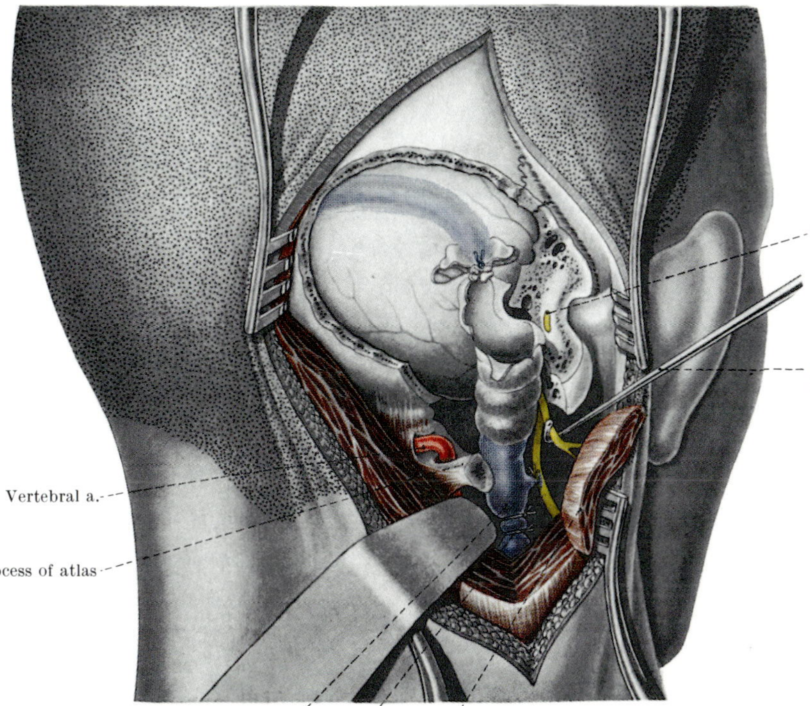

Fig. 91. Glomus jugulare tumor.

Observe: 1. Further removal of petrous bone and the transverse process of the atlas expose the internal jugular bulb and vein. 2. Ligation of the internal jugular vein.

Chapter IX

Meningioma of the Foramen Magnum

The second most frequent location for meningiomas of the posterior fossa is on the anterior rim of the foramen magnum. These tumors may extend for a considerable distance up the clivus or down into the spinal canal. These slow-growing tumors may cause remarkable distortion and compression of the cervicomedullary region. The vertebral artery and its branches, as well as the lower cranial nerves, may be completely enveloped by the tumor (Fig. 92).

Ideally, these patients will have both vertebral arteriography as well as myelography preoperatively. Since myelographic contrast media may obscur the region for a subsequent arteriogram and since the myelogram may suggest the need for urgent operative treatment, it is preferable to do the angiogram first whenever this diagnosis is seriously entertained. Because of the intimate relationship of these firm tumors with the vertebral arteries, any preoperative information that will give the surgeon a three-dimensional concept of the extent of the lesion is important.

The patient is placed in the sitting position and all precautionary measures, as outlined in Chapter I, are observed. A midline incision, as described in Chapter II, is made from above the inion to C_5. The lamina of both C_1 and C_2 are removed and a bilaterally suboccipital craniectomy completes the exposure (Figs. 93 and 94). The dura is incised in the shape of a *Y* and reflected. Fig. 95 illustrates the operative exposure after opening the arachnoid. The tumor depicted descends into the spinal canal on the right side. The highest denticulate ligament is stretched over the tumor. This ligament helps locate the level at which the vertebral artery enters the intrathecal space. In this patient it means that the tumor is covering the right vertebral artery. The dorsal root of C_2 and the highest denticulate ligament are transected, separated from the tumor and reflected medially. The spinal accessory nerve is gently elevated off the tumor capsule (Fig. 96). The tumor capsule is opened inferiorly and gutted. We prefer to use a sharp curette with constant irrigation and suction rather than risk the heat of the cautery loop in this location. The tumor is thus gradually reduced in size. The inferior cerebellum can be elevated and the tumor capsule is gently dissected free of adhesions and feeding vessels. The tumor is removed piecemeal until only the anterior dural attachment remains. This area is then curetted and cauterized using bipolar coagulation.

In large tumors with huge clival extensions, as seen in Fig. 92, this exposure is inadequate. These types of lesions should be approached with a combined foramen magnum — cerebellopontine angle exposure or even occasionally with a supratentorial exposure added to it. In dealing with meningiomas in front of the brain stem, remember that an already-distorted brain stem does not tolerate additional retraction without disasterous results. A multisided exposure will not only give more room but will also help in identifying and protecting important vascular structures and cranial nerves.

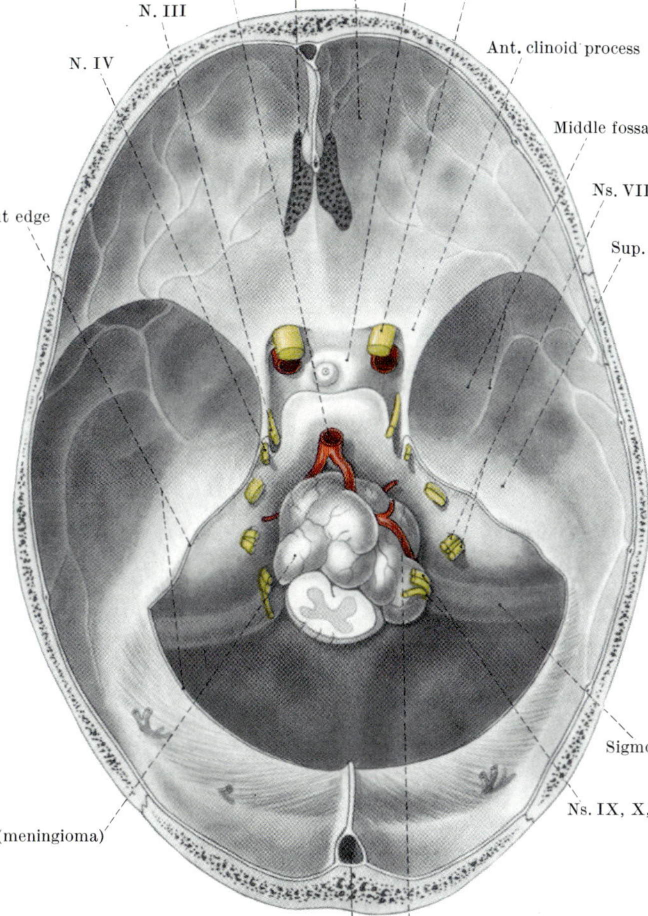

Fig. 92. Anatomico-topographical demonstration of a meningioma of the foramen magnum. The attachment of this tumor is at the anterior rim of the foramen magnum. The tumor extents halfway up the clivus. Its inferior extension reaches to the level of the arch of the atlas (see Figs. 94 and 95).

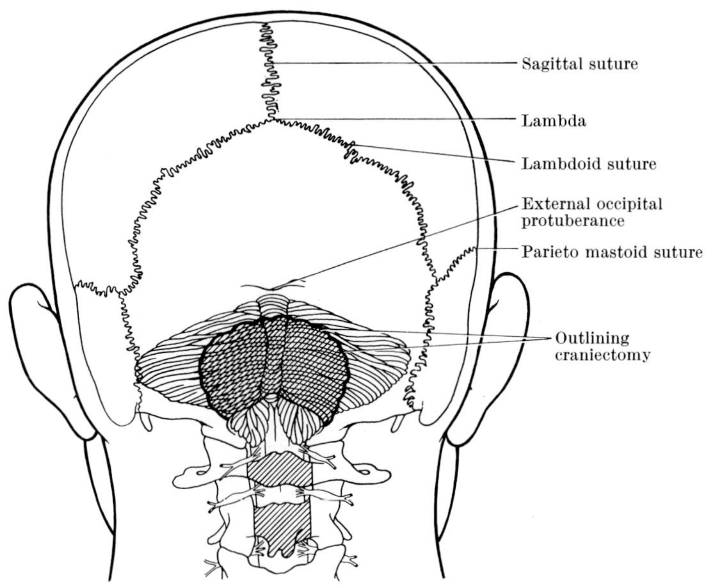

Fig. 93. Craniectomy for a meningioma of the foramen magnum.
Observe. Laminectomy of C_1 and C_2 is also performed.

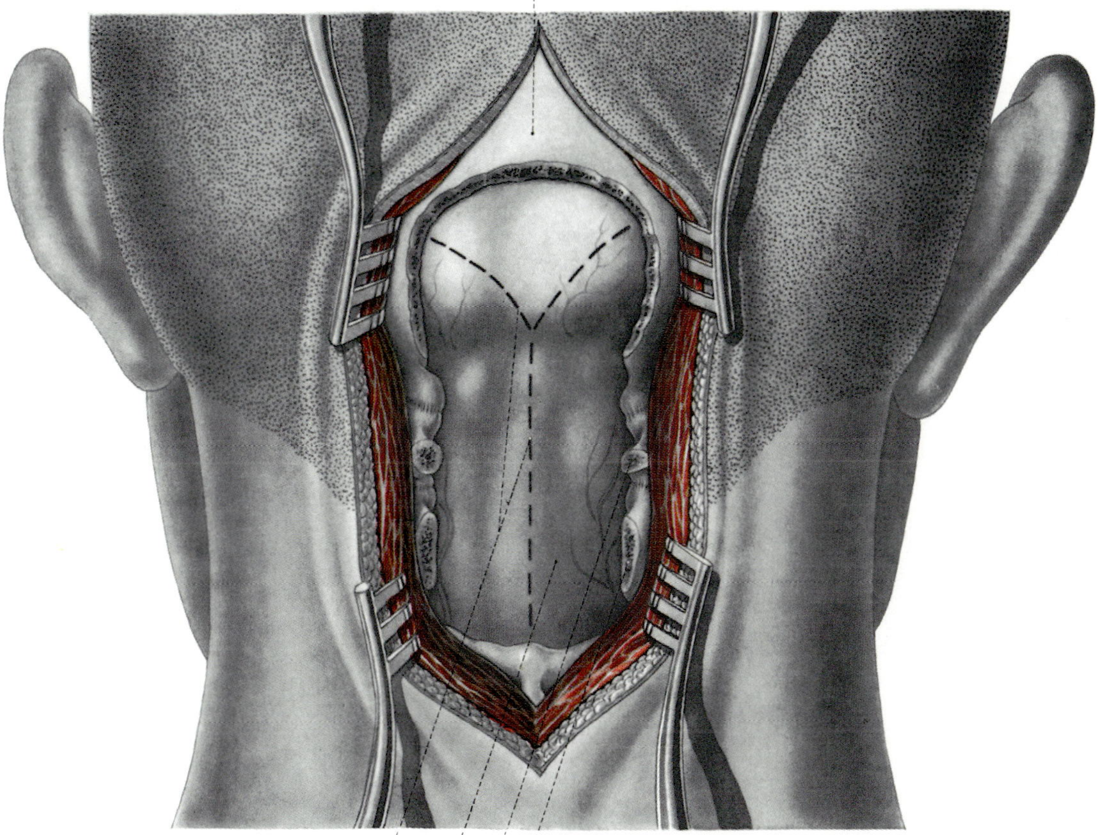

Fig. 94. Meningioma of the foramen magnum: Dural incision.

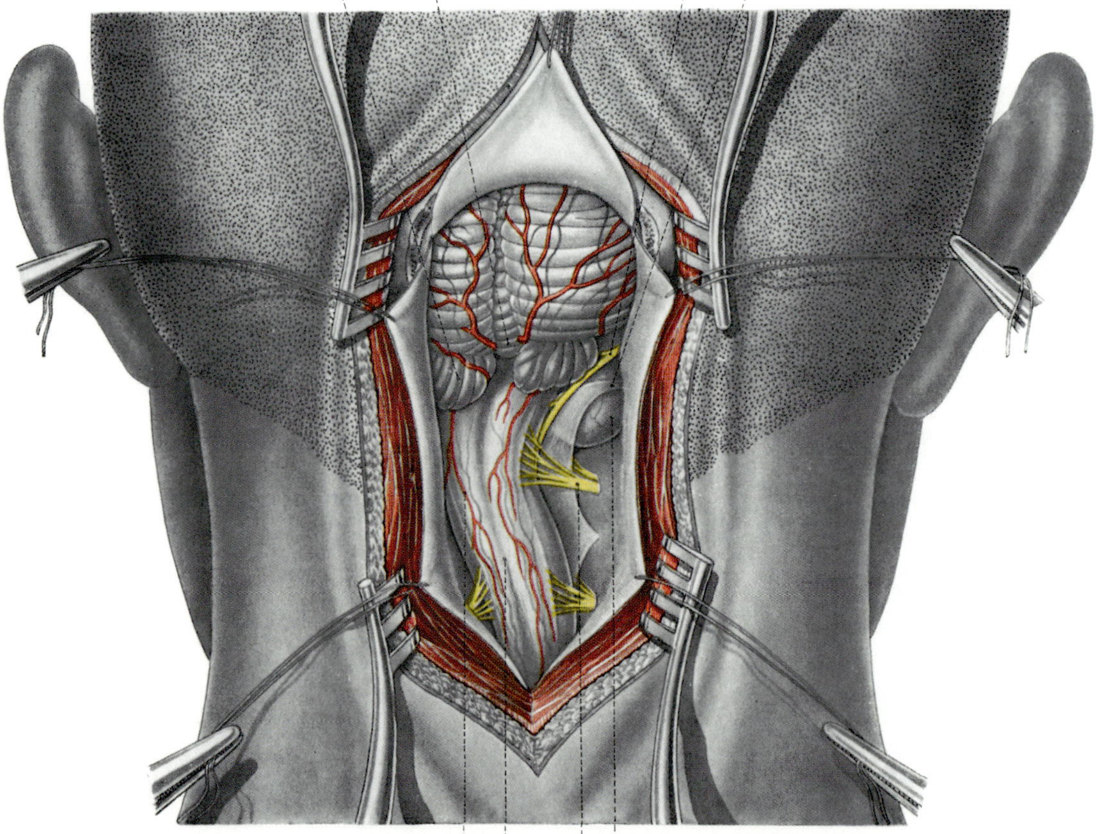

Fig. 95. Meningioma of the foramen magnum: Operative exposure.

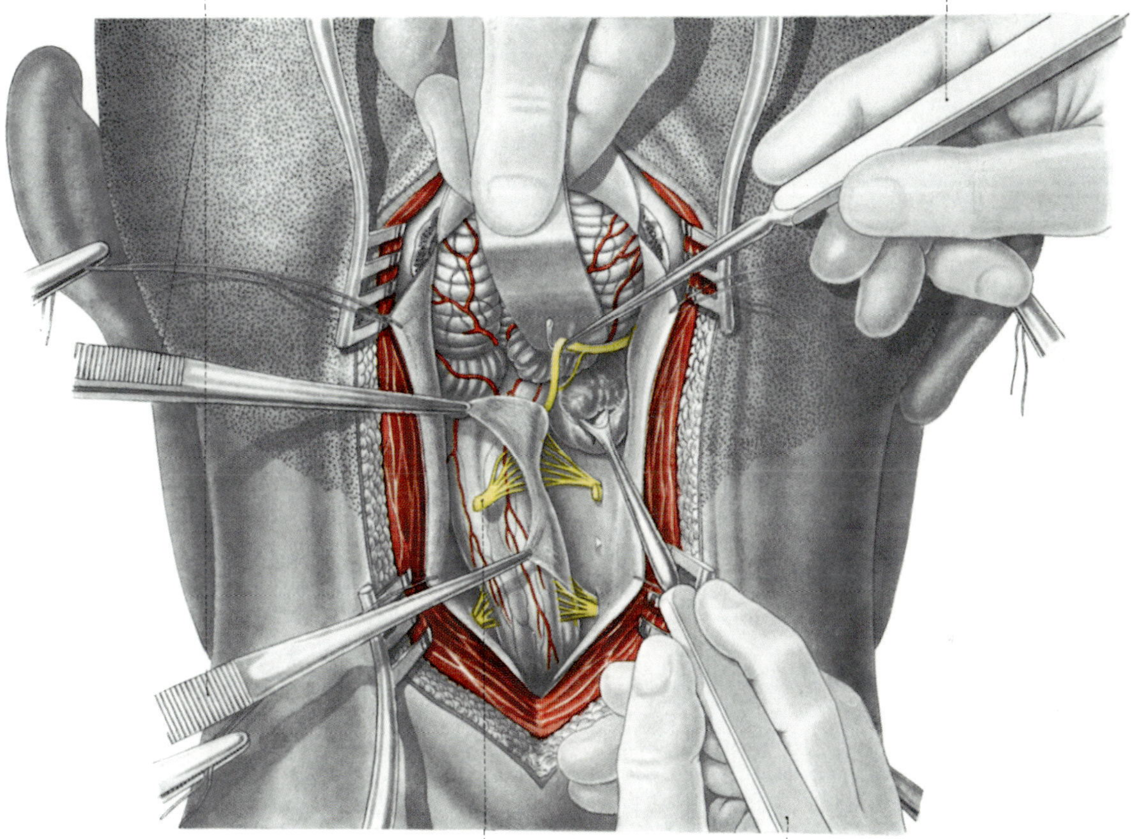

Fig. 96. Meningioma of the foramen magnum: Inferior extent of the tumor is being removed.

Chapter X

Medullary Tractotomy for Facial Pain

A medullary tractotomy is most commonly done for intractable facial pain associated with a malignancy. Occasionally it will be the procedure of choice in trigeminal neuralgia. This operation interrupts the pain fibers in the descending spinal tract of V. Since fibers in this tract carrying pain messages descend as low as C_3, it is possible to abolish pain with an incision five mm. below the obex. Because sensory components of VII, IX and X also descend in the spinal tract of V just medial to the mandibular division, pain deep within the ear can be relieved by this operation. This operation also has the advantage of being technically quite simple.

When general anesthesia is used, the patient is placed in the sitting position. We prefer, if the patient will cooperate, to use local anesthesia and the prone position (Fig. 104). In the prone position the head is kept below the level of the exposure to prevent the intracranial accumulation of air and thus avoid an annoying headache for the patient. Fig. 102 illustrates the placement of needles for deep local anesthesia. Thirty to forty cc. of lidocaine is sufficient to produce analgesia for the entire procedure.

A midline incision beginning at the level of the inion and extending downward approximately 15 cm. will provide adequate exposure of the suboccipital region and the posterior arch of the atlas. Fig. 99 illustrates the area of bone which should be removed. Several burr holes are placed low in the suboccipital region below the inferior nuchal line. The posterior rim of the foramen magnum is removed using a duckbill rongeur. The craniectomy extends superiorly only as far as the inferior nuchal line. The technique for removing the arch of the atlas is described in Chapter I (Figs. 18 and 19). The *Y*-shaped dural incision is illustrated in Fig. 94. A No. 11 scalpel blade is prepared, as shown in Fig. 100, so that five mm. of the cutting edge is exposed. The arachnoid over the cisterna magna is torn and a spatula is inserted below and slightly medial to the cerebellar tonsil. The cerebellum on the side of the patient's pain is gently elevated to expose the dorsomedial surface of the medulla (Figs. 97 and 101). The obex is identified for it is the important landmark determining the level of the tractotomy. Laterally the bulbar rootlets of the accessory nerve are identified leaving the lateral surface of the medulla just anterior to the tuberculum cinereum which is that bulge in the posterolateral surface of the medulla caused by the descending tract of V. Medial to the tuberculum cinereum is a dorsomedial sulcus separating the descending tract of V from the fasciculus gracilis. The region of the tuberculum cinereum may be touched with a fine needle, if the patient is under local anesthesia, and he will varify the proper localization by experiencing increase in his pain.

The knife blade is inserted five mm. below the obex into the tuberculum cinereum at a right angle to the surface (Fig. 101). The incision is made to a depth of five mm. and must include the entire width of the tuberculum cinereum from the bulbar rootlets of XI to the dorsomedial sulcus. To lessen post-operative discomfort, the dorsal roots of C_2 are divided.

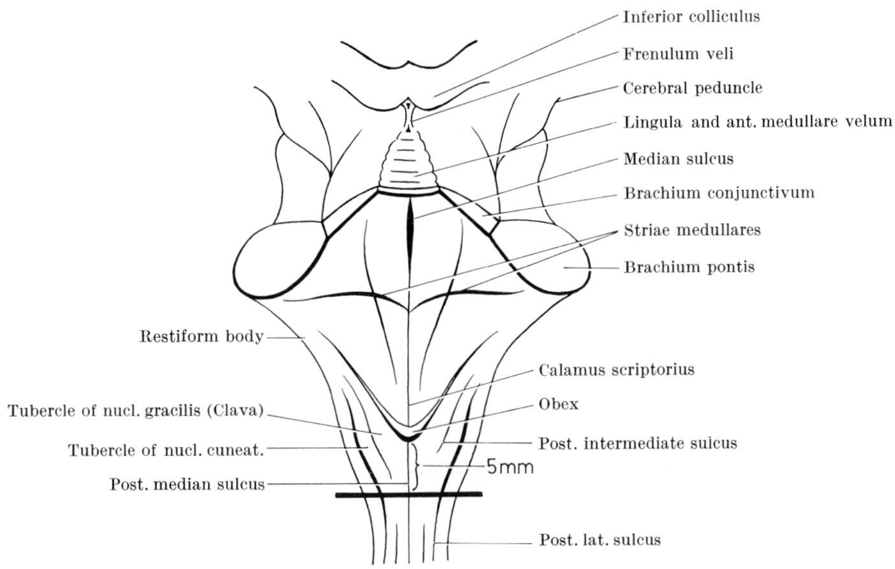

Fig. 97. Medullary tractomy: Dorsal view of the brain stem with cerebellum removed to demonstrate the level of the incision.

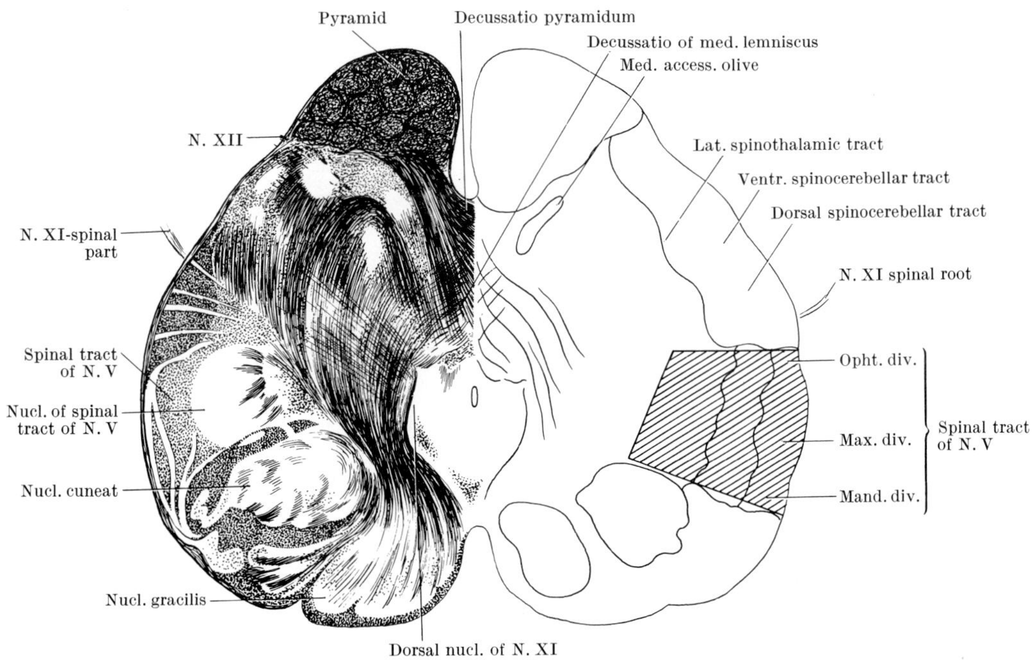

Fig. 98. Medullary tractomy: Cross section of medulla 5 mm below obex showing the area of incision.

Observe: 1. Relationship of the incision to the rootlet of N. XI. 2. Depth of the incision is 5 mm.

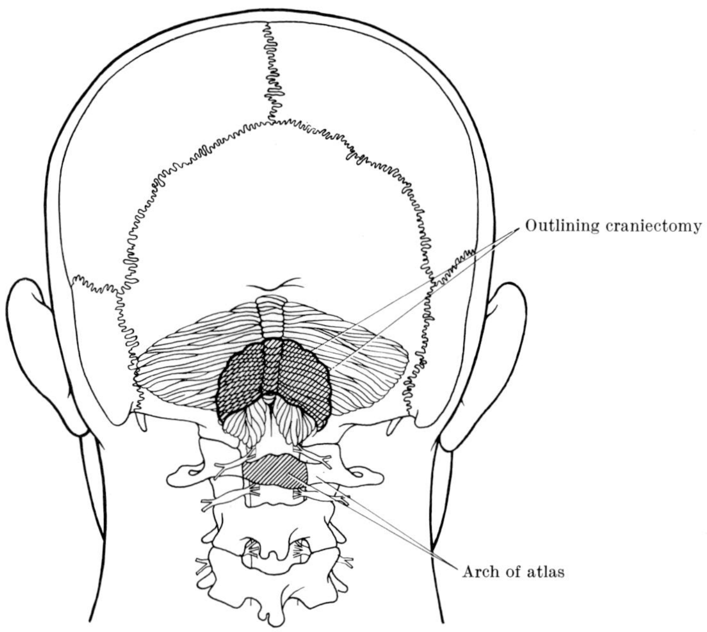

Fig. 99. Medullary tractomy: craniectomy.

Observe: Only small craniectomy is necessary. The arch of the atlas is also removed.

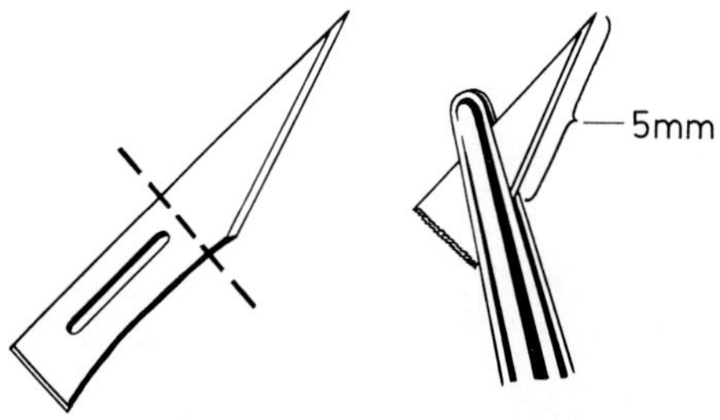

Fig. 100. Medullary tractomy: Use of scalpel blade.

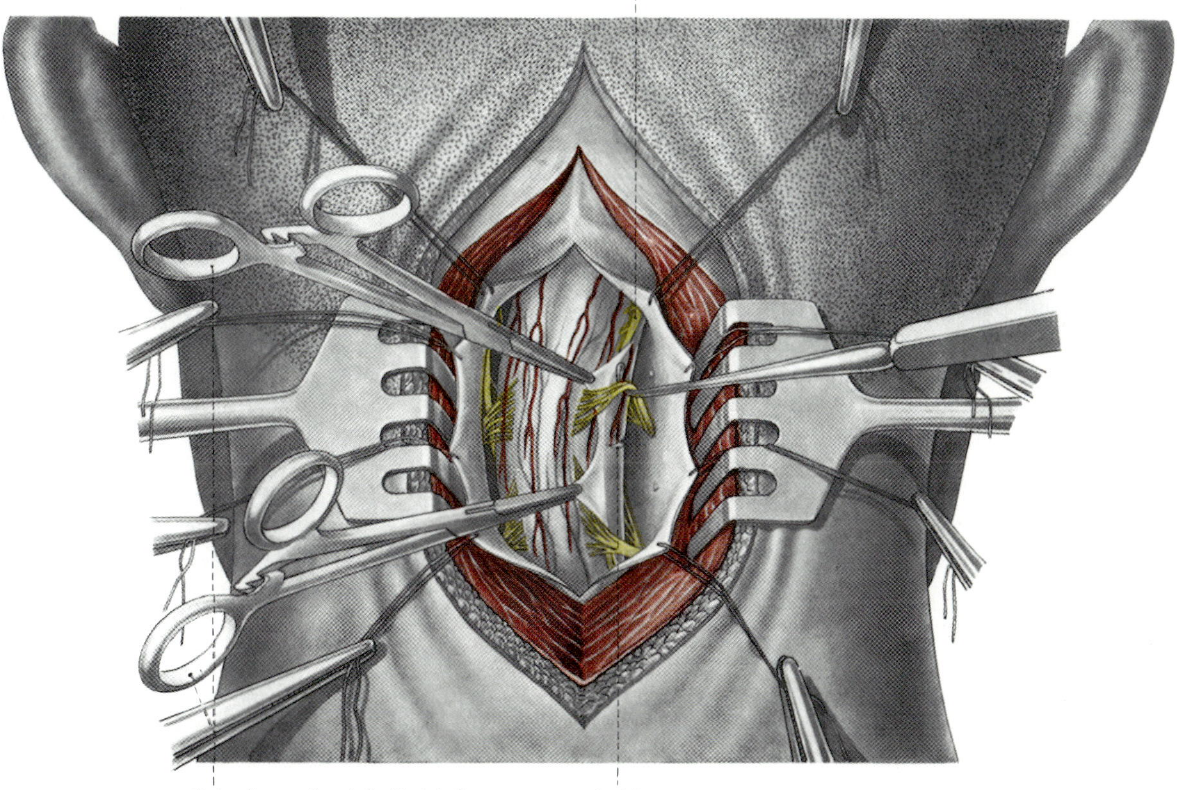

Fig. 106. Cervical cordotomy: Operative view.

Observe: Incision of cord reaches to the insertion of denticulate ligament.

Chapter XII

Cervical Cordotomy — Schwartz Technique[1]

In recent years we have adopted the Schwartz technique of high cervical cordotomy as an improvement on the method described in Chapter XI. This procedure takes much less time and is well tolerated even by very sick patients. Compared to the technique of percutaneous cordotomy, this operation can be done just as quickly and has the advantage of direct visualization.

The patient is placed in the prone position with the head slightly dependent as shown in Figs. 104 and 107. Local anesthesia is used as described in the previous chapter. A midline skin incision is made from the inion to the spinous process of C_3. The muscles are stripped unilaterally from the spinous process and lamina of C_2, the arch of the atlas and the posterior rim of the foramen magnum. A hemilaminectomy retractor is placed between C_2 and the posterior rim of the foramen magnum (see Fig. 108), and the patient's head is flexed. These two maneuvers will widen the interlaminar space between C_1 and C_2. The ligamentum flavum is very thin at this level and usually can be incised and reflected along with the dura. A longitudinal dural incision is made from the lamina of C_1 to the lamina of C_2 in the lateral one third of the dural exposure (Fig. 108). Care must be taken to avoid opening the epidural veins in the lateral gutter. The dural margins are retracted with stay sutures (Fig. 109). The arachnoid is torn and cerebrospinal fluid is aspirated. The denticulate ligament is identified and followed to the cord. This ligament is left attached to the dura to prevent any distortion of the cord. The dentate ligament is then grasped flush with the cord and elevated slightly (Fig. 110). The cordotomy is then completed as described in the previous chapter.

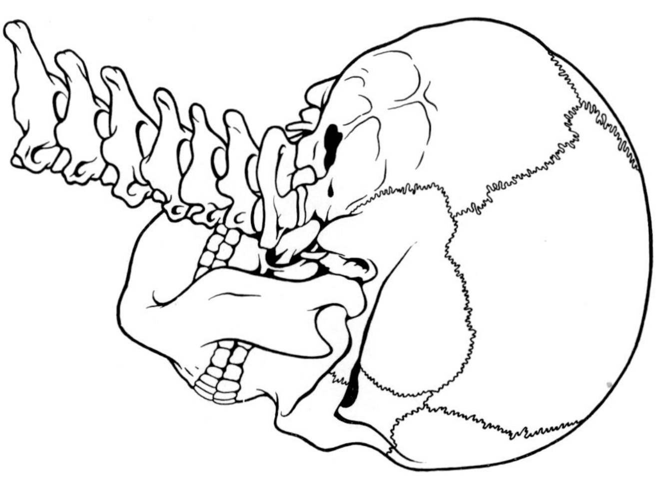

Fig. 107. Cervical cordotomy: Position of skull and spine.

[1] Schwartz, H. G.: High cervical cordotomy. J. Neurosurg. **26**, 452—455 (1967).

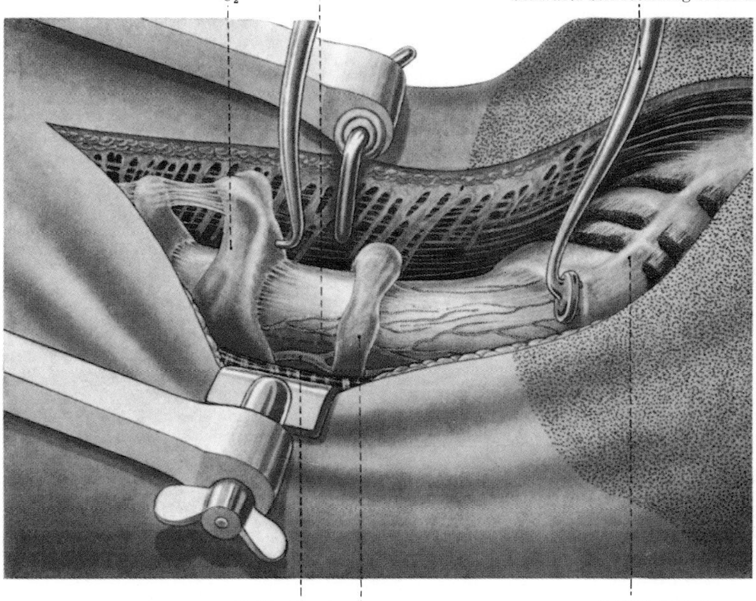

Fig. 108. Cervical cordotomy: Operative view after stripping muscle from the suboccipital squama and lamina of C_1 and C_2.

Observe: 1. The Schwartz self-retaining retractor widens the interlaminar space. The sharp hook is inserted into the spinous process of C_2, and the opposite point is against the occipital bone. 2. Epidural vein. 3. Site of dural incision.

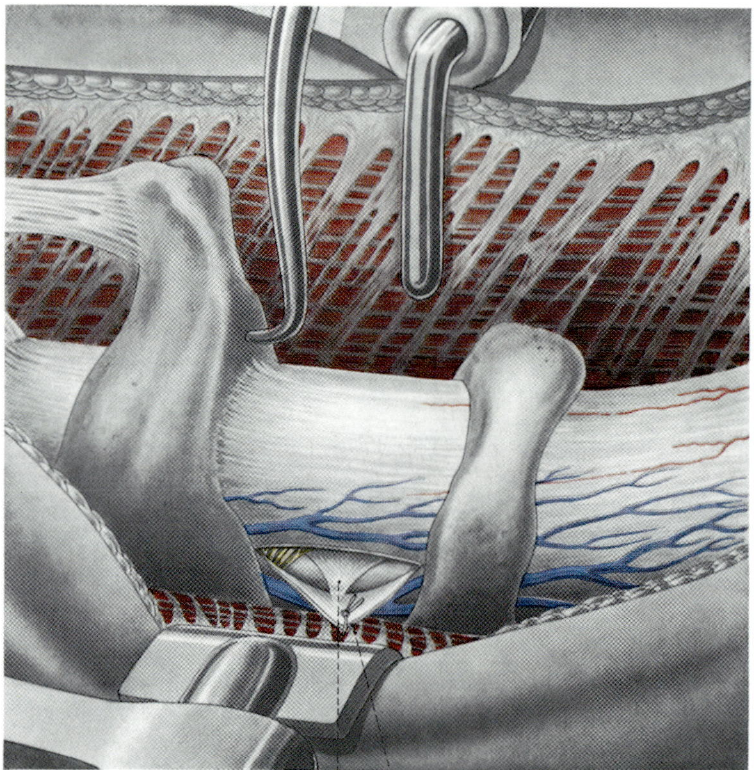

Fig. 109. Cervical cordotomy: Operative exposure after opening the dura between C_1 and C_2.
Observe: 1. Lateral fold reflected over epidural vein. 2. Position of denticulate ligament.

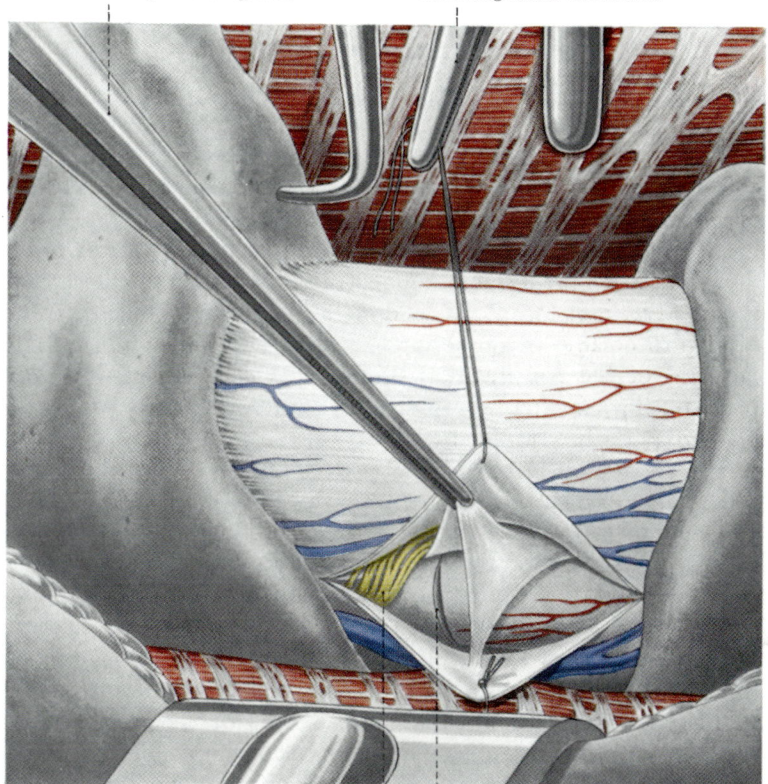

Fig. 110. Cervical cordotomy: Close up view of operative field following incision.

Chapter XIII

Cervical Laminectomy

Syringomyelia

This chapter will describe in detail the technique of cervical laminectomy. Syringomyelia is used as an example to that end; and, as a result, little will be said of syringomyelia as a disease entity. The procedure illustrated in this chapter is a total laminectomy of C_2 through C_5 with a partial laminectomy of C_6. Obviously, the technique of cervical laminectomy is applicable to many different disease processes.

The diagnosis of spinal cord pathology including syringomyelia is most often made by myelography. When a myelogram demonstrates a complete block above the level of the lumbar puncture, a cisternal tap is done and one or two cc. of contrast material is added from above to outline the superior extent of the lesion. A scratch is placed on the skin at the level of the lesion. All patients with a complete block on myelogram should be operated on the same day, preferably within two to three hours. The diagnostic study may precipitate a catastrophe in an already compromised spinal cord. Usually this deterioration is related to ischemia, and it does not matter whether the compressing lesion is intramedullary, extramedullary or extradural.

Cervical laminectomies are most often performed with the patient in the sitting position. Indications for using the prone position include vertebral instability, cordotomy under local anesthesia and any situation in which hypotension would provide a great risk to the patient. In using the sitting position for a cervical laminectomy, the same precautions outlined in Chapter I for suboccipital craniectomy must be taken.

A vertical midline incision is made from two cm. below the inion to over the vertebra prominens (C_7). Figs. 111 and 112 illustrate the extent of the skin incision relative to the topography of the area and the underlying bony landmarks. Because of the downward inclination of the cervical spinous processes, the vertebral bodies are considerably rostral to these spinous processes. Perhaps it is worth interjecting at this point a reminder that the spinal cord segments are even higher than their corresponding vertebral level. The incision is continued in the midline down to the spinous processes. Repeated palpation of the bifid spinous processes of C_2 through C_6 will serve as a guide to the midline. It is easier to stay in the midline if self-retaining retractors are not placed beneath the cervical fascia until the spinous processes have been reached (Figs. 112 and 113). The retractors tend to pull fibers from one side to the other and, thereby, obliterate the median plane.

After reaching the spinous processes, self-retaining retractors are inserted to maintain the exposure. Beginning inferiorly (C_6), the knife is used to transect the muscle attachments of the spinous processes (Fig. 114). The knife blade is always kept against the bone. Because the muscles which insert on the spinous processes predominantly come from an inferolateral direction, separation of these muscles beginning at C_6 and working upward to C_2 will be easier and less bloody. Once the spinous process is exposed, the remaining muscle insertions are elevated by subperiosteal stripping of the spinous process and lamina (Fig. 115). The subperiosteal elevation is carried laterally to the facet, and an opened gauze sponge is then inserted to aid in the blunt elevation of the paravertebral muscles (Fig. 116). This process, for reasons of anatomy and hemostasis, also begins inferiorly and proceeds upward.

The spinous processes are removed with a Horsley bone cutting forceps (Fig. 117). Beginning in the midline the lamina are gradually nibbled away using a rongeur. Extreme care must be taken to avoid pressing the inferior lip of the rongeur against the dura and spinal cord. Removing the lamina with a rongeur requires two hands. One hand maintains pressure on the instrument away from the spinal cord so that if the rongeur slips off the bone it will always be in a direction which will do no harm. Another important point with regard to removing the lamina is that the rongeur is a cutting tool and should be used as such. The rongeur should not be twisted in attempting to cut through a lamina or a whole articular facet is likely to be broken off. The lamina are removed laterally just short of the facet joints bilaterally (Fig. 118). The ligamentum flavum, which becomes very thinned out in the upper cervical levels, is excised along with the lamina. Bone wax is generously applied to the cut lamina to reduce bleeding and prevent air emboli. The laminectomy is extended until a normal pulsating dural sac is encountered superiorly and until a normal dural-epidural relationship is observed inferiorly.

Strips of absorbable gelatin sponges are then placed in the lateral epidural gutters and covered with moist cottonoid strips. Bothersome epidural veins are always encountered laterally and they will bleed even more once the dura is opened and the intrathecal space is decompressed. By covering this area and reflecting the dura over it, hemostasis will be preserved throughout the operation. The dura is opened in the midline over the entire length of the laminectomy (Fig. 120). The dural incision is begun in an area of relative laxness by making fine repeated strokes with a small round-bellied knife blade. In this way the dura can be incised without opening the arachnoid. Once the arachnoid bulges through the small dural opening, a fine instrument is inserted to separate the arachnoid from the dura. We prefer to complete the dural incision using a specially designed blade holder with a protecting footplate (Fig. 119). Multiple stay sutures are placed in the dural margin bilaterally after dissecting the arachnoid free of the dura. Lateral extensions at the extremes of the dural incision are not made in those operations in which a water-tight dural closure is important. If the laminectomy has been carried above and below the pathology, there is no need for these lateral incisions.

Opening the dura separate from the arachnoid has many advantages. It affords a beautiful undisturbed picture of the underlying pathology. It lessens the chance of a post operative pseudo-meningocele because the dura can be reapproximated without having the arachnoid membrane in the suture line. It is very important in the surgical treatment of syringomyelia since, as will be illustrated in this chapter, a catheter is placed into the subarachnoid space.

As illustrated in Fig. 121, the markedly widened spinal cord is now exposed. Gentle palpation suggests that the cord contains a cyst. A fine gauged needle is inserted through an avascular area over one dorsal columns just to the side of the midline. A small amount of fluid is aspirated (Fig. 121) to establish the cystic nature of the lesion. A one to two cm. incision is then made in this same avascular area into the cystic cavity. A small soft blunt-tipped catheter is passed both superiorly and inferiorly in the cystic cavity to determine its dimensions. If the catheter encounters abnormal resistance or if the spinal cord does not collapse after opening the cyst, a tumor should be suspected, and the myelotomy is enlarged to visualize the lesion. Chapter XV deals with the removal of such a lesion. Having ascertained that we are dealing with idiopathic syringomyelia, one end of the soft silastic catheter is placed superiorly into the cyst cavity. The distal catheter is cut so that five or six cm. of catheter protrudes from the cavity. This end of the catheter is then placed inferiorly into the subarachnoid space anterior to the dentate ligament. The catheter is attached to the dura with a fine silk suture to prevent migration (Fig. 122). This catheter not only functions as a shunt but also acts as a wick to keep the cystic cavity open.

The dura is reapproximated so that it is water tight. The wound is closed in layers. A few sutures in the muscle will decrease the dead space but the fascia must be meticulously closed using heavy silk, nylon or wire sutures. The subcutaneous tissue is closed with inverted sutures. The skin is reapproximated with fine silk or wire. Application of the dressings in these wounds is important, particularly when the incision reaches below C_7. The patient's shoulders should be held back, and broad pieces of tape applied from shoulder to shoulder. This will keep tension off of the wound in the post operative period.

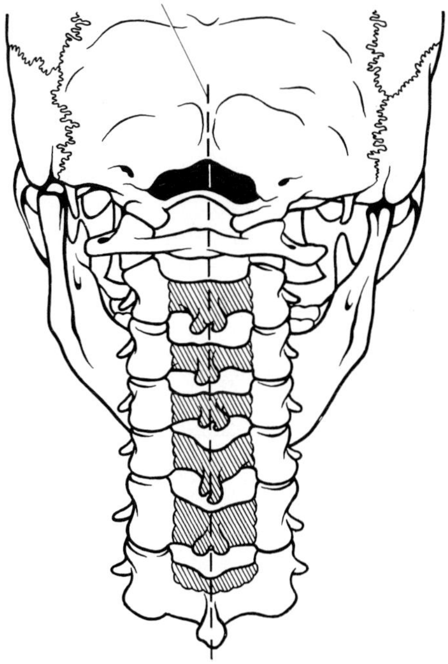

Fig. 111. Cervical syringomyelia: Skin incision and area of laminectomy. *Observe:* Total laminectomy of C_2 through C_6 and partial laminectomy of C_7.

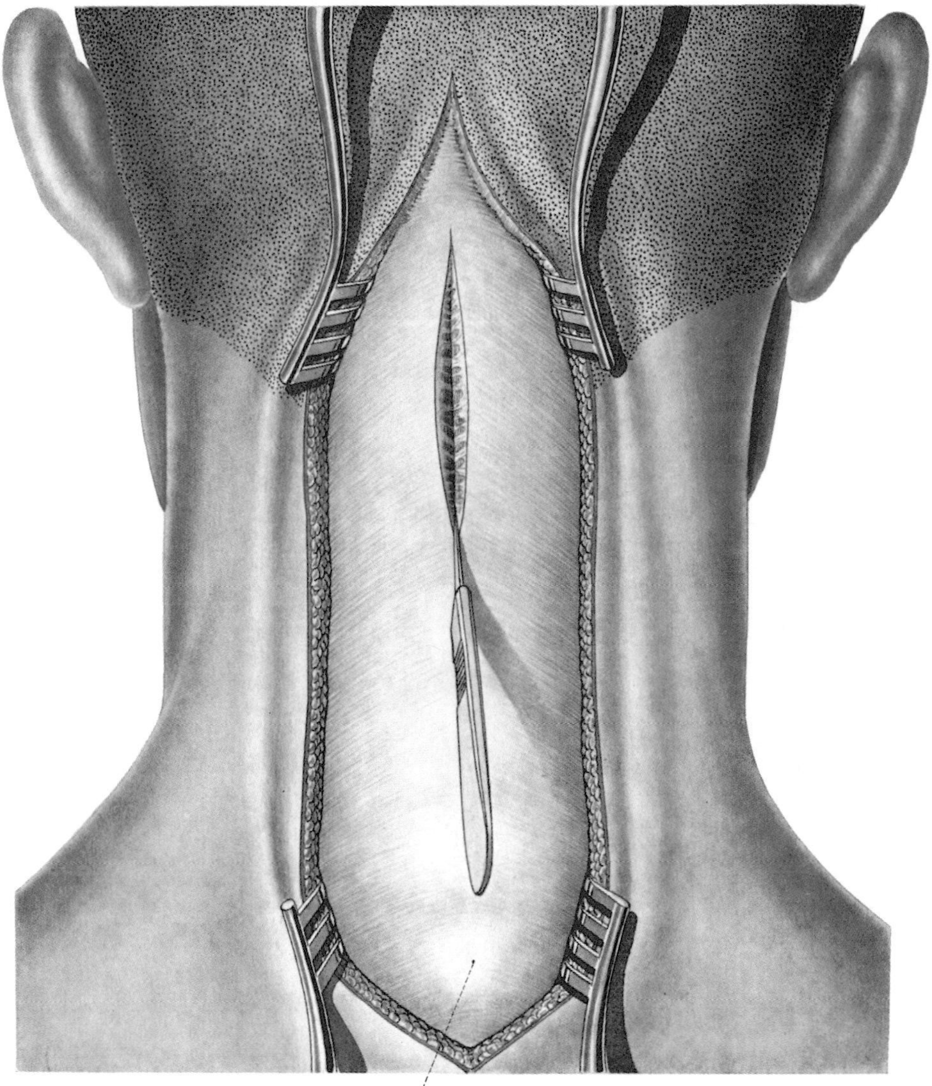

Fig 112. Cervical syringomyelia. After the skin is opened, the superficial cervical fascia is incised staying within the ligamentum nuchae over the suboccipital and upper cervical areas (compare with Fig. 115).

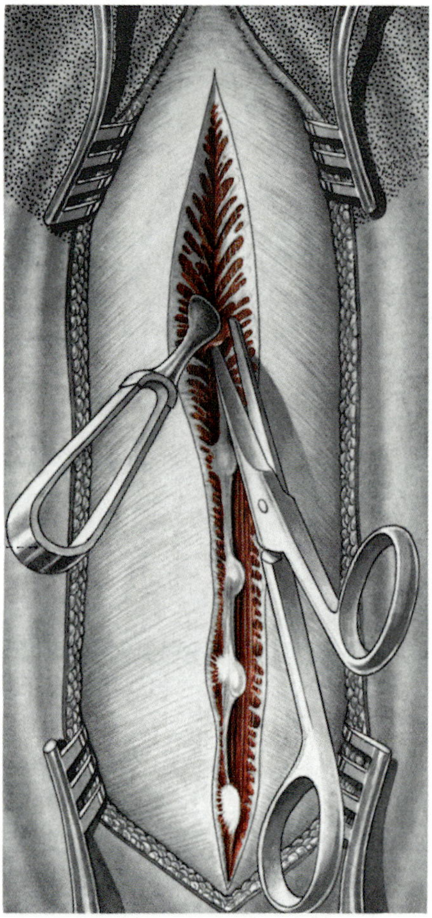

Fig. 113.

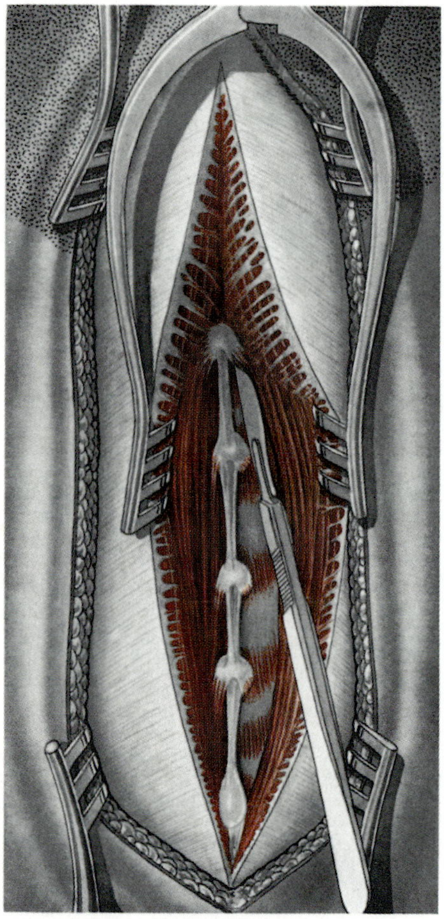

Fig. 114.

Fig. 113. Cervical laminectomy for syringomyelia.

Observe: The incision is made deeper using a periosteal elevator to retract and the straight scissors to cut muscle fibers and fibrous tissue while staying in midline. The midline incision is continued using a straight scissors as the muscles are retracted with periosteal elevators.

Fig. 114. Cervical laminectomy for syringomyelia: Cutting muscle insertions close to the bifid processes.

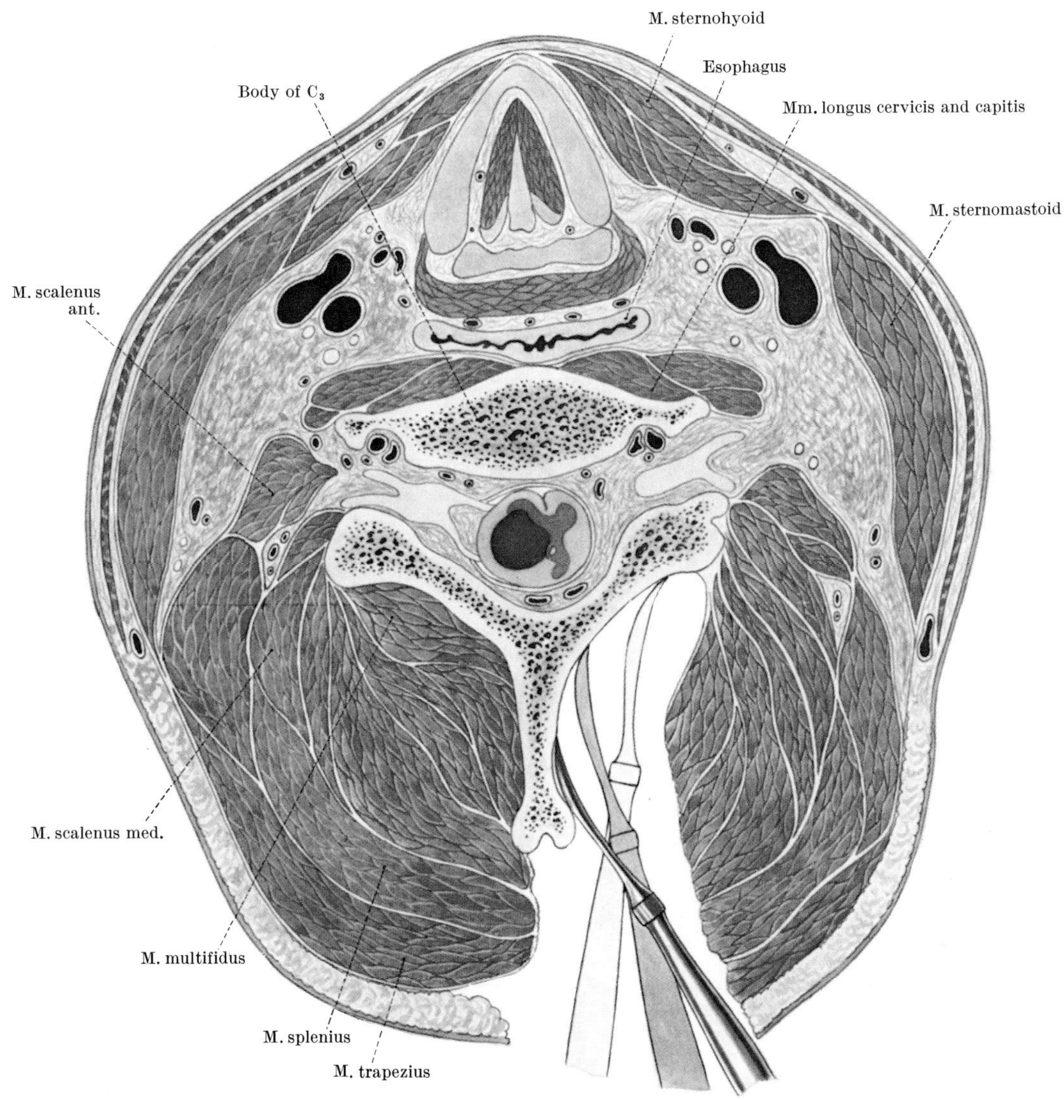

Fig. 115. Cervical laminectomy for syringomyelia: Cross section of the neck to demonstrate subperiosteal stripping of the cervical spinous processes and laminae.

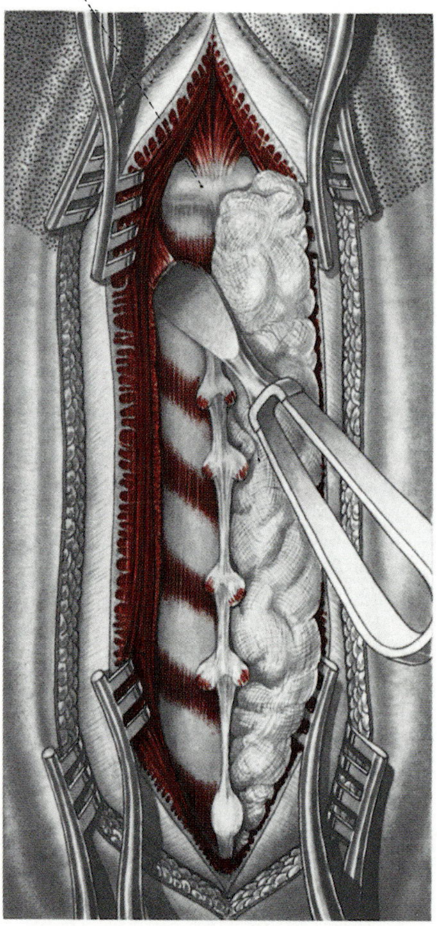

Fig. 116.

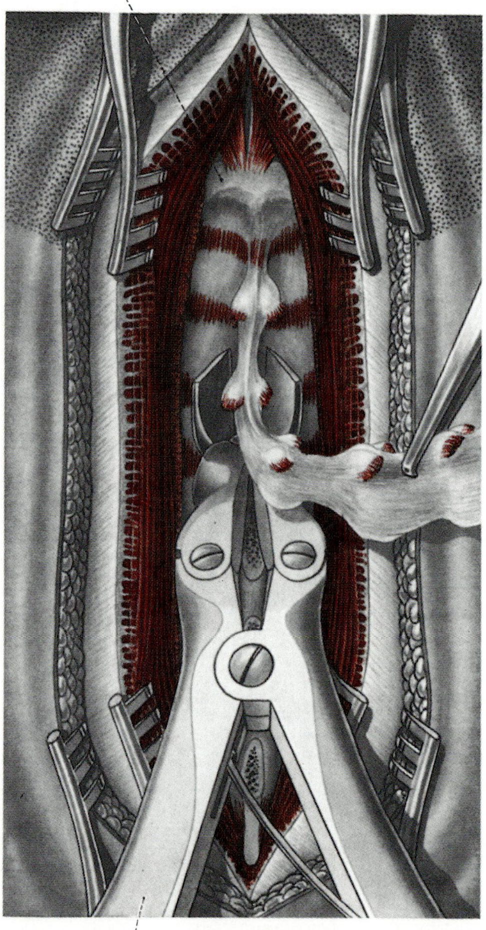

Fig. 117.

Fig. 116. Cervical laminectomy for syringomyelia: Operative view of muscle stripping.

Fig. 117. Cervical laminectomy for syringomyelia: Removal of spinous processes using double action bone cutting forceps.

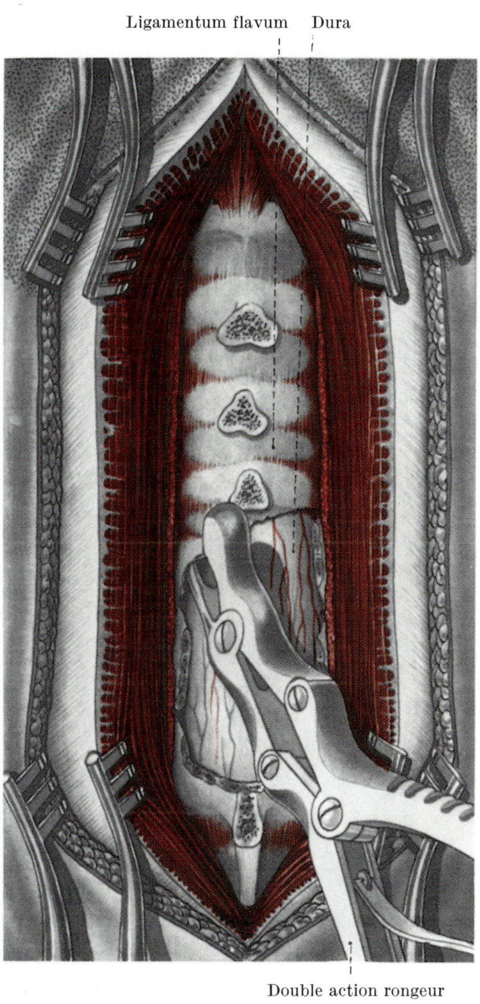

Fig. 118.

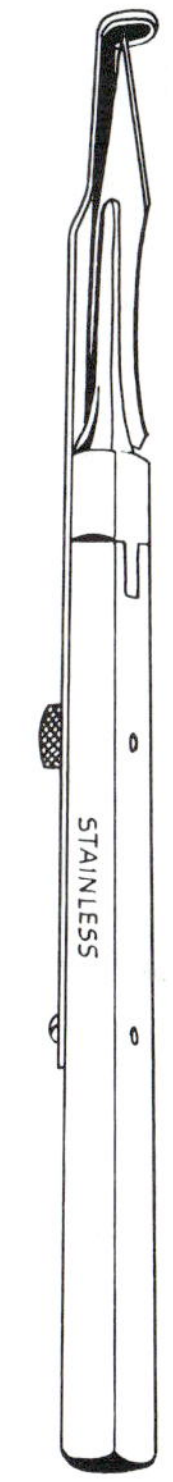

Fig. 119.

Fig. 118. Cervical laminectomy for syringomyelia: Removal of laminae.

Fig. 119. Cervical laminectomy for syringomyelia: Knife-blade-holder for opening of dura.

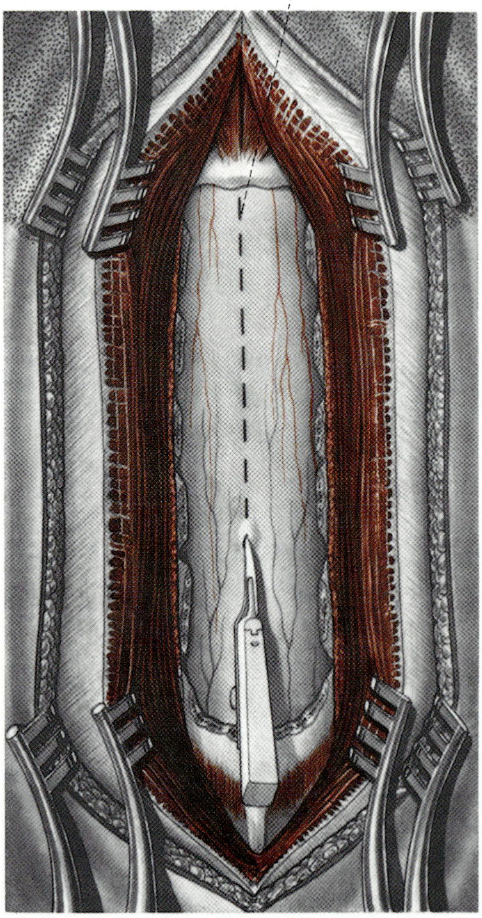

Fig. 120.

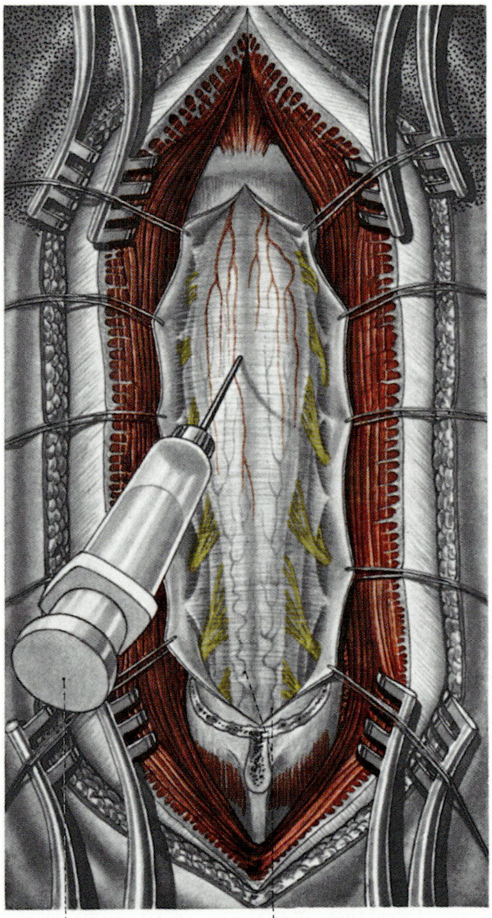

Fig. 121.

Fig. 120. Cervical laminectomy for syringomyelia: Dural incision.

Fig. 121. Cervical laminectomy for syringomyelia: Operative view showing aspiration of intramedullary cyst.

Observe: 1. Dural stay sutures are held taut by hemostats not seen here. 2. Large cottonoids are placed epidurally surrounding the entire opened dura. These are not shown here to avoid obliterating anatomical landmarks. 3. Insertion of needle over avascular paramedian area. 4. Congested vasculature below widened cord.

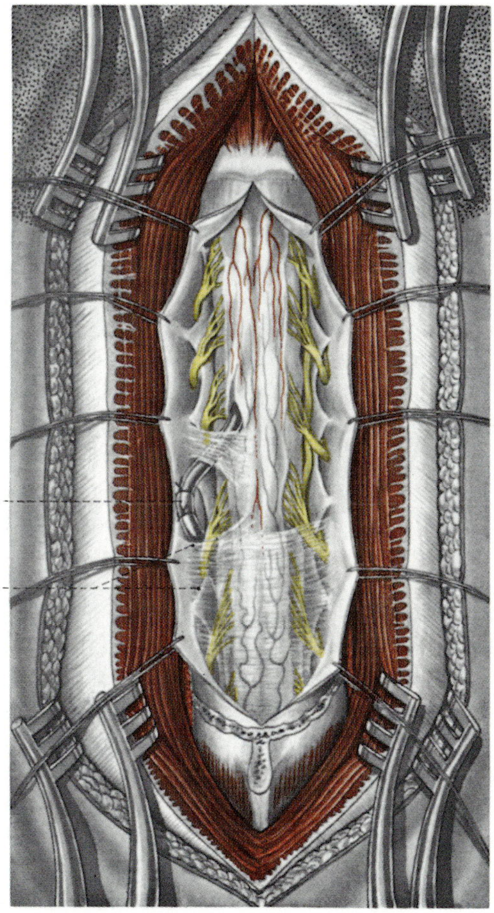

Fig. 122. Cervical laminectomy for syringomyelia: Catheter drainage tube inserted into the cyst, fastened to inside of dura and passed into subarachnoid space.

Observe: 1. Collapsed spinal cord. 2. The catheter is passed into the subarachnoid space ventral to anterior thoracic nerve roots.

Chapter XIV

Spinal Cord Arterio-Venous Malformation

The natural history of spinal cord arterio-venous (A-V) malformations, once the lesion has become symptomatic, is slow progression. The increasing neurological dysfunction is related to repeated hemorrhage and progressive ischemia.

Fortunately, the majority of spinal cord A-V malformations appear to be situated over the dorsal surface of the cord. This finding may be only apparent since it makes the lesion easier to detect by myelography. As a result, when this lesion is suspected it is important to use the supine as well as the prone position during the myelogram. It also should be emphasized that 15 to 20 cc. of contrast material are often necessary to demonstrate the thoracic subarachnoid space. A-V malformations occupying the parenchyma of the cord may not cause any myelographic abnormality. The myelogram, for example, in the patient whose arteriogram is illustrated in Figs. 123a—125b, was interpreted as normal. When possible these lesions should always be studied by selective arteriography. This study provides the information necessary to determine the type and operability of the lesion.

The treatment of choice of A-V malformations is surgical excision. The ligation of selective arterial feeders can hardly be expected to be of any lasting value. At surgery it is often surprising to see many feeding vessels and anastomotic channels under magnification which were not detected by pre-operative arteriography. When an A-V malformation occupies a considerable portion of the parenchyma of the cord, surgical excision is not possible. All other lesions are operable in this age of improved neurosurgical instrumentation and technique. Figs. 123a—125b illustrate an inoperable lesion involving the entire width of the spinal cord. Angiograms in at least two planes are essential to reveal the extent of the parenchymal involvement. The lateral view will help to demonstrate any ventrally located feeding vessels.

The technique of operative excision of a spinal cord A-V malformation will be illustrated using a cervical cord lesion as the example. The myelogram (Fig. 126) shows a typical tortuous, dilated dorsal draining vein. Selective arteriography, via retrograde femoral catheterization, demonstrates arterial feeders from the vertebral artery and the thyrocervical trunk (Fig. 127a—b). A later phase of the lateral arteriogram (Fig. 128a—b) shows the same dorsal vein demonstrated by the myelogram.

Essential surgical tools for this operation include magnification, fine bipolar coagulation forceps and an assortment of metallic clips. Various other microsurgical instruments are also helpful.

The patient is placed in the sitting position. A total laminectomy over the entire length of the malformation is carried out as described in the previous chapter. The dura is carefully opened in the midline. The arachnoid may be rather adherent to the dura in those patients who have had repeated hemorrhages. Therefore, prior to reflecting the dura, the arachnoid is separated from it with a small blunt elevator. Fig. 129 illustrated the operative exposure at this point. Because the largest arterial feeders are coming from inferiorly and the largest vein is draining superiorly on the angiogram, the surgical removal begins inferiorly. The lowest feeding vessels are exposed and clipped. These vessels have thinner walls than normal arteries and, therefore, are very fragile. Tiny clips which approximate perfectly are essential. After coagulating the vessel with a bipolar forceps, it is divided on the malformation side of the clip. As feeding vessels are transected, the malformation can be dissected off the surface of the cord and gently elevated. This will expose arteries coming from the parenchyma of the cord which enter the malformation. They must be divided in the same manner (Fig. 130). A very fine spatula will aid in dissecting the malformation from the cord parenchyma but leptomeningeal adhesions must be divided using a fine microsurgical scissors. At this stage of the procedure, magnification is essential. Many tiny vessels, otherwise invisible, can be cauterized and cut. The malformation will gradually shrink in size as dissection proceeds upward. Finally, only the large draining vein remains and it is also clipped and divided. Meticulous hemostasis is essential before the wound is reapproximated.

Figs. 131 and 132 demonstrate the post-operative arteriogram in this patient.

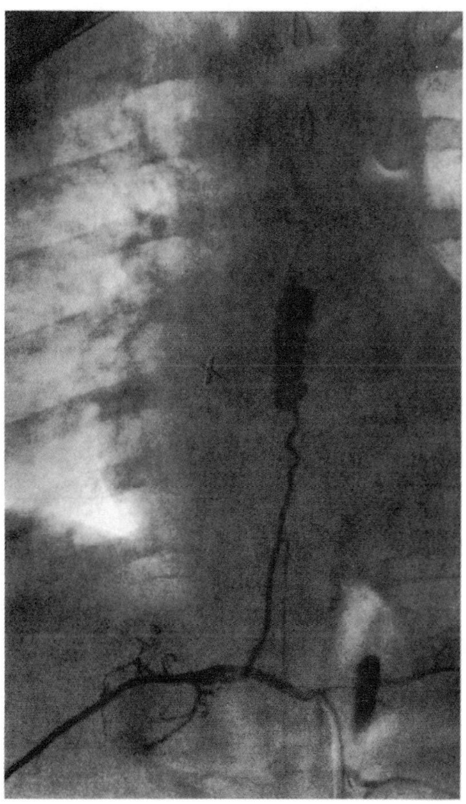

Fig. 123a.

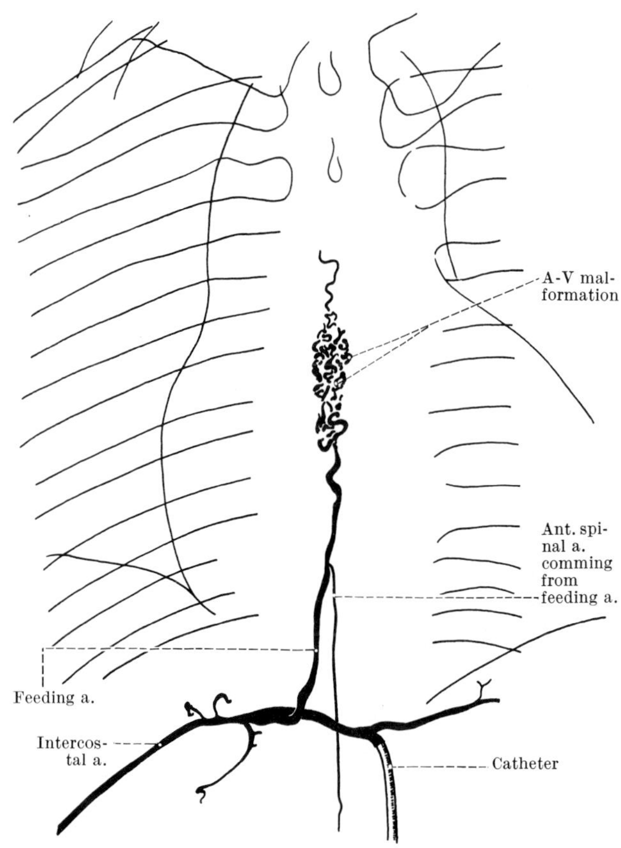

Fig. 123b.

Fig. 123a. Angiography of an angioma of the thoracic cord (substraction film).

Fig. 123b. Line drawing elucidating Fig. 123a.

Observe: Major feeding vessel is the artery of ADAMKIEWICZ.

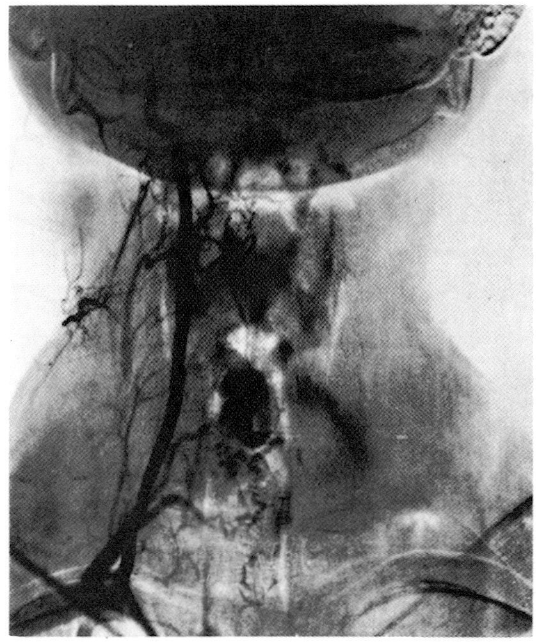

Fig. 127a. Angiography of an arterio-venous malformation of spinal cord at the cervical level (a.-p. view, substraction film).

Observe: Arterial feeders arise from the right vertebral artery and thyrocervical trunk.

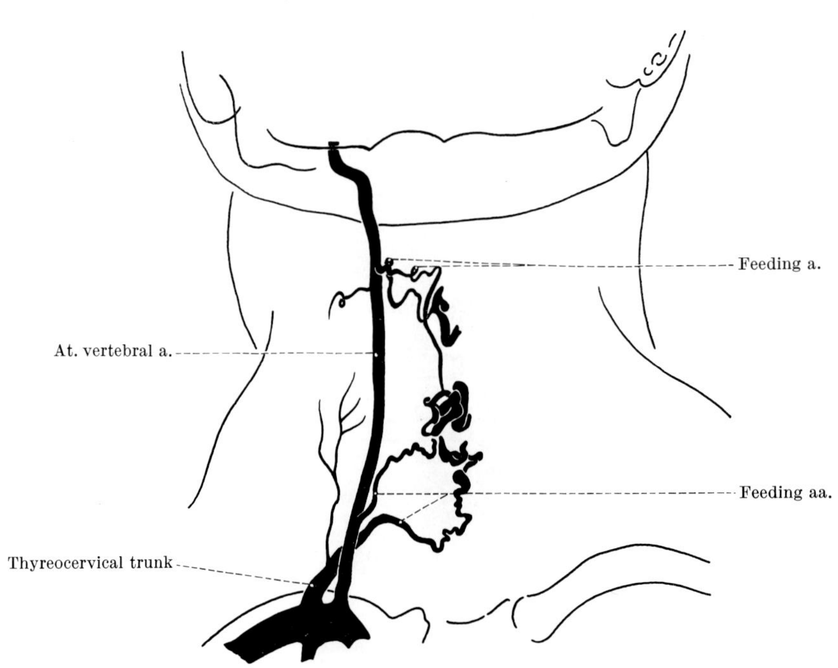

Fig. 127b. Line drawing elucidating Fig. 127a.

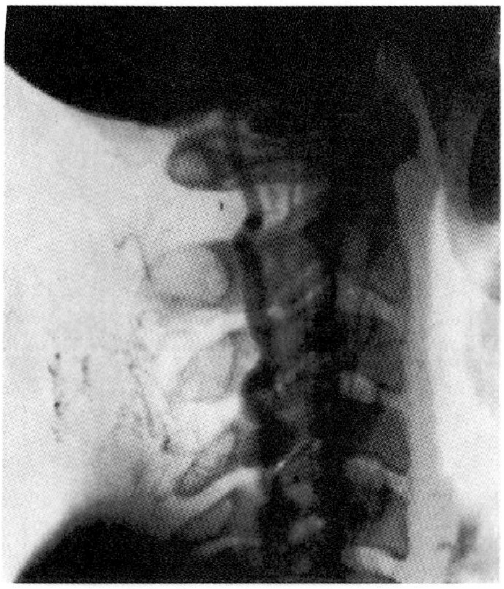

Fig. 128a. Angiography of an arterio-venous malformation of the cervical cord (lateral view).

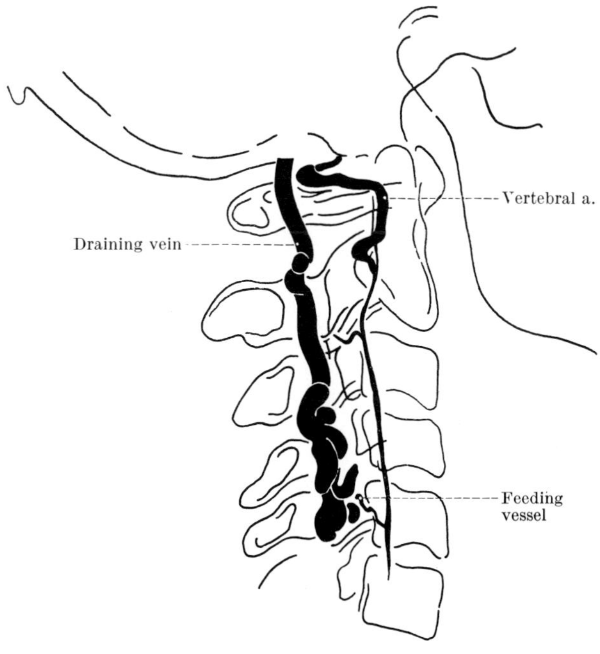

Fig. 128b. Line drawing elucidating X-ray Fig. 128a.

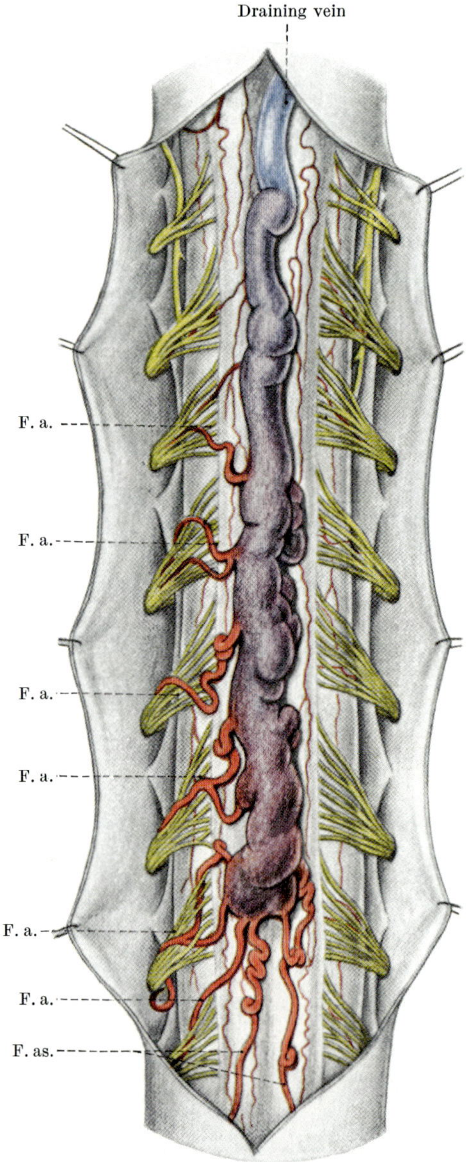

Fig. 129.

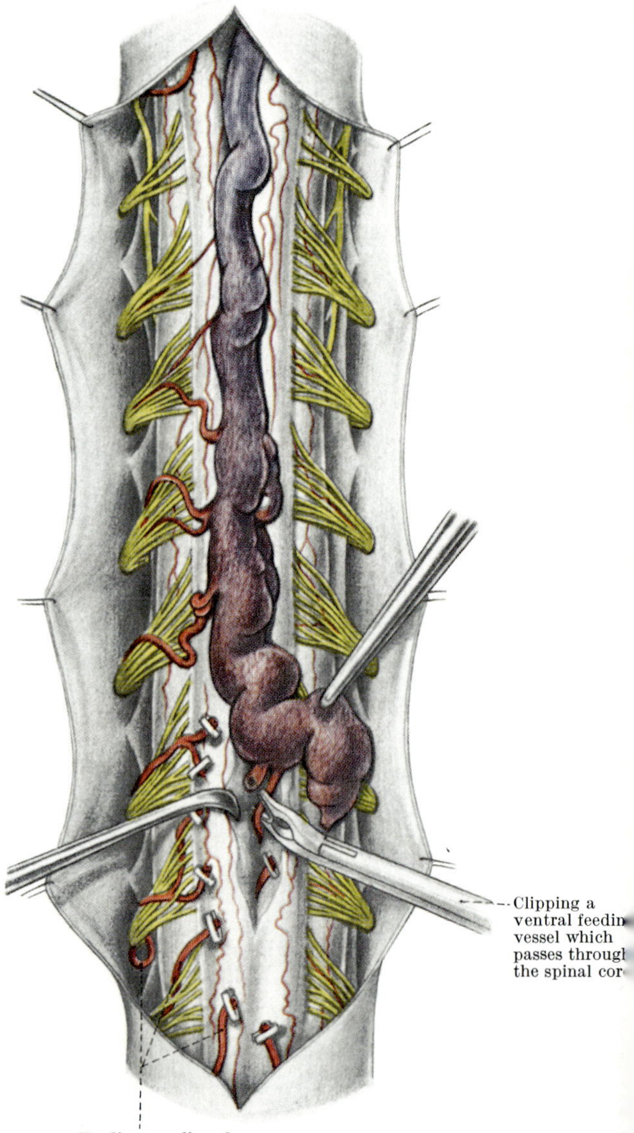

Fig. 130.

Fig. 129. Operative view of arterio-venous malformation of cervical cord. Compare with angiographic demonstration. *F.a.* feeding artery.

Fig. 130. Operative view of arterio-venous malformation of cervical cord.

Observe: 1. The malformation is situated over the dorsal surface of the cord. 2. A myelotomy was necessary to expose and transect feeding vessels passing through the parenchym of the cord.

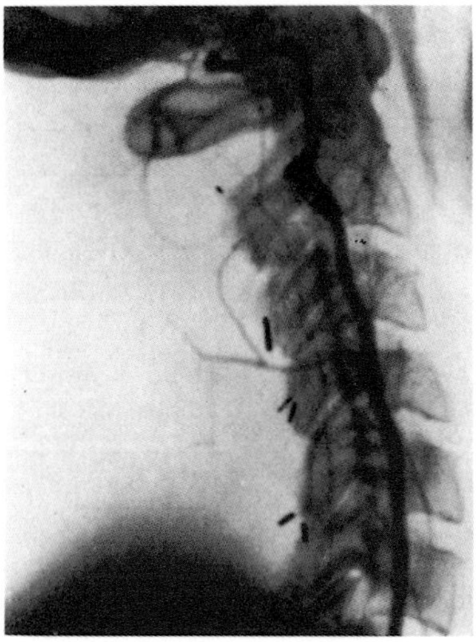

Fig. 131. Postoperative angiogram of an arterio-venous malformation of the cervical cord (lateral view).

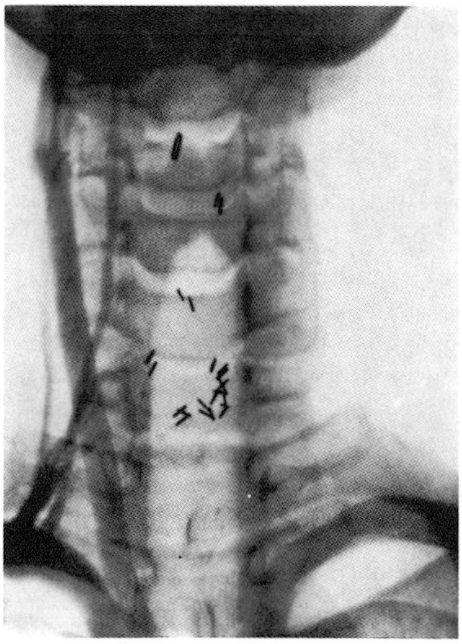

Fig. 132. Postoperative angiogram of an arterio-venous malformation of the cervical cord (a.-p. view).

Chapter XV

Intramedullary Spinal Cord Tumor — Ependymoma

Ependymomas are the most common intramedullary spinal cord tumors. They constitute 65% of gliomas of the spinal cord and filum terminale seen at Walter Reed General Hospital.

Myelography in patients with intramedullary spinal cord tumors often reveals a complete block. In this situation, 2 cc. of contrast material should be added from above via a cisternal puncture to delineate the extent of the lesion. As previously emphasized, when a complete block is demonstrated on myelography, surgery should follow as soon as possible. In addition to myelography, angiography is sometimes a useful diagnostic tool in spinal cord tumors as, for example, in a patient with Von Hippel-Lindau's Disease.

The operation illustrated is for an intramedullary ependymoma of the cervical cord. The patient is in the sitting position. A laminectomy, as described in Chapter XIII, is performed from well above to well below the extent of the tumor. A normally pulsating dural column is exposed superiorly, and inferiorly there should be a normal dural-epidural anatomical relationship. Fig. 133 illustrates the exposure after the dura has been opened in the midline. Note the tortuosity of the surface vessels especially below the fusiform enlargement of the spinal cord. The arachnoid is opened along the lateral aspect of the cord on either side. The spinal cord is gently palpated to determine whether the mass is cystic or solid. A thin-walled 22 gauge needle can be inserted into the caudal one-third of the enlargement in an attempt to find a cystic cavity. Cysts within spinal cord ependymomas are usually located at the inferior pole of the tumor. A myelotomy is then made just lateral to the midline over the entire length of the spinal cord enlargement (Fig. 133). After incising the pia in an avascular plane, the posterior column on the side of the myelotomy is split longitudinally using a fine spatula. Thin strips of absorbable gelatin sponges can be placed on each side of the incision for hemostasis. Intramedullary ependymomas usually present as well-defined greyish, granular tumors. They may have a very extensive caudal cyst. Despite the lack of a capsule, these lesions are so circumscribed that surgical removal is often possible. Dissection should begin inferiorly. Fine spatulas are used to define the margins of the tumor. Bipolar coagulation forceps are used as feeding vessels are encountered. The blood supply to these lesions is often primarily at the rostral end. Fig. 134 illustrates the tumor after its inferior and dorsal surfaces have been defined. The inferior pole of the tumor is then gently lifted so that dissection can proceed superiorly (Fig. 135). In lifting the tumor, traction should not be applied to the spinal cord. The tumor is held up to facilitate vision and not to extract the tumor. If an area is encountered where the tumor margin is not definable, the lesion must be transected even though some tumor tissue will be left behind. After removing the mass (Fig. 136), the tumor cavity is irrigated with copious amounts of isotonic, isothermic saline. Meticulous hemostasis must be attained. If the tumor has been totally removed, the dura is reapproximated. If the tumor has not been totally removed, the dura is left open and covered with an absorbable gelatin sponge. Patients with intramedullary tumors are given systemic steroids to reduce post-operative spinal cord edema.

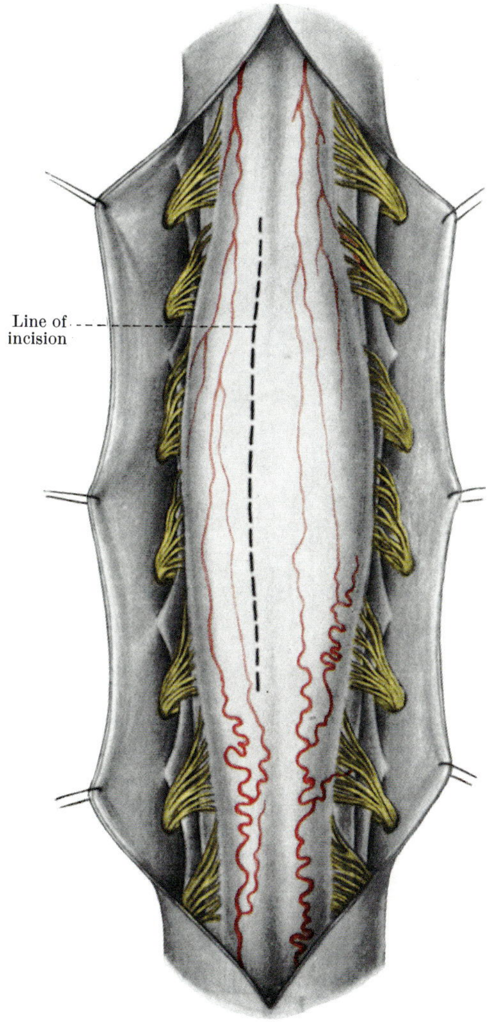

Fig. 133.

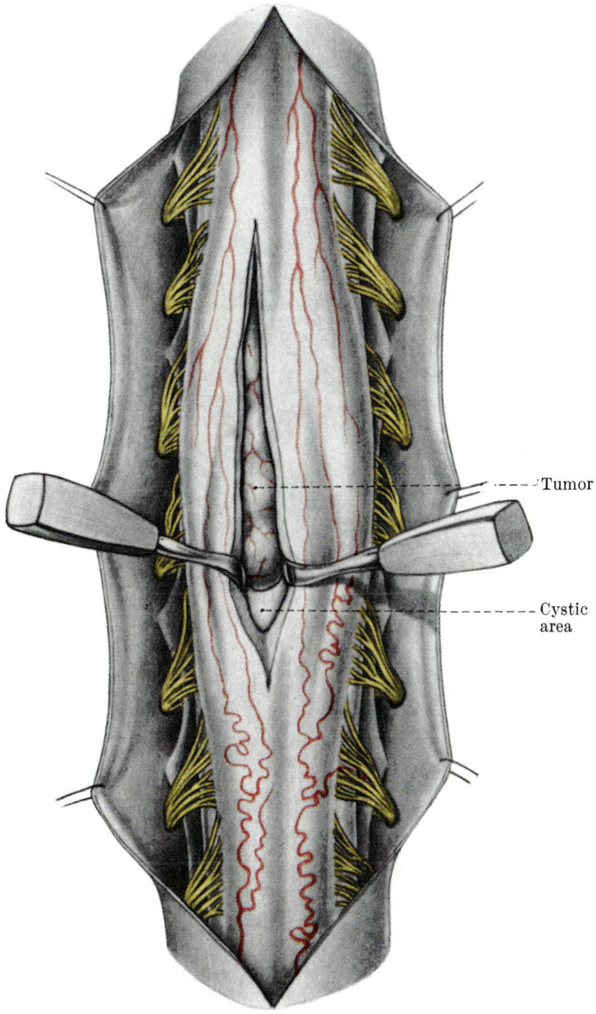

Fig. 134.

Fig. 133. Intramedullary tumor of the cervical cord.

Observe: 1. Paramedian line of incision over avascular dorsal surface of spinal cord. 2. Fusiform enlargement of spinal cord. 3. Tortuosity of surface vessels below lesion. 4. Laminectomy is well above and below the area of the tumor.

Fig. 134. Intramedullary tumor of the cervical cord.

Observe: Adequate length of incision over the tumor allows exposure by gentle retraction.

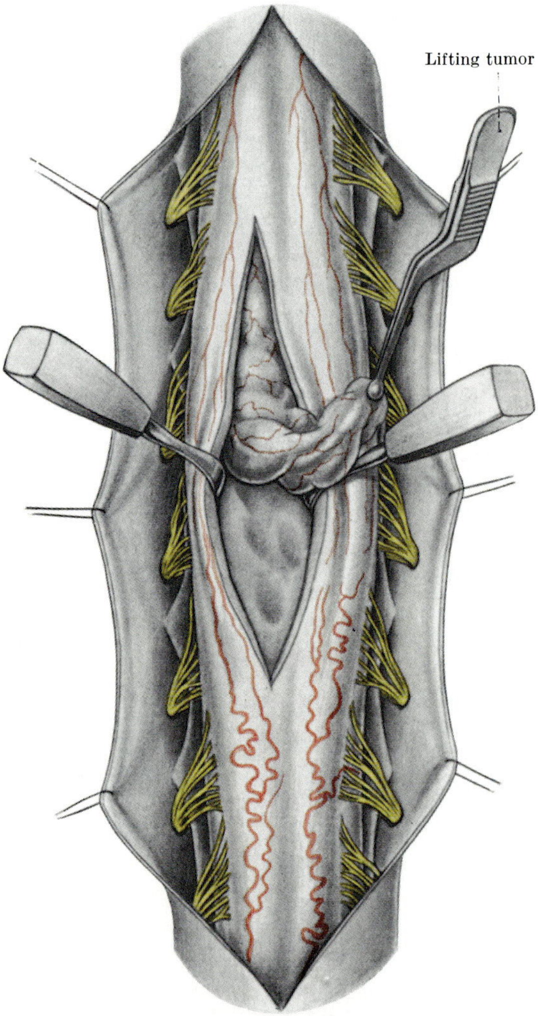

Fig. 135.

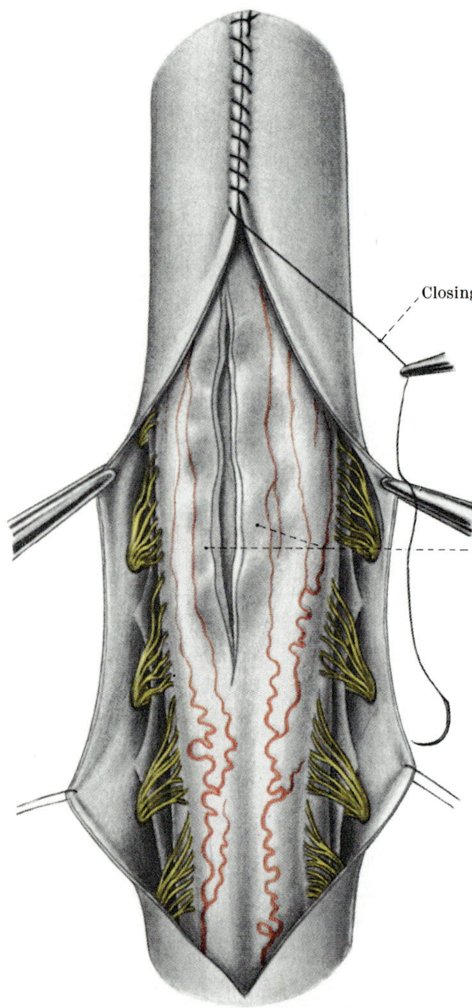

Fig. 136.

Fig. 135. Intramedullary tumor of the cervical cord.

Observe: By gentle upward traction the solid tumor can be carefully dissected from the cystic cavity.

Fig. 136. Intramedullary tumor of the cervical cord.

Observe: Because removal of the tumor resulted in decompression of the spinal cord the dura is reapproximated.

Chapter XVI

Cauda Equina — Conus Medullaris Ependymoma

Ependymomas of the cauda equina — conus medullaris region are often well-defined, sausage-shaped, small tumors attached to the filum terminale. These lesions are easily separable from the nerve roots and the tip of the spinal cord. On the other hand, the tumor may envelope the nerve roots and conus so that the origin of the lesion is questionable and its total removal may be impossible. Occasionally this type of tumor will reach tremendous size and exhibit marked erosion of the surrounding bony structures. When this tumor cannot be totally removed, the goal of surgery becomes decompression of the nervous elements which it surrounds. With the aid of magnification and microsurgical instruments, more neoplasm can be resected with less damage to the cord and nerve roots than was previously thought possible. In dealing with these tumors it is imperative that the blood supply to the conus is preserved. Large vessels often accompany sacral nerve roots upward to supply not only the tumor but the conus as well.

Ependymomas in this region cause a lower motor neuron type of neurological deficit. The tumor may initially causes symptoms referrible to only one or two nerve roots. In this situation this lesion may be clinically misinterpreted as a radiculopathy secondary to a herniated intervertebral disc. It is a good rule to always include the area of the conus in a myelographic study done for lower motor neuron disease.

When a tumor of the cauda equina — conus medullaris region is suspected, it is wise to attempt the myelogram with a lumbar puncture as low as possible; i.e., L-5—S-1. If this tap reveals only blood and no spinal fluid, a suboccipital puncture is done and two cc. of contrast material are added from above.

The operation illustrated is for a typical well-defined myxo-papillary ependymoma which arises from the filum terminale. The patient is placed in the prone position on the operating table (see Figs. 282 and 283). The lesion is exposed by means of a midline incision and total laminectomy well above and below the level of the tumor. Fig. 137 illustrates the exposure after the dura and arachnoid have been opened. The filum terminale is identified in the midline by gently separating the nerve roots just below the tip of the conus. Compared to the rootlets, the filum terminale is fibrous and firm due to the continuation of the pia of the conus upon it. The filum terminale is clipped at its origin (Fig. 138) and divided. Beginning the dissection at this end of the mass prevents any possibility of traction and injury to the conus medullaris. The nerve roots are dissected free of the tumor surface and the tumor is gradually delivered (Fig. 139).

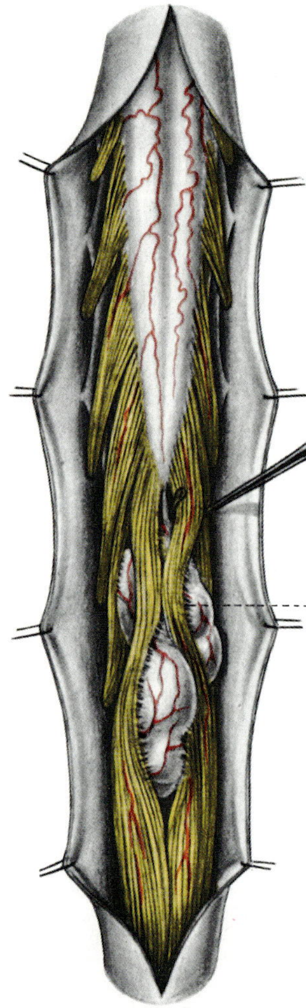

Fig. 137. Ependymoma of the filum terminale.

Observe: 1. Extensive exposure both above and below the level of the tumor. 2. The arachnoid is not shown. 3. Tumor exposure begins rostrally by identifying the conus medullaris and the filum terminale. 3. Nerve roots must be separated to identify the origin of the filum terminale.

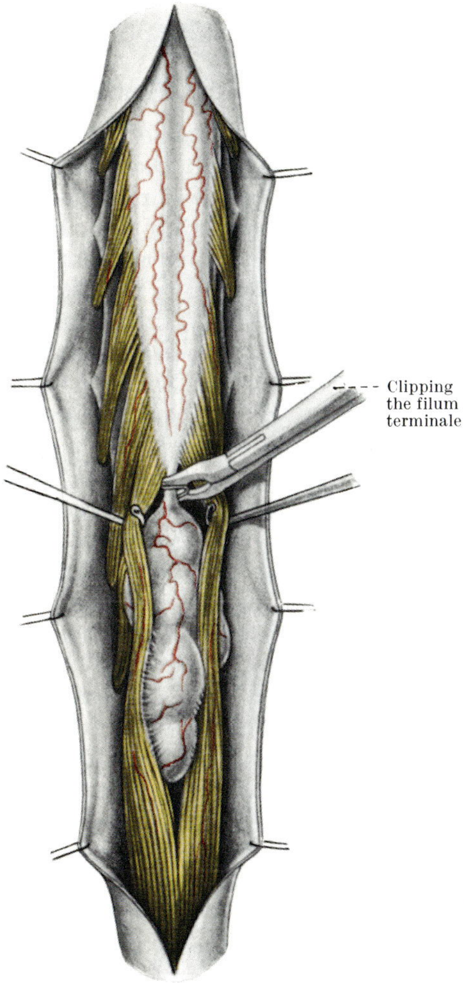

Fig. 138.

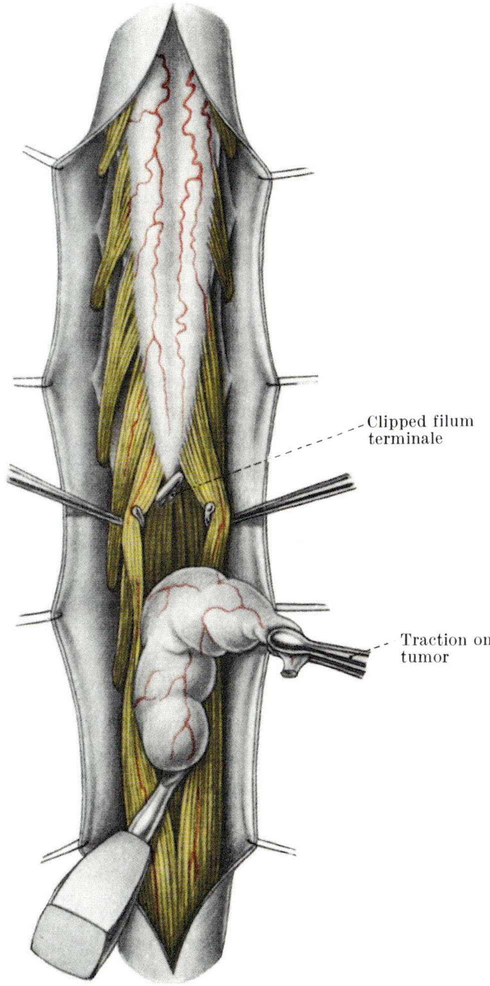

Fig. 139.

Fig. 138. Ependymoma of the filum terminale.

Observe: The filum terminale is clipped at its origin prior to dissection of the tumor from surrounding nerve roots.

Fig. 139. Ependymoma of the filum terminale.

Observe: Tumor removal begins rostrally and preceeds caudally to prevent injury of the conus medullaris.

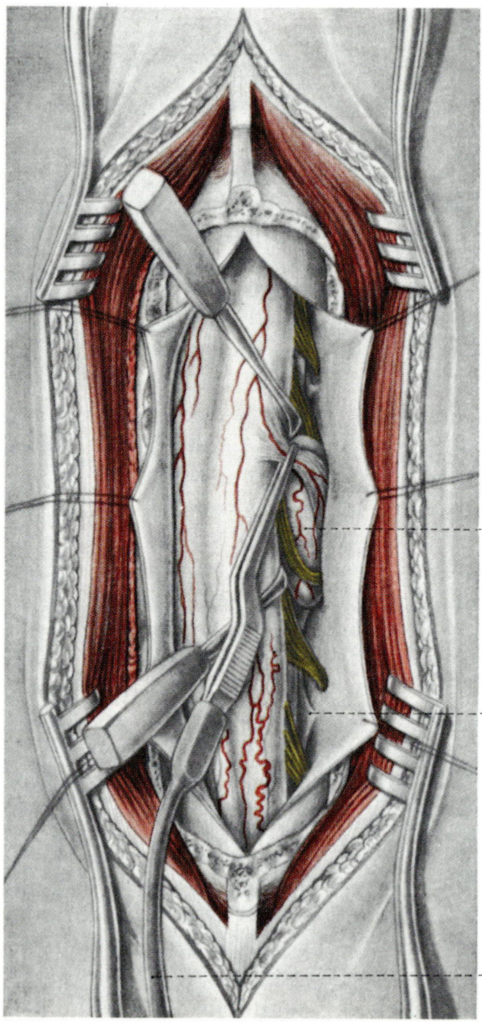

Fig. 141. Intrathecal extramedullary tumor (Meningioma of the thoracic cord): Dissection.

Observe: 1. The arachnoid is opened allowing retraction of the cord. 2. The tumor lies dorsal to the denticulate ligament. 3. The dorsal root is being divided to permit removal of the tumor without undue retraction of the cord.

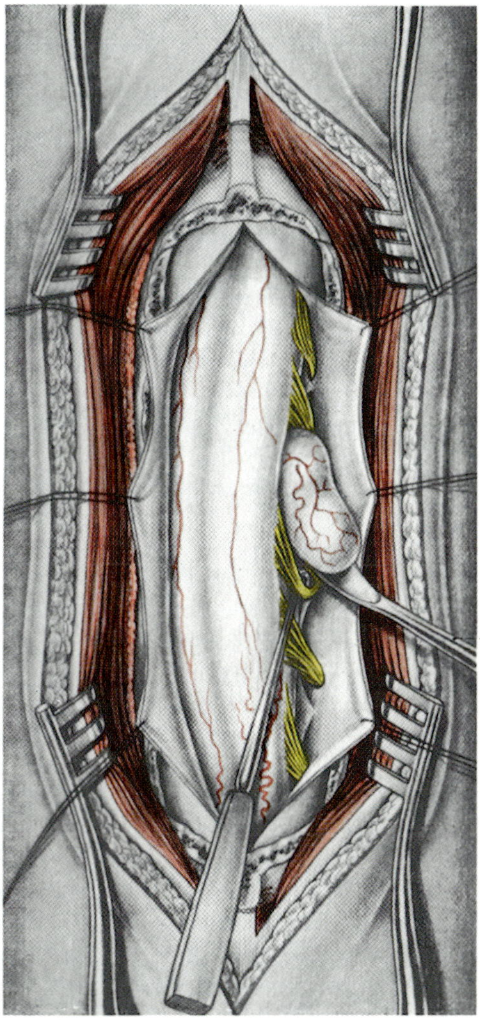

Fig. 142. Intrathecal extramedullary tumor (Meningioma of the thoracic cord): Excision.

Observe: Traction on the tumor is always away from the cord.

Chapter XVIII

Intra- and Extradural Tumor — Dumbbell Schwannoma

Schwannomas (neurolemmomas) constitute 33 percent of the spinal cord tumors seen during the last 20 years at Walter Reed General Hospital. Characteristically these tumors originate from a dorsal thoracic nerve root intrathecally. The tumor may extend along the nerve peripherally through the intervertebral neural foramina. The extradural portion of this well-encapsulated lesion may reach tremendous size. X-rays of the spine may show erosion around the foramina or even complete absence of the pedicles and lamina on the side of the tumor. When a mediastinal tumor is thought to be a Schwannoma, a myelogram should be performed even in the absence of any neuropathy or myelopathy. The intradural portion of this tumor should always be removed prior to surgical treatment of a mediastinal extension to avoid damage to the spinal cord during manipulation of the extradural portion of the lesion.

The operation for thoracic tumors is performed with the patient in the prone position; whereas, the sitting position is preferable for cervical lesions. A total laminectomy is done from one segment above the tumor to one segment below. Fig. 143 illustrates the exposure after the laminectomy is completed. The lamina over the extradural portion of the tumor may be paper-thin. The dura is opened in the midline and the arachnoid is torn laterally. The smooth, encapsulated tumor is traced to its dural exit. The lesion is usually constricted at this point giving a dumbbell configuration to the tumor. The dura is incised perpendicular to the original midline incision laterally to the waist of the tumor (Fig. 144). The intradural portion of the tumor is gently freed from any adherent nerve roots or arachnoidal adhesions between the tumor capsule and the spinal cord. Any retraction on the tumor must always be in a direction away from the spinal cord (Fig. 145). If the tumor is too large to permit easy dissection of its borders, the capsule is opened and the tumor is gutted using a curette. Once the intradural portion of the tumor is mobilized, the tumor is transected at its waist and the intradural portion of the tumor is removed (Fig. 146). The extradural portion of the Schwannoma is dissected free of surrounding structures. The tumor can be elevated, as in Fig. 147, to aid in identifying its distal boundaries and the normal nerve root coming from it. It is advisable to clip the nerve root distal to the tumor before it is transected. Once it is cut, the nerve will retract and bleeding from small nutrient vessels may be difficult to control. The tumor removal is then completed (Fig. 148). When a nerve root tumor is located at the fifth to eighth thoracic levels, it may be important to identify and preserve important radicular arteries arising from posterior branches of the intercostal arteries. At lower thoracic and upper lumbar levels it is essential that the artery of Adamkiewicz be kept in mind and preserved. The dural defect is closed using a periosteal or fascial graft (Fig. 148). The dura in older patients can often be reapproximated by using a book flap of the outer layer of dura. The dural closure should be water-tight and without constriction of the spinal cord. The dural closure is important in preventing a postoperative hydrothorax or pseudo-meningocele.

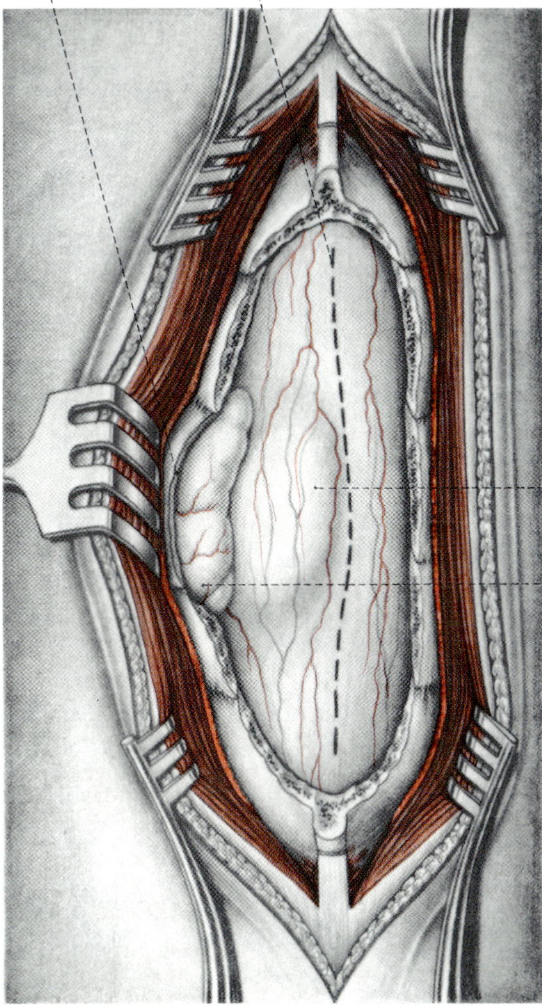

Fig. 143. Intra- and extrathecal tumor (Dumbbell neurofibroma of a thoracic nerve root): Exposure.

Observe: 1. Generous laminectomy above and below the tumor. 2. Extradural tumor extends through neural foramen. 3. The dura is tense and bulging from the intradural portion of the tumor.

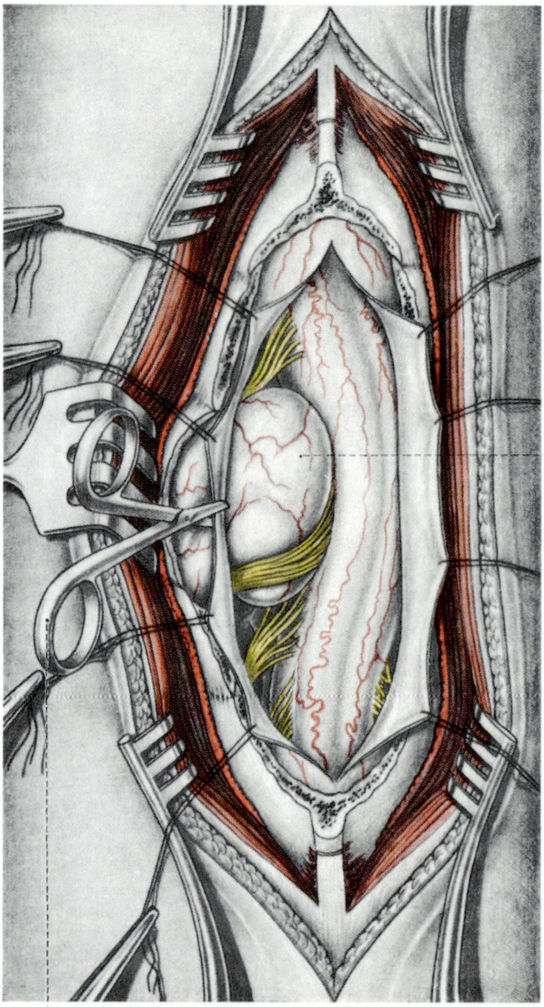

Fig. 144. Intra- and extrathecal tumor (Dumbbell neurofibroma of a thoracic nerve root): Intradural dissection.

Observe: 1. Displacement of cord and nerve root. 2. The dura is incised immediately over the extradural portion of the tumor perpendicular to the original dural opening.

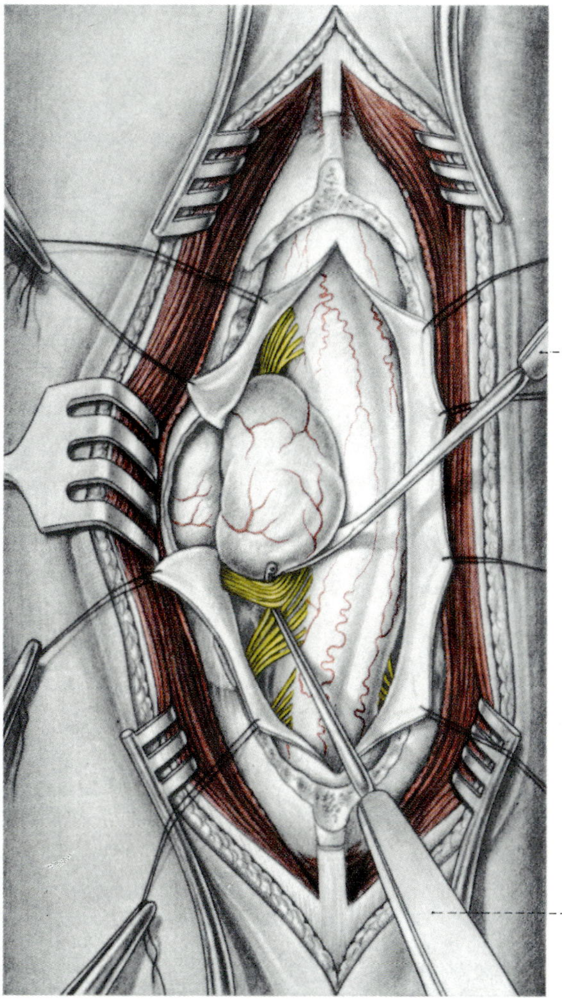

Fig. 145. Intra- and extrathecal tumor (Dumbbell neurofibroma of a thoracic nerve root): Intradural excision.

Observe: Traction on the tumor must be away from the spinal cord.

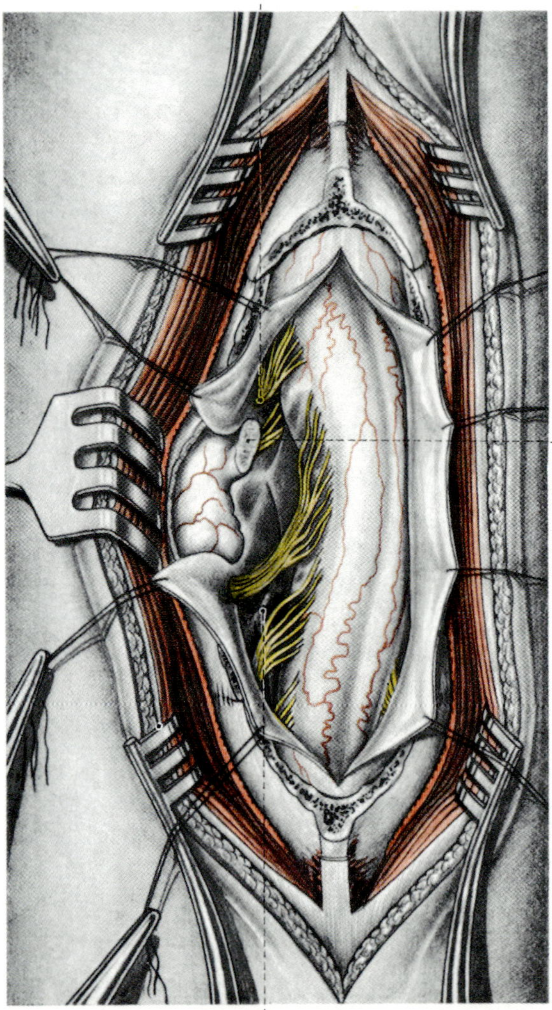

Fig. 146. Intra- and extrathecal tumor (Dumbbell neurofibroma of a thoracic nerve root): After removal of intradural portion of the tumor.

Observe: Deformation of spinal cord and elongation of nerve root.

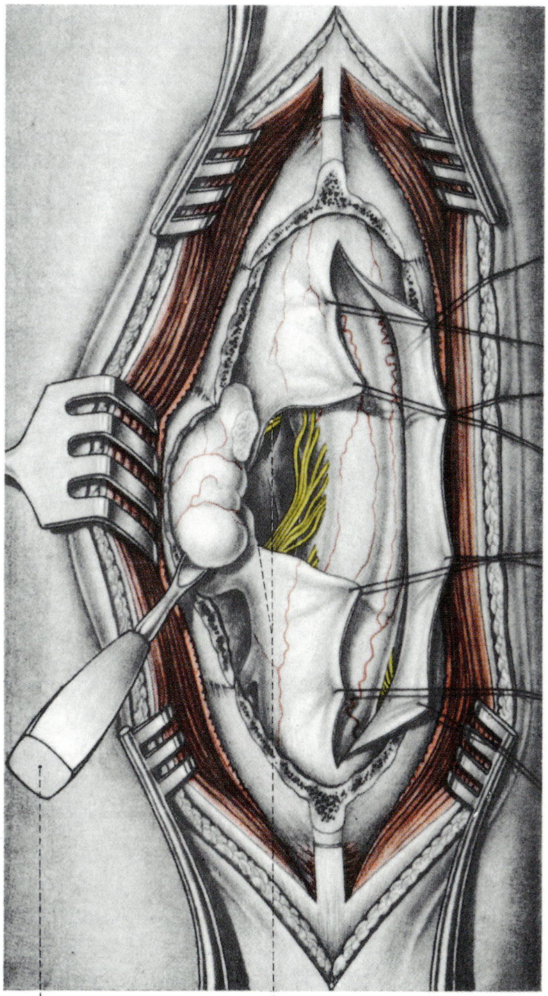

Fig. 147. Intra- and extrathecal tumor (Dumbbell neurofibroma of a thoracic nerve root): Excision of extradural tumor.

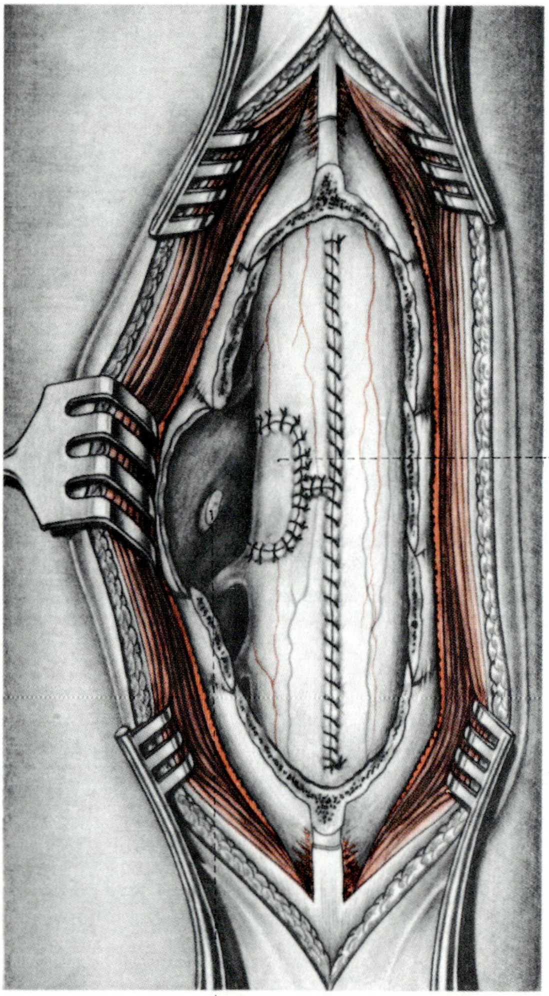

Fig. 148. Intra- and extrathecal tumor (Dumbbell neurofibroma of a thoracic nerve root): Operative field following removal of the tumor.

Observe: 1. Watertight but not constricting dural closure using dural graft which prevents a postoperative hydrothorax or meningocele. 2. Cavity formed by pressure erosion of lamina and pedicle.

Chapter XIX

Cervical Laminectomy for Trauma

The *sine qua non* in the management of cervical spinal cord injuries is immobilization. The patient should not be moved from the stretcher on which he is carried to the Emergency Room until an examination is performed, x-rays are taken and skeletal traction is instituted. In a restless patient, temporary head holder traction may be used to immobilize the patient's neck during the physical and x-ray examinations. If the patient with multiple injuries including a cervical cord injury has any air way difficulties, a tracheostomy is much safer than endotracheal intubation.

Stereoscopic roentgenograms are preferred in evaluating cervical spine injuries. They provide more knowledge of the extent of the fracture than just routine views. However, even with this aid, the extent of bony damage seen at surgery usually exceeds the radiological prediction by 50 percent.

The proper application of skeletal traction should be based on the type of fracture demonstrated on x-ray. When a cervical fracture is not associated with luxation, the skull tractor should be placed directly above the ear (Fig. 149). In a hyperextention injury with a posterior luxation, the skull tractors are inserted an inch behind the ear (Fig. 150). In a flexion injury with anterior luxation, the skull tractors are inserted an inch in front of the ear (Fig. 151). The skull tractors must be inserted an equidistance above the ear on each side to provide traction in the long axis of the spine (Fig. 152). The Vinke tongs are personally preferred because they require less constant attention. In military casualties with evacuation of the patients from hospital to hospital, this factor is important. The mechanism by which the Vinke tongs are held in the skull, as illustrated in Fig. 153, prevents any movement of the part of the instrument in contact with bone.

Once the skull tractor is in place, the patient is transferred to a Stryker or Foster rotating frame. Fifteen pounds of skeletal traction is applied and a lateral x-ray is again taken. If reduction of the luxation has not occurred, the traction is increased by five pounds every half-hour. Before each weight is added, another lateral x-ray is obtained. Occasionally 40 to 50 pounds are required to obtain reduction. Once proper alignment is achieved, the weight of traction is reduced to 15 pounds. When an operation is performed for an injury to the cervical spinal cord, the patient should remain in traction on the frame.

The indications for cervical laminectomy in patients with cervical spine and spinal cord trauma have been debated by neurosurgeons for many years. It is not within the scope of this book to enter this argument except to state that as a policy in the Army all cervical spinal cord injuries are surgically explored at some point in their course. This philosophy was expressed by Meirowsky at the conclusion of the Korean conflict when he said:

. . . *decompressive laminectomy should be done in every case so as to give the patient every possible opportunity to regain whatever function can be regained. In cervical cord injury, the function of one or two pairs of cervical roots above the level of transection may be interfered with by depressed bone fragments. Restoration of function of those roots, as can be accomplished frequently by decompression, may make the difference between permanent quadriplegia or permanent paraplegia*[1].

[1] Meirowsky, Arnold M., in: Neurological surgery of trauma, ed. Meirowsky, Arnold M., Office of the Surgeon General, Dept. of the Army, Washington, D.C., 1965, p. 307.

Certainly all cervical cord injuries in patients with penetrating wounds, neurological progression or bone fragments in the spinal canal should be operated on as soon as possible. This chapter will illustrate and discuss a cervical laminectomy performed for a closed fracture of the cervical spine.

Except in contaminated compound wounds, patients with cervical cord injuries are given systemic steroids in large doses as soon as possible following the injury. Fluids must be judiciously replaced. During the period of spinal shock, low blood pressure recordings should not be interpreted as an indication for massive administration of electrolyte solutions since this may lead to tragic respiratory complications.

When operative treatment is indicated the patient is anesthetized and entubated while lying supine on the frame with skeletal traction in place. The patient is then turned prone on the frame for surgery. In penetrating wounds of the cervical spine, local anesthesia may sometimes be preferable. In this case, great care must be taken to prevent infiltration of the local anesthetic near a dural laceration.

A laminectomy for a traumatic injury differs from that described in Chapter XIII in that sharp, rather than blunt, dissection is used in the subperiosteal stripping of the lamina. With the type of injury illustrated in Fig. 154, it is easy to visualize how a blunt instrument could drive bone fragments into the spinal cord. While gently elevating and retracting the paravertebral muscles, a knife is used to clear the lamina laterally to the facet (Fig. 155). After the muscles have been stripped back, the exposure is maintained with self-retaining retractors. Before removing the spinous processes and lamina, the degree of bony injury is evaluated (Fig. 156). The spinous processes are grasped with a towel-clip, and the stability of the vertebra is ascertained by gentle movement. The laminectomy should extend at least one level above and below the site of injury. All loose fragments of bone are carefully removed. Repeated irrigation with isothermic saline will help to keep the field clear of blood so that normal landmarks can be seen. The facets are palpated for fractures and to evaluate their stability. The facets should be preserved whenever possible; however, if a fractured facet is compressing a nerve root, it should be sacrificed. Decompression of injured nerve roots, especially above the level of cord injury, can be crucial in rehabilitation of a quadraplegic patient. Instability can always be taken care of later by an anterior fusion (see Chapter XXIV). The dura is opened even if a laceration, as seen in Fig. 157, is not present. Absorbable gelatin strips are placed in the lateral epidural spaces and the dura is incised in the midline. The dural margins are retracted by stay sutures. The injury to the spinal cord is then evaluated (Fig. 158). If debridement of the cord is necessary, it should be performed using magnification. If subpial discoloration or marked swelling are present, hematomyelia should be suspected. In this situation, a fine 23 gauge needle is inserted and a two cc. syringe is used to gently aspirate. The pia is then incised over the swelling and a myelotomy is made through a posterior column to decompress a hematomyelic or myelomalacic cavity. The dura is debrided. If the dura is reapproximated, it must not cause constriction of the spinal cord. Fig. 159 illustrates closure of the dura using a fascial graft. The alternative to this type of reapproximation is to leave the dura open and cover the spinal cord with an absorbable gelatin strip. A meticulous closure of the wound in layers is important.

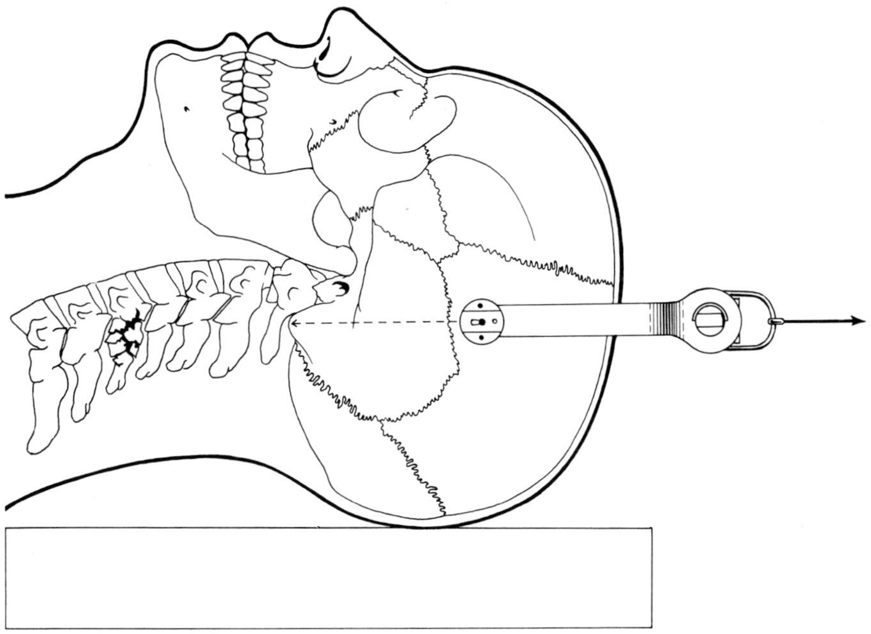

Fig. 149. Skeletal traction in fractures of the cervical spine: Position of Vinke tongs in fractures without dislocation.

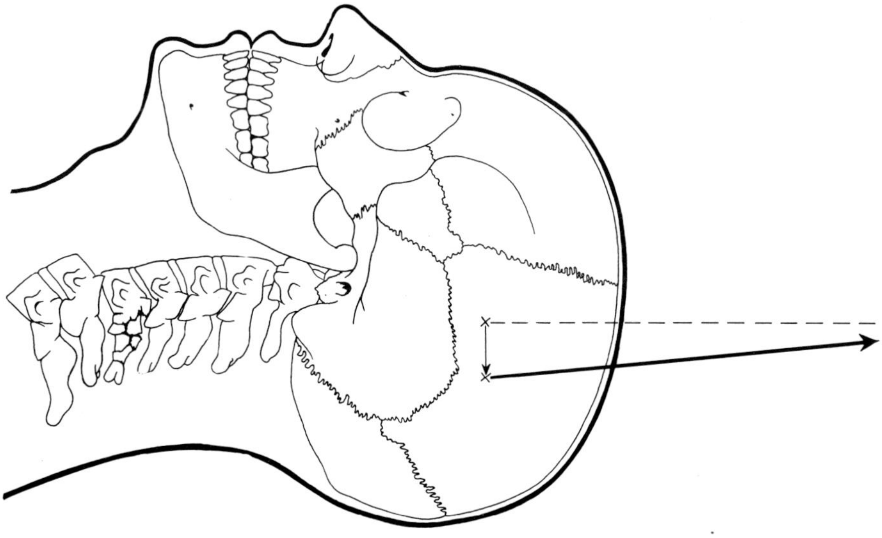

Fig. 150. Skeletal traction in fractures of the cervical spine: Position of the Vinke tongs in fractures with posterior dislocation (flexion injury).

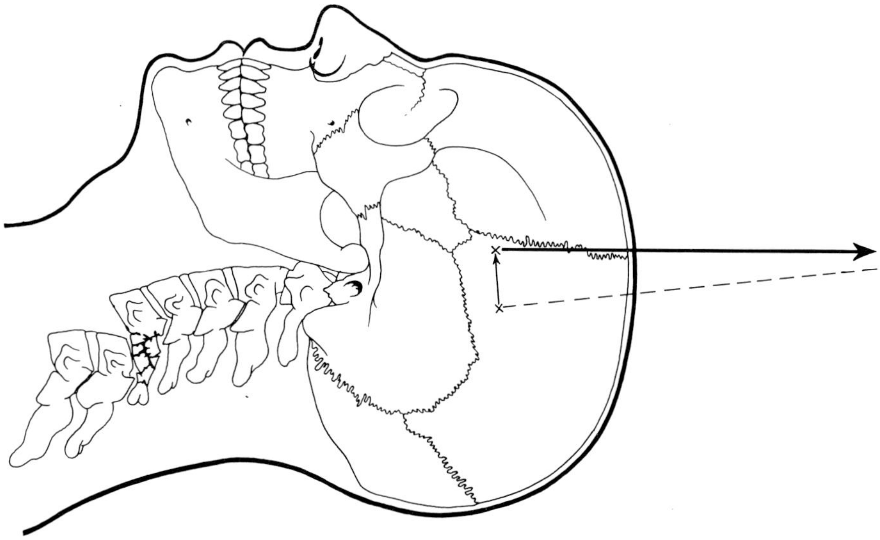

Fig. 151. Skeletal traction in fractures of the cervical spine: Position of Vinke tongs in fractures with anterior dislocation (hyperextension injury).

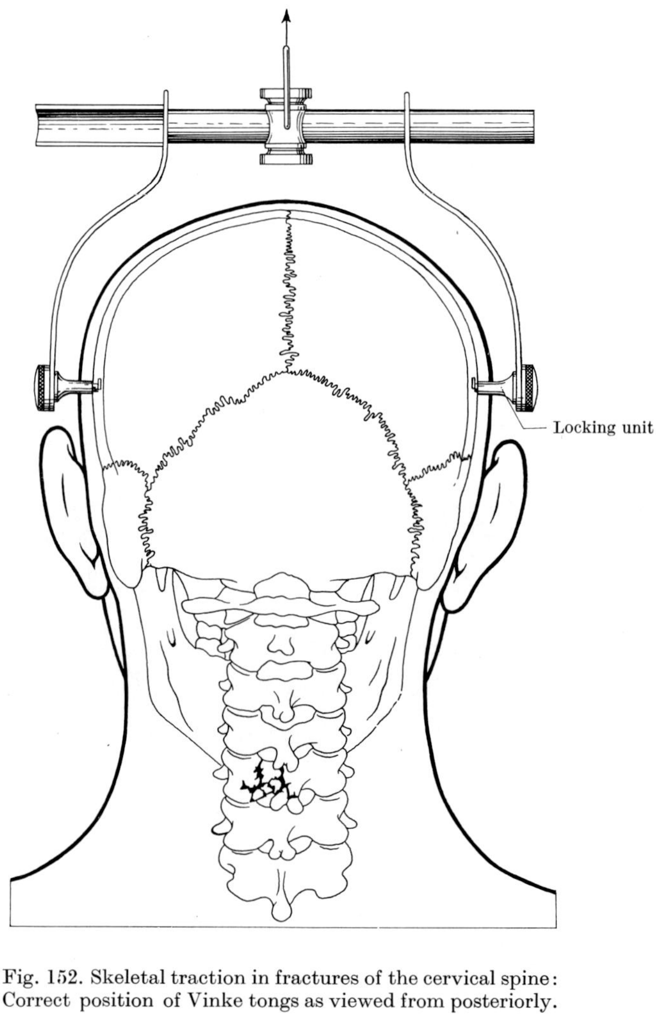

Fig. 152. Skeletal traction in fractures of the cervical spine: Correct position of Vinke tongs as viewed from posteriorly.

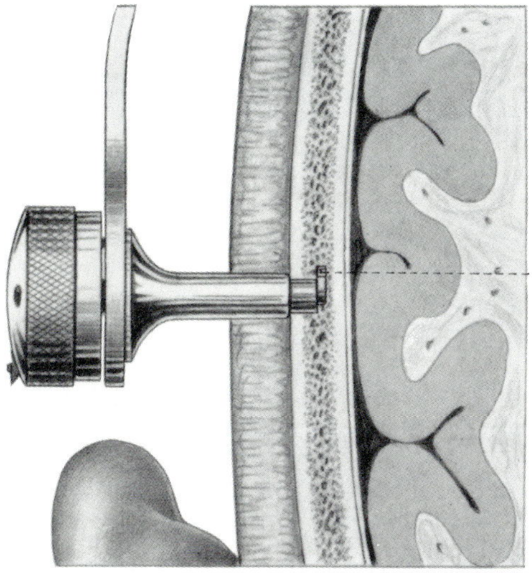

Fig. 153. Skeletal traction in fractures of the cervical spine: Proper position of Vinke tong locking unit in the skull.

Observe: Flange of locking unit secured between inner and outer table.

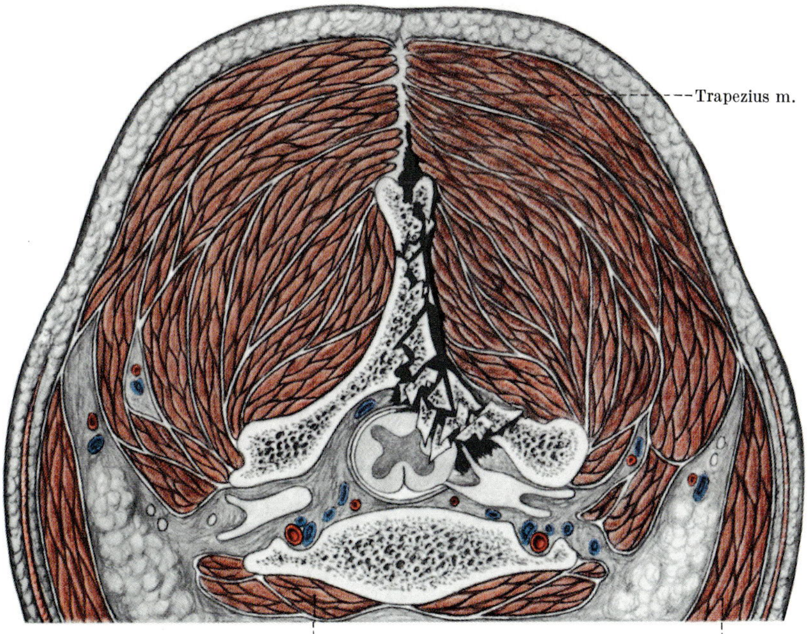

Fig. 154. Transverse section through the neck at C VI level to illustrate topographical anatomy in a compound fracture of the cervical spine.

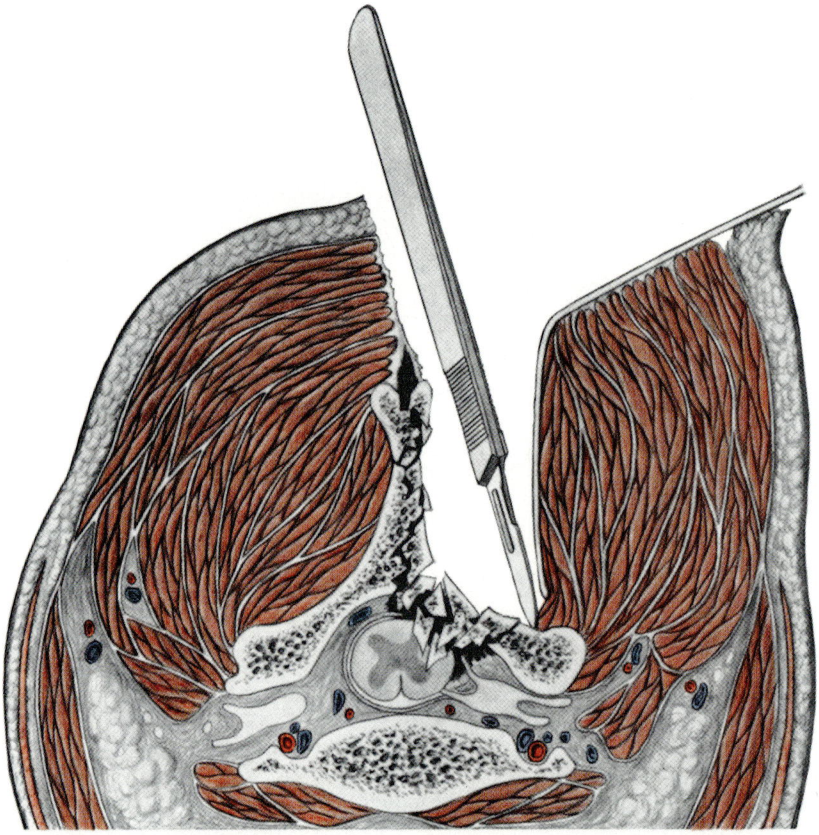

Fig. 155. Laminectomy for compound fracture of the cervical spine: Transverse section through the neck at C VI level.

Observe: Separation of the muscles from fractured spinous processes and laminae is done by *sharp* dissection.

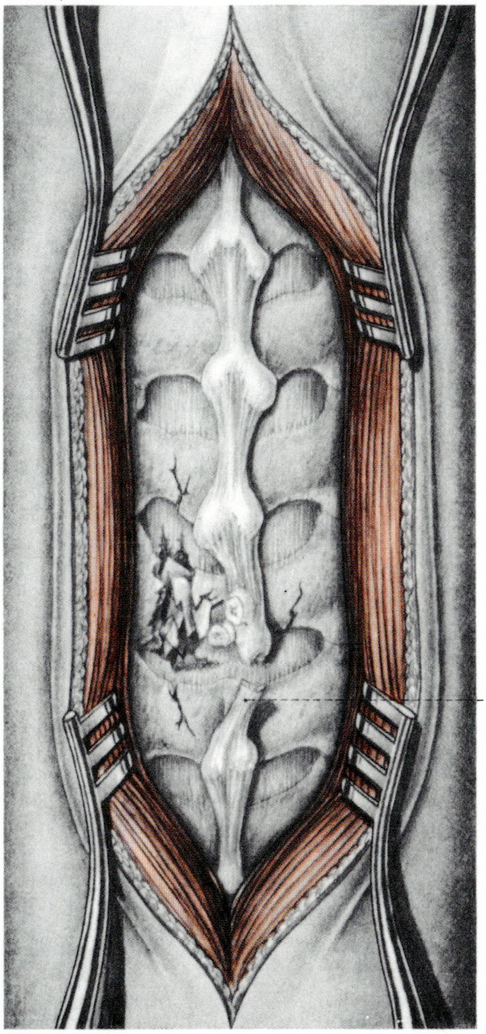

Fig. 156. Laminectomy for compound fracture of the cervical spine: Operative view following sharp dissection of muscle from spinous processes and laminae.

Observe: Ruptured interspinous ligament.

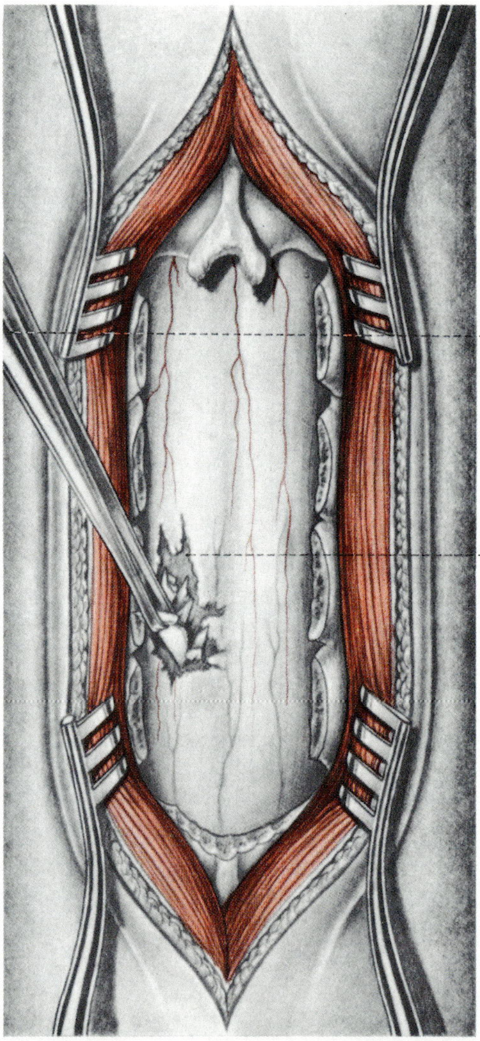

Fig. 157. Laminectomy for compound fracture of the cervical spine: Operative view following removal of spinous processes and laminae.

Observe: The laminectomy extends well above and below the area of fracture.

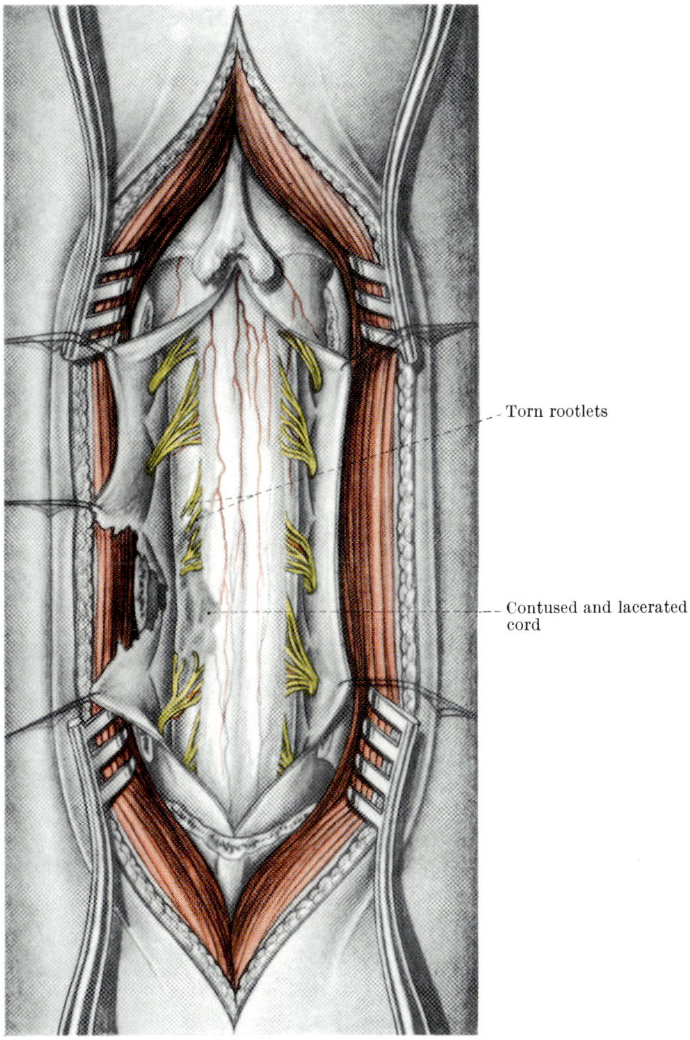

Fig. 158. Laminectomy of compound fracture of the cervical spine: Operative view following debridement.

Observe: The dura is opened over the entire extent of the laminectomy.

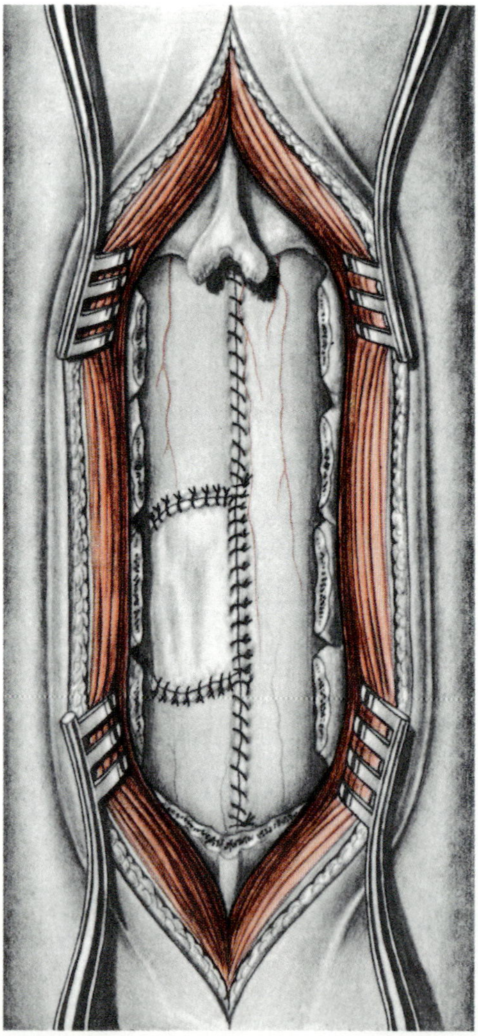

Fig. 159. Laminectomy for compound fracture of the cervical spine: Operative view following dural closure.

Observe: A patch graft is used so that the dura can be reapproximated without causing any constriction of the site of injury.

Chapter XX

Myelomeningocele Repair

Spina bifida may be associated with a tremendous spectrum of meningeal and neural herniation varying from a small outpouching of meninges to complete rachischisis. Meningoceles and myelomeningoceles present with a great variety of locations, forms, sizes and coverings. Neurological function varies from complete paralysis below the level of the lesion to neurological intactness. The most common location of these congenital anomalies is over the lumbosacral region. Many other congenital abnormalities may also be found in these children.

Indications for surgery in myelodysplasia continue to be debated by neurosurgeons. The author believes that there is no justification for operation in the presence of total paralysis of the lower extremities, bowel and bladder. It is increasingly apparent that if surgery is contemplated it should be done early. Meningoceles that rupture at the time of delivery must be operated on as soon as possible or overwhelming sepsis will usually occur. Surgical correction of myeloschisis must be done within hours of birth or total paralysis will result.

The goals of surgery are to remove the mass lesion and obtain a water-tight dural closure without increasing the neurological deficit. The repair of a lumbar myelomeningocele (Fig. 160) is presented in this chapter.

The baby is placed prone on the operating table with the head slightly lower than the back so that the cerebrospinal fluid will not be replaced by air (Fig. 161). The newborn will tolerate the operative procedure well with only a brandy and sugar nipple. One percent lidocaine with epinephrine is diluted 1:10 with saline and used for local anesthesia. Older infants and children require endotracheal anesthesia. The skin is cleansed with mild soap and water. The anal area is sealed off from the operative field by proper draping. The drapes are applied with a generous area exposed so that mobilization of extensive skin flaps is possible. Before the incision is made, blood replacement is begun. Ten cc. of whole blood per pound is given. As blood loss exceeds this amount, it is replaced cc. for cc. The skin incision is sketched on the baby's back with methylene blue (Fig. 162). Transverse extentions of the circular incision must be planned before the lesion is excised. An incision is made into the skin immediately adjacent to the exposed meninges. Even if the skin extends well on to the dome of the lesion, it should be preserved. Redundant skin can always be excised later. The incision is carried down to the meningeal sac which is stripped from the subcutaneous tissue and lumbosacral fascia much the way an inguinal hernia sac is dissected. The base of the defect is identified (Fig. 163). The sac is then opened beginning dorsally in the midline in an area free of neural elements. The nerve roots in the wall of the sac are mobilized and placed back into the spinal canal. Within the spinal canal the filum terminale can often be identified. It should be sectioned to prevent tethering of the spinal cord later in life. Some neural elements will end in the sac itself and may be sacrificed. Redundant dura is excised (Fig. 164). A water-tight closure is essential. After the dura has been closed, jugular compression by the anesthetist will test the quality of the closure. To reinforce the dural suture line, semilunar flaps of lumbosacral fascia are swung across the midline and sutured to the base of the opposite side (Figs. 165, 166). The skin margins are undermined to the extent that the wound can be reapproximated without tension. Figs. 162 and 167 illustrate the extent of subcutaneous dissection. Stainless steel wire is used for the skin closure and the stitches are left in place for 10 to 14 days. The dressing must remain dry and isolate the wound from feces.

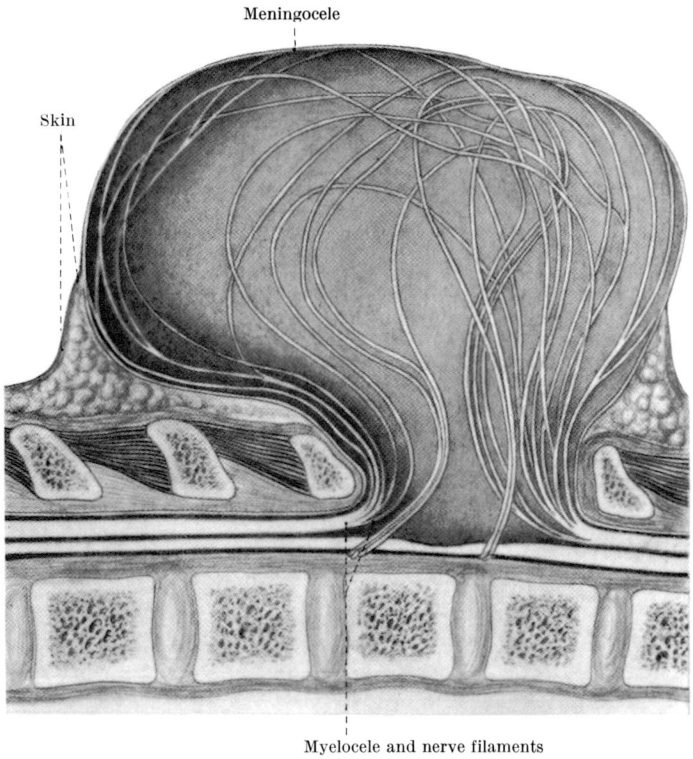

Fig. 160. Lumbar myelomeningocele: Sagittal section.

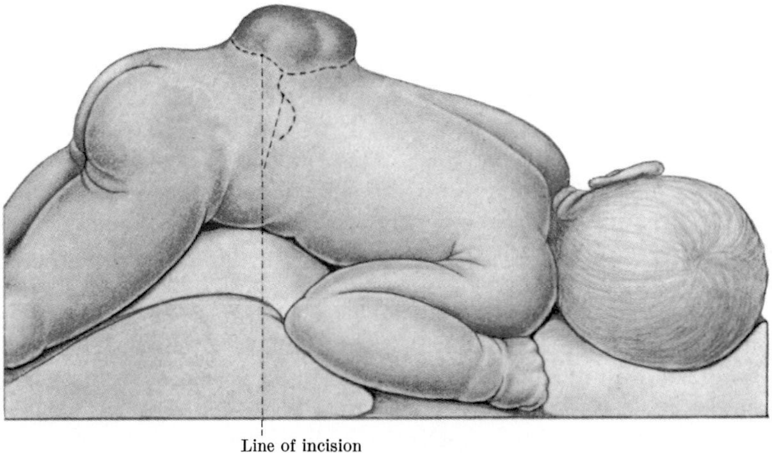

Fig. 161. Lumbar myelomeningocele: Operative position of patient.

Observe: 1. Elevation of lumbar area to reduce escape of cerebral spinal fluid. 2. Circumferential line of incision which saves as much healthy skin as possible.

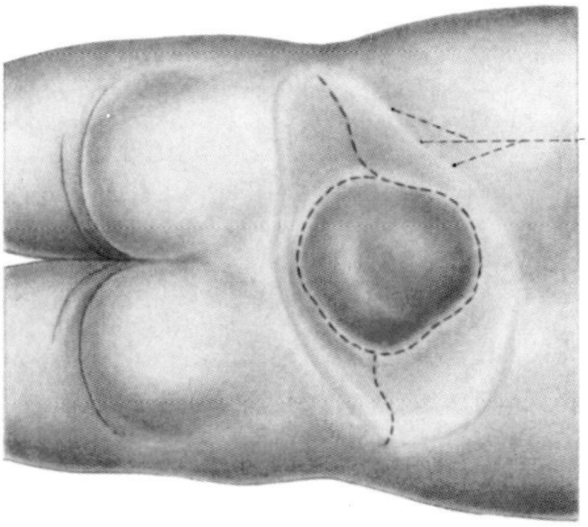

Fig. 162. Lumbar myelomeningocele: Operative field as viewed by the surgeon.

Observe: Shaded area indicates extent of undermined skin to accomplish closure.

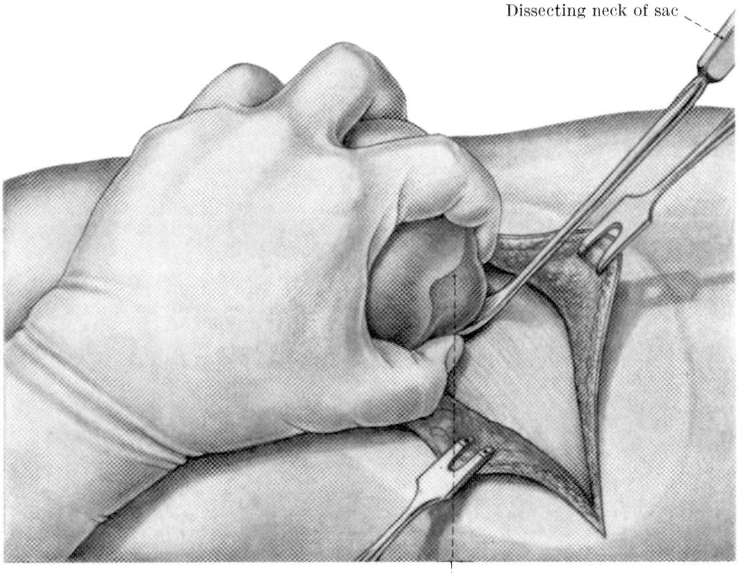

Fig. 163. Lumbar myelomeningocele: Dissecting neck of dural pedicle.

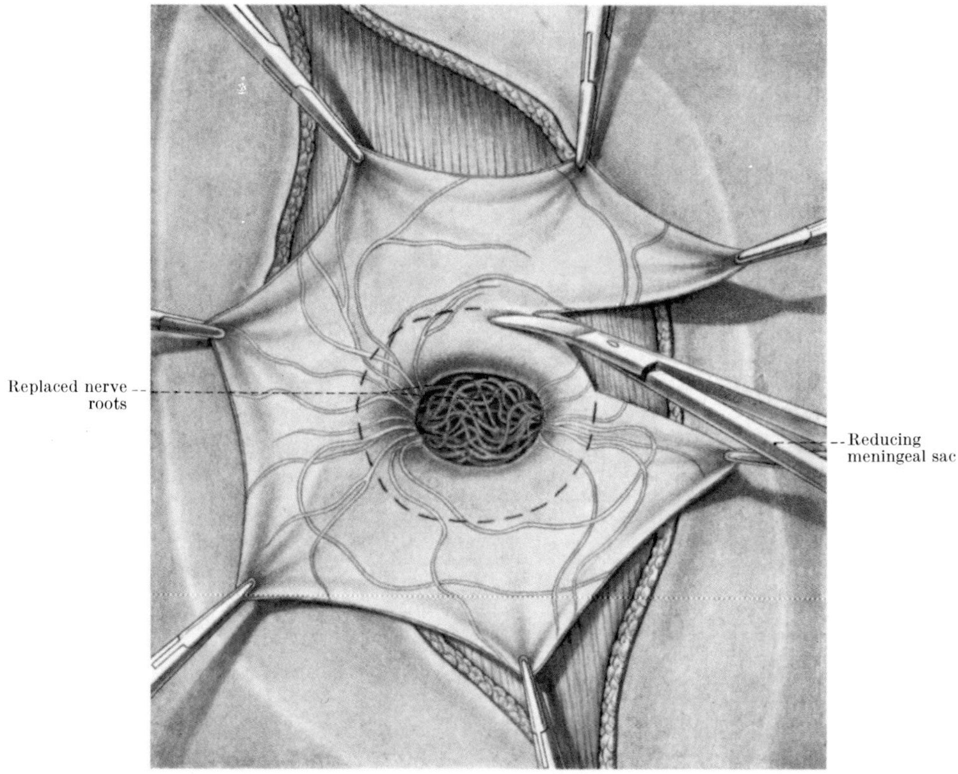

Fig. 164. Lumbar myelomeningocele: Excising redundant dura.

Observe: All potentially viable nervous elements have been stripped from the meninges and replaced into the spinal canal.

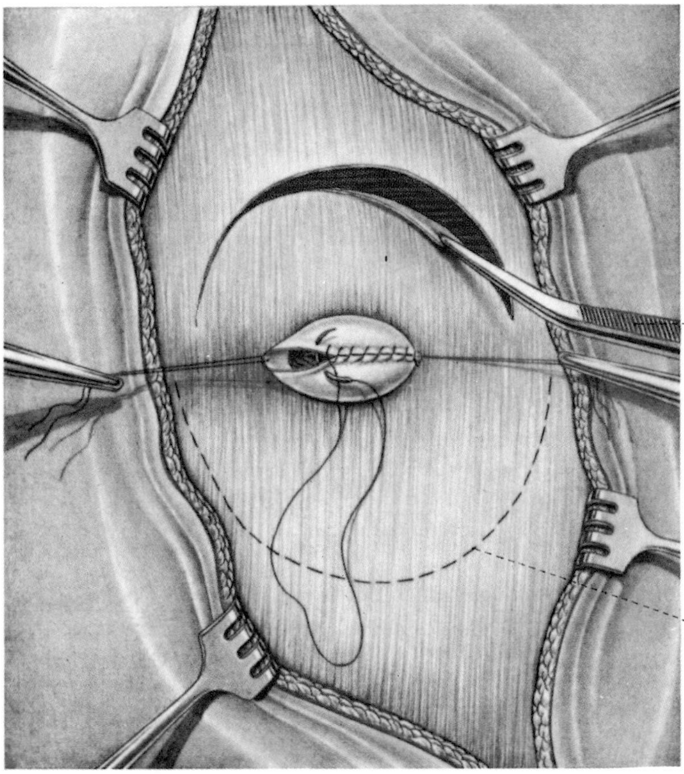

Fig. 165. Lumbar myelomeningocele: Dural closure.

Observe: 1. Following excision of the redundant dura a watertight closure is performed. 2. Paravertebral fascia is elevated and used to reinforce the dural closure. 3. The fascial incision is not the same on both sides.

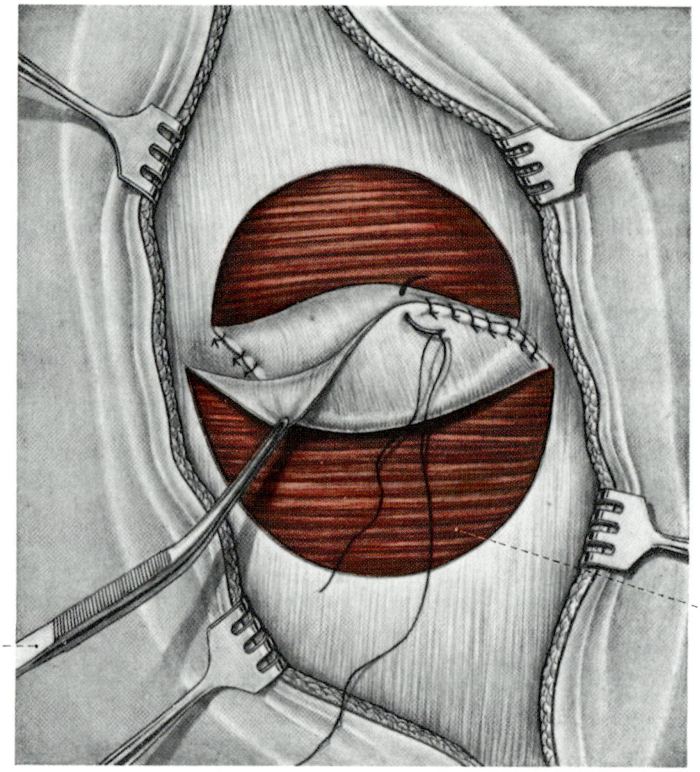

Fig. 166. Lumbar myelomeningocele: Fascial closure.

Observe: The fascial flap on each side is then folded across the midline and sutured to the base of the opposite side.

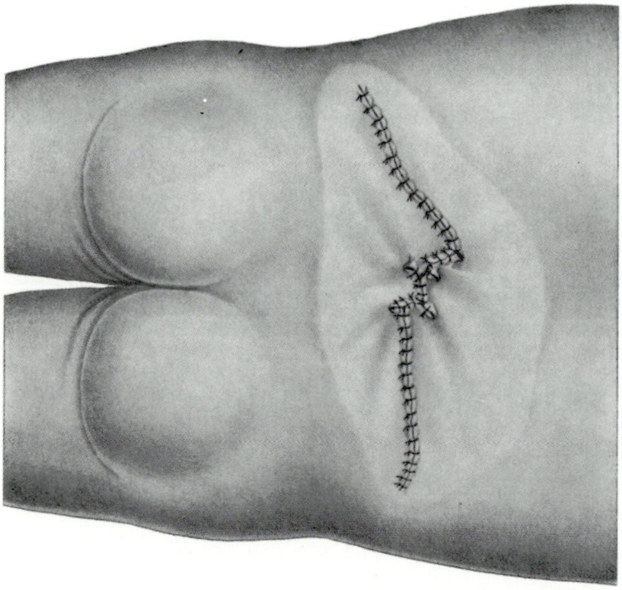

Fig. 167. Lumbar myelomeningocele: Skin closure.

Observe: Sufficient subcutaneous undermining allows a tension-free closure.

Chapter XXI

Surgery of Peripheral Nerves

A. Principles of Peripheral Nerve Surgery

Because trauma is responsible for peripheral nerve injuries requiring operative treatment, it is understandable that times of war have produced most of the knowledge upon which the principles of peripheral nerve surgery is based. Experience gained during two world wars in the treatment of peripheral nerve injuries still guides the handling of injured nerves.

Since peripheral nerve injuries are not life threatening, other system injuries are usually of primary concern. Having stabilized the cardiorespiratory condition of the patient, attention may then be directed to compound extremity injuries. Prior to any operative debridement, a careful examination should be done to ascertain the extent of neurological dysfunction. At the time of this initial surgery, the nerve injury is inspected and described as to its nature, location and severity. Surgical repair of the nerve is deferred at the time of this initial surgery. Combat wounds are all contaminated; and today's improved surgical technique with aseptic and antiseptic measures has not decreased the risk of an apparently "clean" wound becoming infected with extensive secondary loss of tissue, making reconstructive surgery even more difficult. Separated nerve ends may be tagged with radio-opaque sutures to aid localization at the time of a delayed neurorrhaphy. Other methods of marking the cut ends of a divided nerve are superfluous.

In any patient awaiting delayed nerve repair, the care of denervated tissue is of paramount importance. The paralyzed muscle must not be overstretched. Thermal and pressure injuries must be prevented. Unnecessary long-term immobilization with attendant stasis, degeneration of muscle fibers, formation of excessive fibrous tissue and adhesions are to be avoided. Patients with fractures requiring immobilization benefit from physiotherapeutic measures such as massage and from rotating beds to prevent circulatory stasis. All of these efforts will result in a more normal limb at the time of reinnervation. If, at the time of initial debridement, the nerve was found to be severed, the eventual surgical repair is obviously indicated. Patho-anatomical studies have shown that the ideal time for secondary suture is about 20 days following injury. The neurorrhaphy can be done at that time only if no evidence of local or systemic sepsis is present and no other injury precludes operative intervention.

The surgical treatment of an injured nerve is also required when the pathology of the lesion is unknown and clinical evidence points to a complete or partial nerve lesion. It is re-emphasized that the clinical assessment of such situations requires accurate anatomical knowledge of the level of the nerve branches to various muscle groups. Electrodiagnostic studies are also important in the evaluation of questionably complete nerve injuries. Electromyography with search for denervation fibrillations, positive sharp waves and other muscle action potentials as well as the determination of chronaxie and strength-duration curves is often of value. Nerve conduction velocities are sometimes of aid in partial nerve injuries. An uncommonly used, but reliable, tool is testing of the galvanic skin response (GSR) to map areas of cutaneous sensory denervation. For more details the reader is referred to one of the standard texts on electrodiagnosis.

The often discussed Tinel's sign provides an opportunity to observe the rate of growth of some regenerating sensory fibers. However, a positive Tinel's sign tells us only that some sensory axons are moving peripherally from the proximal side of an area of trauma. A positive sign is no justification for delay of surgical exploration if other evidence of motor or sensory reinnervation fails to appear within the expected time.

The operative approach to the traumatized nerve must provide a wide exposure, and the preoperative skin preparation should allow for extension of the incision either proximally or distally. Skin scars should be excised or avoided, and the skin incision is made in normal skin creases over joints. The incision is planned so that the nerve repair does not lie directly beneath the suture line. Local infiltration with 1:200,000 epinephrine in normal saline is helpful to reduce oozing. The use of a tourniquet is not necessary. Thorough anatomical knowledge, delicate handling of tissues and dissection parallel to normal tissue planes will reduce blood loss and obviate the need for a tourniquet. The risk of postoperative hematoma formation and ischemic necrosis in using a tourniquet far outweigh the danger of intraoperative hemorrhage especially by the less experienced surgeon.

The surgical exposure at the time of a delayed nerve repair must be done through normal anatomical planes above and below the area of injury. Having identified the nerve proximal and distal to the lesion, dissection is carried into the area of injury. A detailed understanding of the regional anatomy is imperative. Without this knowledge there is great danger of further damage to the nerve trunk or its branches. Electrical stimulation may be of help in locating functional nerve fibers within a large mass of scar tissue, thus guiding further dissection. After the nerve has been completely freed from surrounding scar tissue, an often difficult decision must be made as to whether or not a neuroma in continuity should be resected or not. Inspection and palpation, although helpful, may be misleading in this regard. The presence of a neuroma is not incompatible with excellent spontaneous recovery. Conversely, a nerve which appears normal may have severe intrafascicular damage precluding regeneration. In these situations electrical stimulation, with or without *in vivo* recording of evoked potentials, is a valuable guide. Such stimulation actually can most reliably be done above and below the area of injury before the neurolysis is completed since manipulation can cause a temporary conduction block. Surgeons most experienced in peripheral nerve surgery agree that the results of incision and end-to-end anastomosis of peripheral nerves are not good enough to justify the risk of performing such a procedure on a nerve that might recover spontaneously.

The underlying pathology necessitating surgical intervention may be pressure on or tension of the nerve with impairment of function and a variable potential for recovery. The indicated surgical procedure for such lesions is a neurolysis with rerouting of the nerve and removal of constricting bone or ligament. Neurolysis is defined as the removal of constricting scar which has been preventing regenerating axons from growing through the area of constriction or causing a physiological conduction block at the area of constriction. A neurolysis may be either external or internal.

In performing an external neurolysis the entire nerve trunk is dissected carefully from its surrounding bed of scar tissue. Again it is emphasized that this procedure is done after first exposing the nerve through normal anatomical planes both above the below the site of injury while sparing all branches by dissecting with the aid of magnifying lenses. Bleeding points on the nerve proper are not electrocoagulated. If the neurolysis obviously interferes with the vascular supply of the nerve, no benefit can be expected from the surgical procedure.

The performance of a proper internal neurolysis is most difficult. The objective is to free the individual fascicles within the nerve. This is done either by microscopic dissection or by injection of warm saline solution. Both techniques are designed to disrupt constricting scar tissue. Avoiding damage to the delicate intrafascicular vascular network is most difficult. Only the epineurium is incised while avoiding disruption of the perineurium and especially avoiding injection of saline into a fascicle.

A majority of traumatized nerves, however, require more than either an internal or an external neurolysis and need to be repaired by an end-to-end anastomosis. To obtain a tension-free anastomosis, an extensive mobilization of a nerve may be required. Transposition of the nerve to a new bed may also be necessary. Effective mobilization may necessitate stripping of branches from the parent nerve even though this may cause a loss of some blood supply to the nerve (Figs. 173 and 174). To prevent damage to adjacent fascicles, this stripping is done only under magnification and only as far as the branch can be easily separated. Ease of dissection alone is not a sufficient guide for this procedure. Magnification is essential because without it small fascicles may be overlooked. In mobilization of a nerve, nutrient vessels are encountered which unavoidably must be sacrificed. In this situation the nutrient vessel must be ligated well away from the nerve trunk to prevent damage to the intrinsic vessels of the nerve. The longitudinally oriented superficial arterial system cannot be adequately visualized and preserved if the limb is made ischemic by the use of a tourniquet. The tourniquet also enhances the risk of postoperative bleeding from these vessels with attendant hematoma and scar formation.

Correct axial orientation of nerve ends prior to neurorrhaphy is essential for optimal apposition of fascicles (Fig. 168). Nerve ends must be cut at precise right angles as the distal and proximal ends are resected back to healthy appearing bundles. Ideally a similar cross-sectional arrangement of the bundles can be recognized in the two ends. Reapproximation is performed using the suture material, such as 5—0 to 8—0 nylon, which causes the least fibroblastic proliferation.

To facilitate apposition of nerve ends, various joints of the extremity may be flexed. Experience gained from two World Wars, Korean and Vietnam, has established that flexion of greater than 90 degrees at the elbow and knee must be strictly avoided. Flexion should not exceed 40 degrees at the wrist nor 10 degrees at the ankle.

Whenever possible a direct end-to-end anastomosis of the nerve should be performed. However, nerve autografting has proved to be a preferable method of treatment than the archaic procedure of shortening long bones. Until homografts have been more intensely evaluated, autografting is the procedure of choice in bridging irreparable gaps.

The ideal autograft is one with a similar size and fascicular pattern. This is rarely possible, however, so that a nerve with a simple parallel fascicular pattern is most often used. Thin grafts are more successful than thick ones because vascularization is more easily achieved. The shorter the graft the better the chance will be of it being bridged by sprouting axons. Grafts greater than 15 cm. in length universally fail. The superficial radial and the sural nerves are the best donors for free nerve grafts. The medial and lateral antebrachial cutaneous nerves as well as the lateral femoral cutaneous nerve are often used.

Pedicle grafting is also a valuable adjunct in the repair of peripheral nerves. In Fig. 169, an adjacent uninjured nerve serves as a pedicle graft. The dorsal cutaneous nerve, a branch of the ulnar nerve, may serve as a donor for a median nerve injured in the forearm. This procedure has not been of great value in our experience. On the other hand, the use of a full thickness pedicle graft from the ulnar nerve to repair a median nerve when both nerves have been injured, has resulted in good sensory recovery. Fig. 170 demonstrates this technique. The ulnar and median nerves are both cut back to normal appearing fascicules and are then sutured together. The gap in the injured median nerve is measured and the ulnar nerve is then transected this same distance proximal to the ulnar-median anastomosis. The ulnar nerve is not further dissected at this time, but rather the distal anastomosis is delayed for a three-week period. This delay allows development of new vasculature to the pedicle graft and also gives time for Wallerian degeneration to occur in the graft. By this same method the common peroneal nerve may be used to repair the tibial nerve.

A pedicle graft using a cutaneous forearm nerve may also be used to bridge a gap in the median nerve. In Fig. 171 the lateral antebrachial cutaneous nerve serves as the donor. To accommodate the larger median nerve, a double strand of graft is used.

Another method of repairing injured nerves is illustrated by the nerve crossing procedure used in repairing the facial nerve. Fig. 172 demonstrates a hypoglossal-facial nerve anastomosis in which the descendens hypoglossi is anastomosed to the distal hypoglossal nerve.

The results of peripheral nerve repair are dependent on many factors which have already been mentioned. The additional well-recognized variables of age of the patient and site of the lesion must also be considered. The younger the patient, the better the return of function will be. The more distal a nerve is injured, the more effective regeneration will be. The closer a lesion is to the nerve cell body, the more profound will be the effect on this trophic center. Sensory nerve cells are affected more by this retrograde phenomenon than are motor nerve cells.

The surgeon is often confronted with a patient whose injury is many months old. The question then arises as to whether surgical repair is still justified. From our experience it can be said that good results are commonly observed with repair of nerves after delays of 12 to 14 months. This in no way, however, should be construed as evidence that a much earlier repair is not preferable.

Fig. 168a—d. Technique of nerve suture.

a Tension sutures are placed into the epineurium to approximate the nerve ends during the anastomosis and to aid in proper alignment.

b Traction and tension sutures apposes the nerve ends. The anastomosis is done with 5—0 to 8—0 nylon or silk depending on the size of the injured nerve.

c and d Rotation of the tension sutures permit completion of suture line.

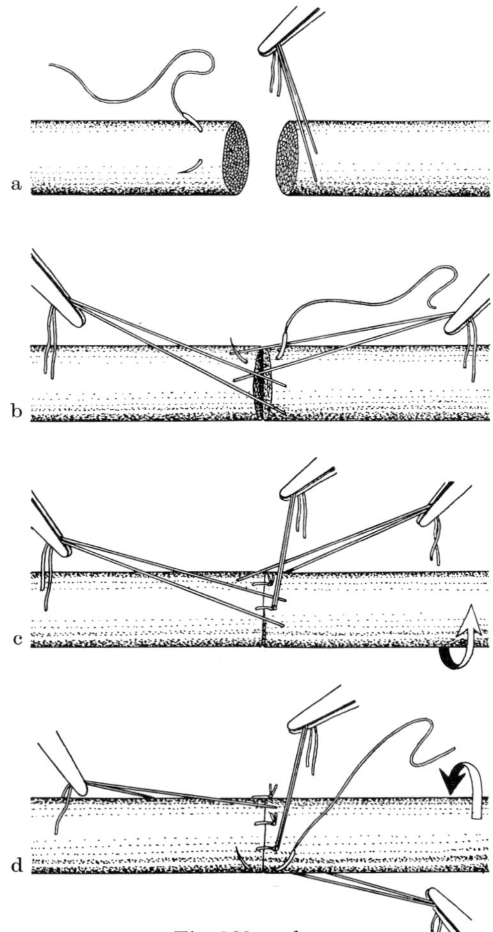

Fig. 168a—d.

Fig. 169. Methods of bridging gaps: Lateral pedicle grafting from adjacent normal nerve.

Observe: Cutaneous nerves provide the most readily available donors. In this instance the dorsal cutaneous branch of the ulnar nerve is used to repair a defect in the median nerve.

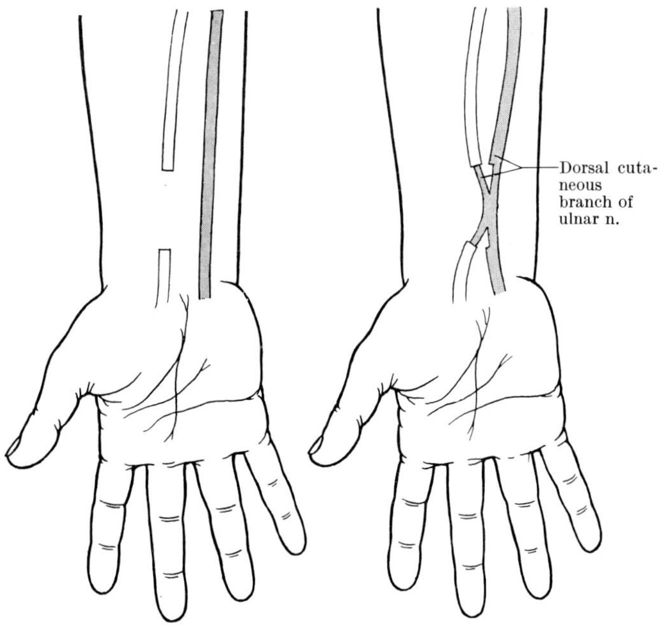

Fig. 169.

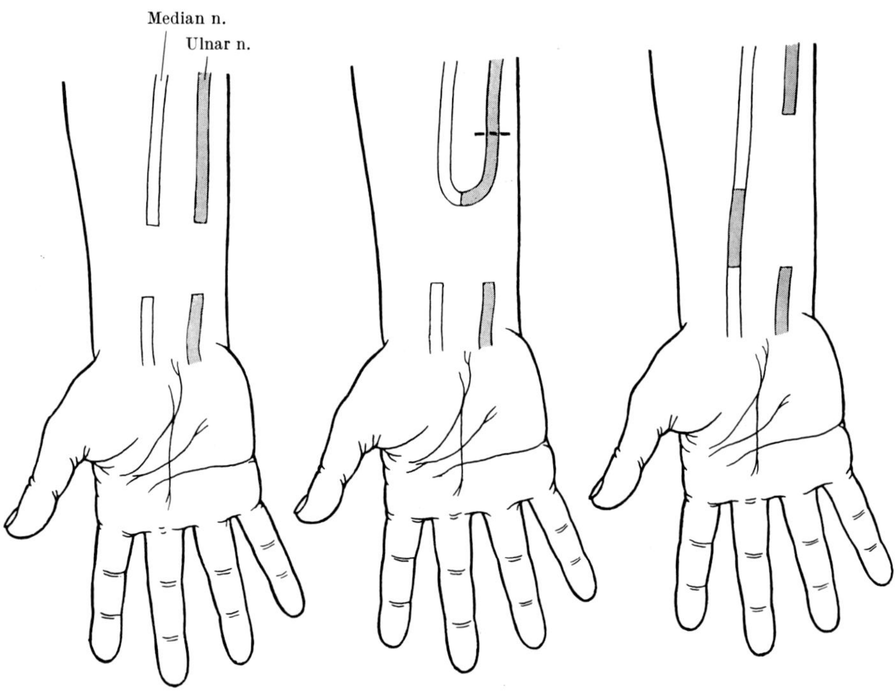

Fig. 170. Methods of bridging gaps: Full thickness pedicle grafting from adjacent injured nerve.

Observe: 1. In this example both the ulnar and median nerves have been damaged to the extent that neither are reparable by the end to end anastomosis. 2. The ulnar nerve is sacrificed in favor of the median nerve because of their respective sensory and motor distributions. 3. The proximal stump of the ulnar nerve is used as a full-thickness pedicle graft.

Fig. 171. Methods of bridging gaps: Full thickness pedicle grafting from an adjacent normal nerve.

Observe: 1. A less important uninjured nerve, i.e. the lateral antebrachial cutaneous nerve, is sacrificed. 2. The donor nerve is divided at the level of the gap. 3. These ends are then sutured into the proximal and distal stumps of the injured nerve, i.e. the median nerve. 4. A length of graft is taken both distally and proximally from the donor nerve and fashioned into a cable graft.

Fig. 172. Methods of bridging gaps: Full thickness nerve crossing graft as in facial-hypoglossal anastomosis.

Observe: Not only is the hypoglossal nerve anastomosed to the distal facial stump but the descendens hypoglossi is sutured to the distal hypoglossal nerve (compare Fig. 251).

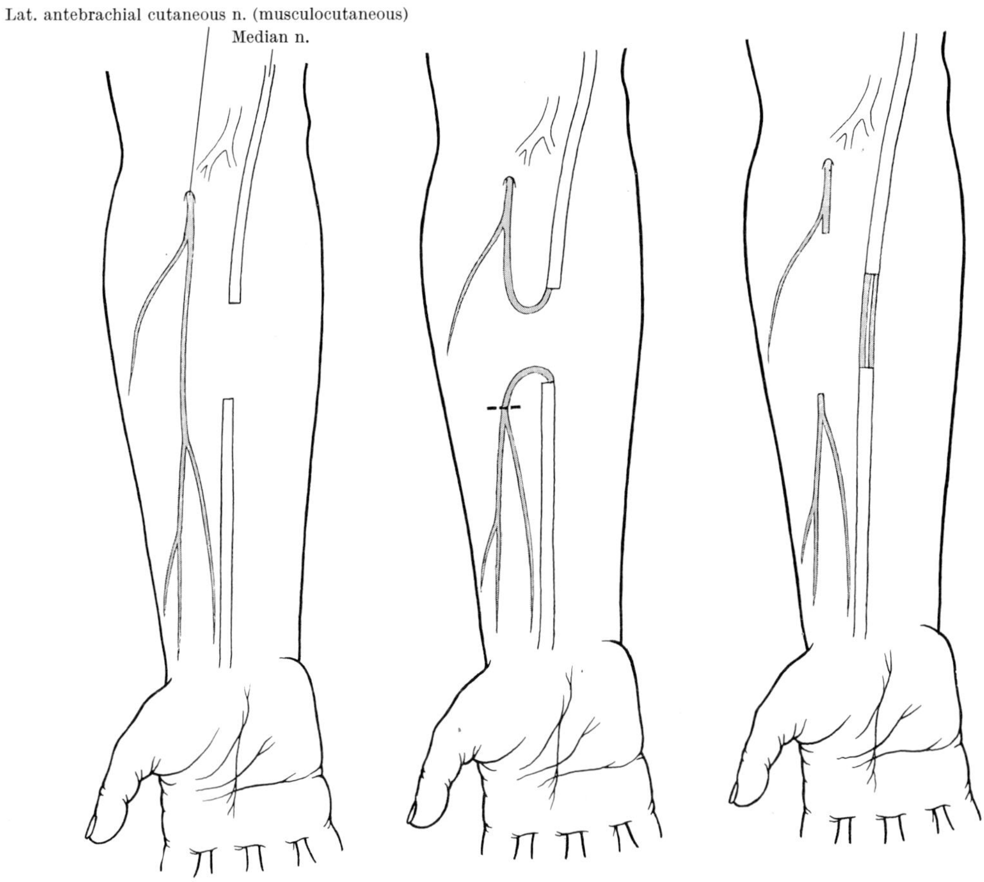

Fig. 171.

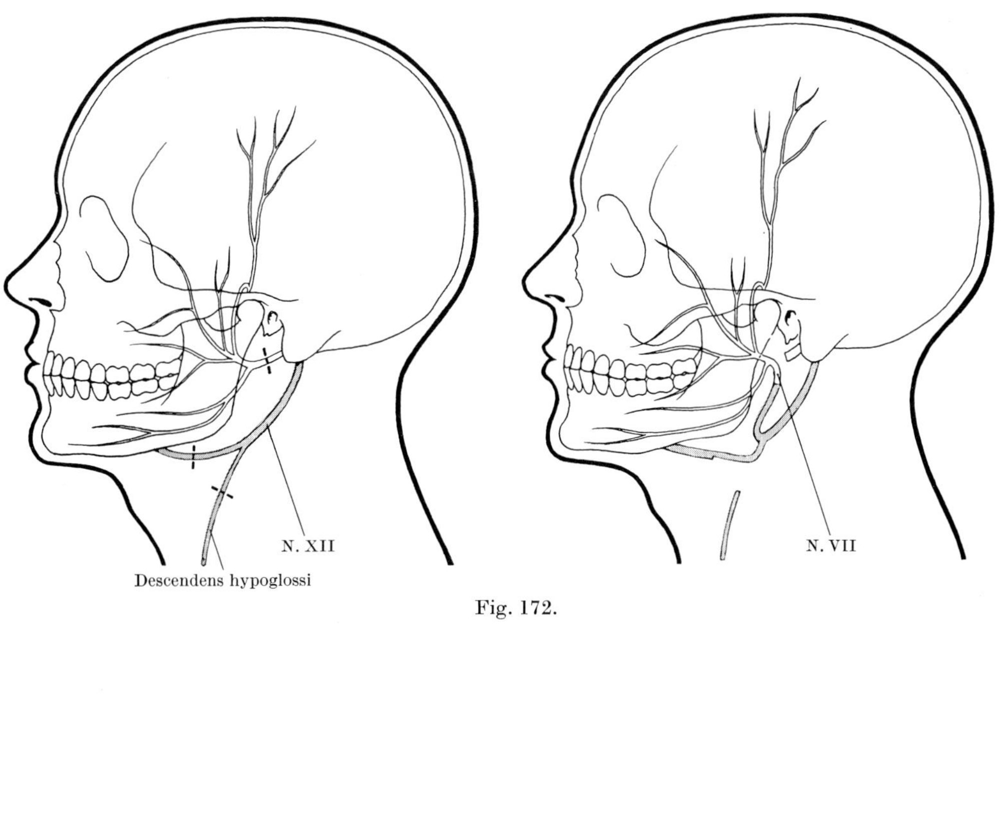

Fig. 172.

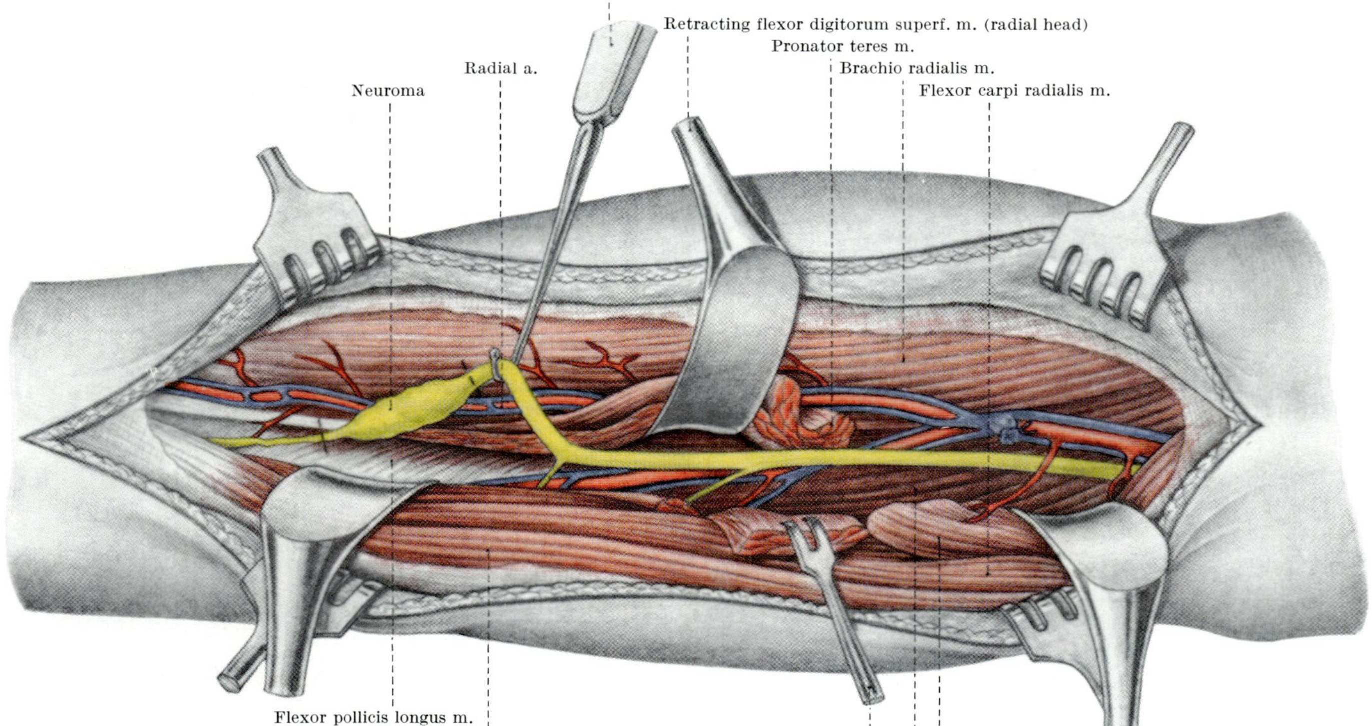

Fig. 173. Methods of bridging gaps: Mobilization. The median nerve in the forearm serves as an example to illustrate this method.

Observe: 1. The median nerve is freed throughout its course in the forearm. 2. The pronator teres muscle is divided without injury to its innervation. 3. The flexor digitorum superficialis muscle is divided at the fibrous arch between the humeral and radial heads. 4. The lacertus fibrosus is incised parallel to the pronator teres muscle and retracted with the skin.

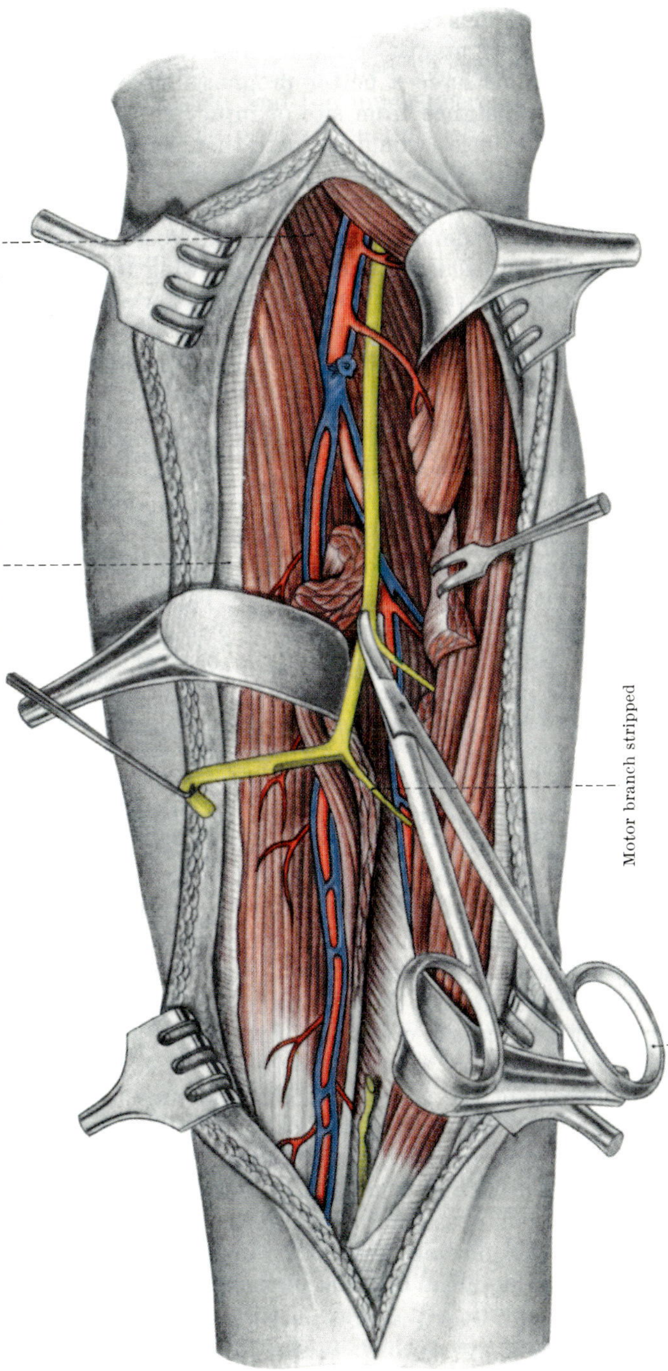

Fig. 174. Methods of bridging gaps: Mobilization. Stripping of the branches mobilizes the nerve from its muscular bed. Stripping is always done under magnification to prevent fascicular damage and to preserve the longitudinal blood supply.

is made along the posterior margin of the deltoid muscle. The nerve is located on the inferior surface of the deltoid muscle where it lies between the teres major and minor muscles. If a neurorrhaphy is performed, the shoulder joint is immobilized with the arm abducted. Surgical results have been gratifying, but return of function may require six to seven months.

3. Musculocutaneous Nerve. The transaxillary incision (Fig. 183) may also be used to expose the musculocutaneous nerve. This nerve is the continuation of the lateral cord of the brachial plexus after its contribution to the median nerve is given off. In exposing the musculocutaneous nerve surgically (Fig. 184), it can most easily be located by following the median nerve proximally. Close to its origin this nerve gives off one or two branches to the coracobrachialis muscle, and these branches may be easily injured if dissection is not begun high enough in the axilla. The nerve pierces the coracobrachialis muscle only a few centimeters later and then descends in the arm between the biceps and brachialis muscles.

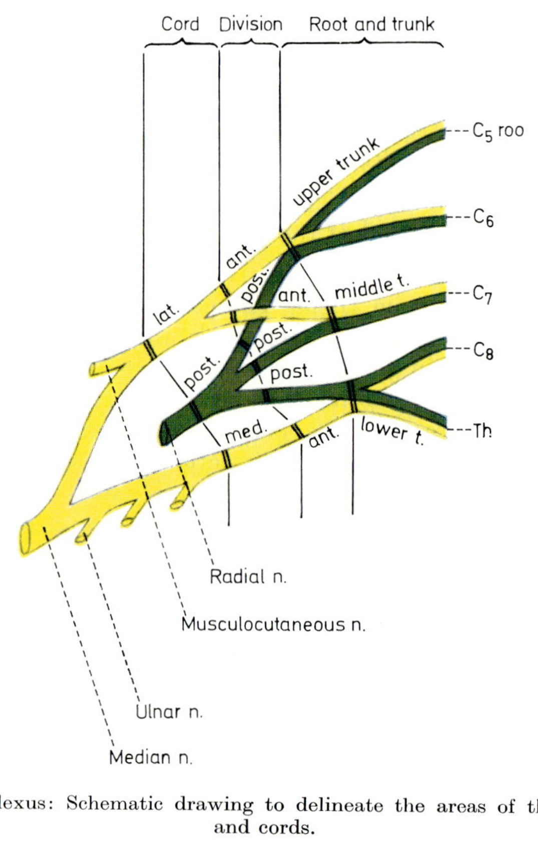

Fig. 175 b. The brachial plexus: Schematic drawing to delineate the areas of the roots, trunks, divisions and cords.

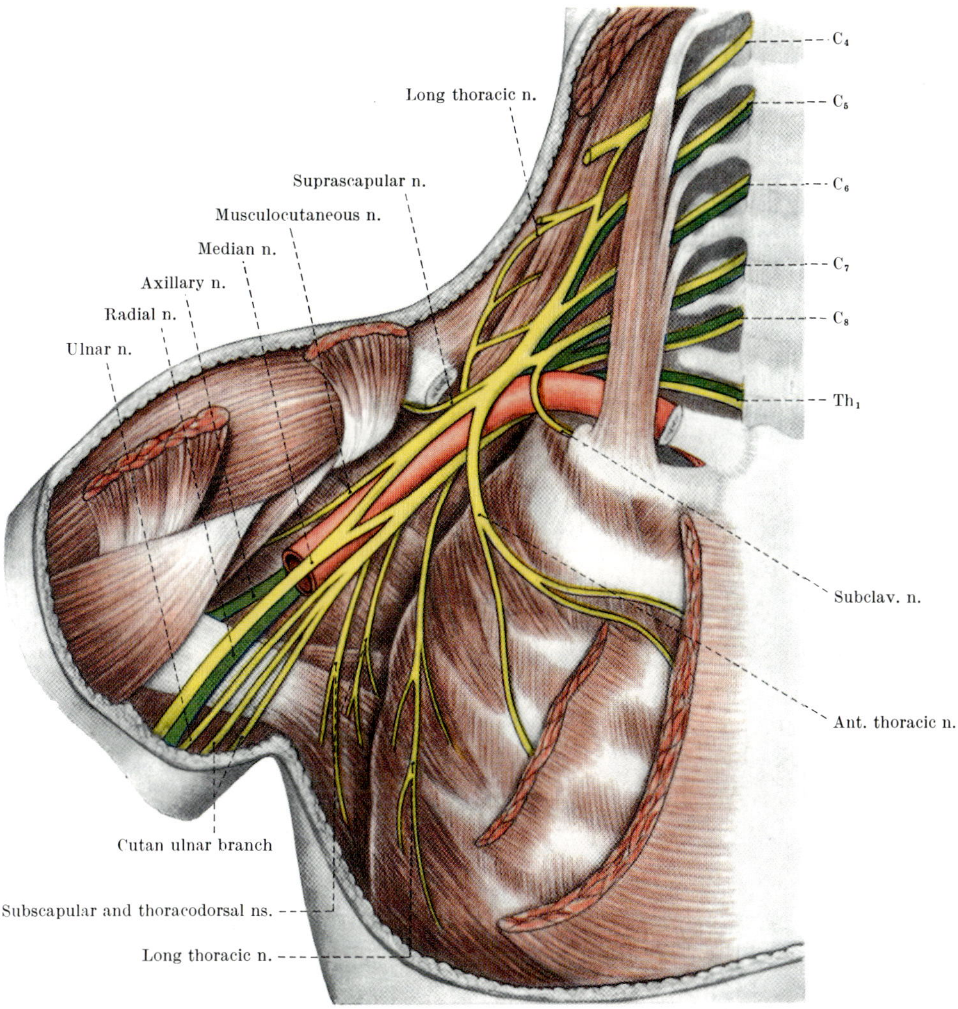

Fig. 175a. The brachial plexus: Anatomy.

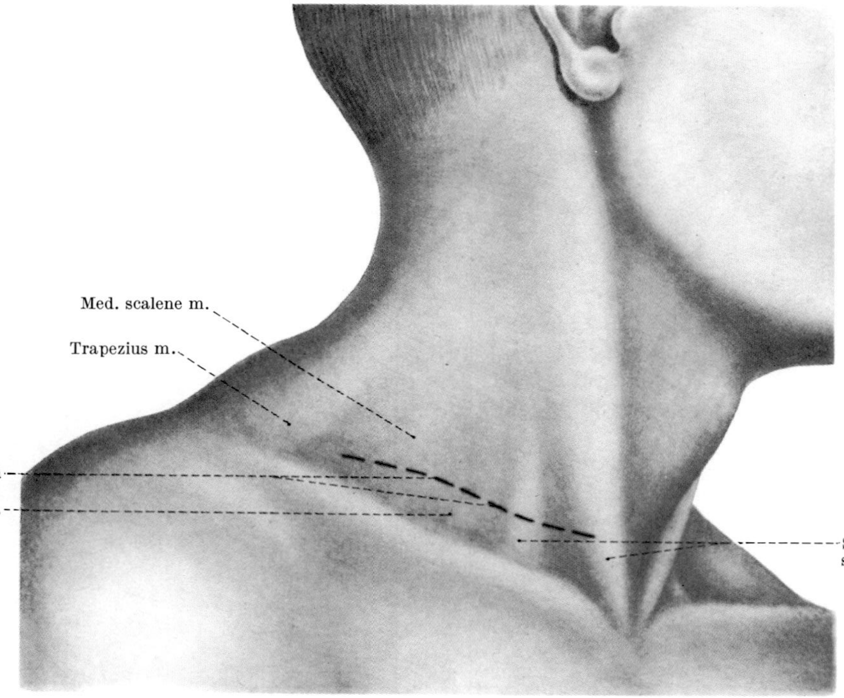

Fig. 176. Exploration of the brachial plexus: Supraclavicular incision.

Observe: 1. The position of the patient for supraclavicular exposure of the proximal brachial plexus. 2. A 6 cm. incision is made 2 cm. above and parallel to the clavicle.

Fig. 177. Exploration of the brachial plexus: Exposure of the posterior cervical triangle.

Observe: 1. The relationship of the phrenic nerve to the anterior scalene muscle. 2. The long thoracic nerve, after being formed by branches from C_5, C_6 and C_7, emerges between the fibers of the medial scalene muscle. 3. The fifth and sixth cervical nerve roots converge and join to form the *upper trunk* (compare Fig. 175a and b). 4. The seventh cervical nerve root appears from behind the lateral rim of the anterior scalene muscle to become the *middle trunk* as it crosses the medial scalene muscle. 5. The *lower trunk* is formed by the union of the eighth cervical and first thoracic nerve roots and is not seen in this supraclavicular exposure (compare Fig. 179). The structures being held posteriorly by Sibson's fascia (see text) are behind and occasionally beneath the subclavian artery.

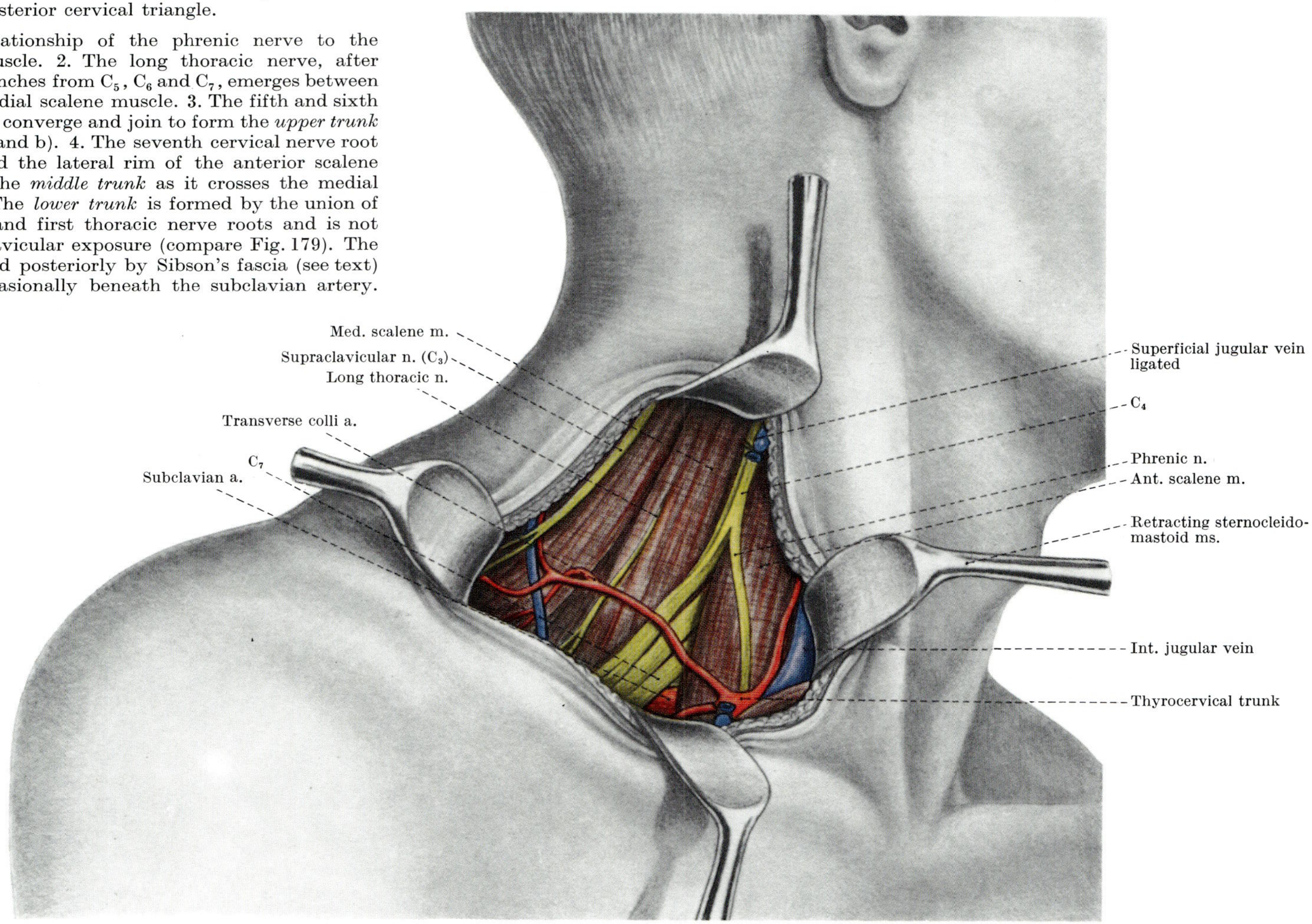

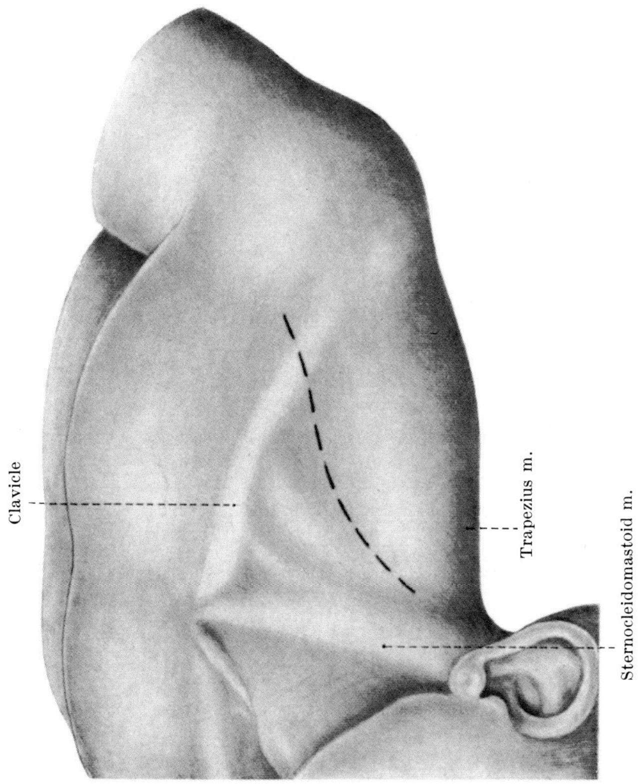

Fig. 178. Exploration of brachial plexus: Transclavicular approach: Skin incision.

Observe: The incision crosses the clavicle in its outer third.

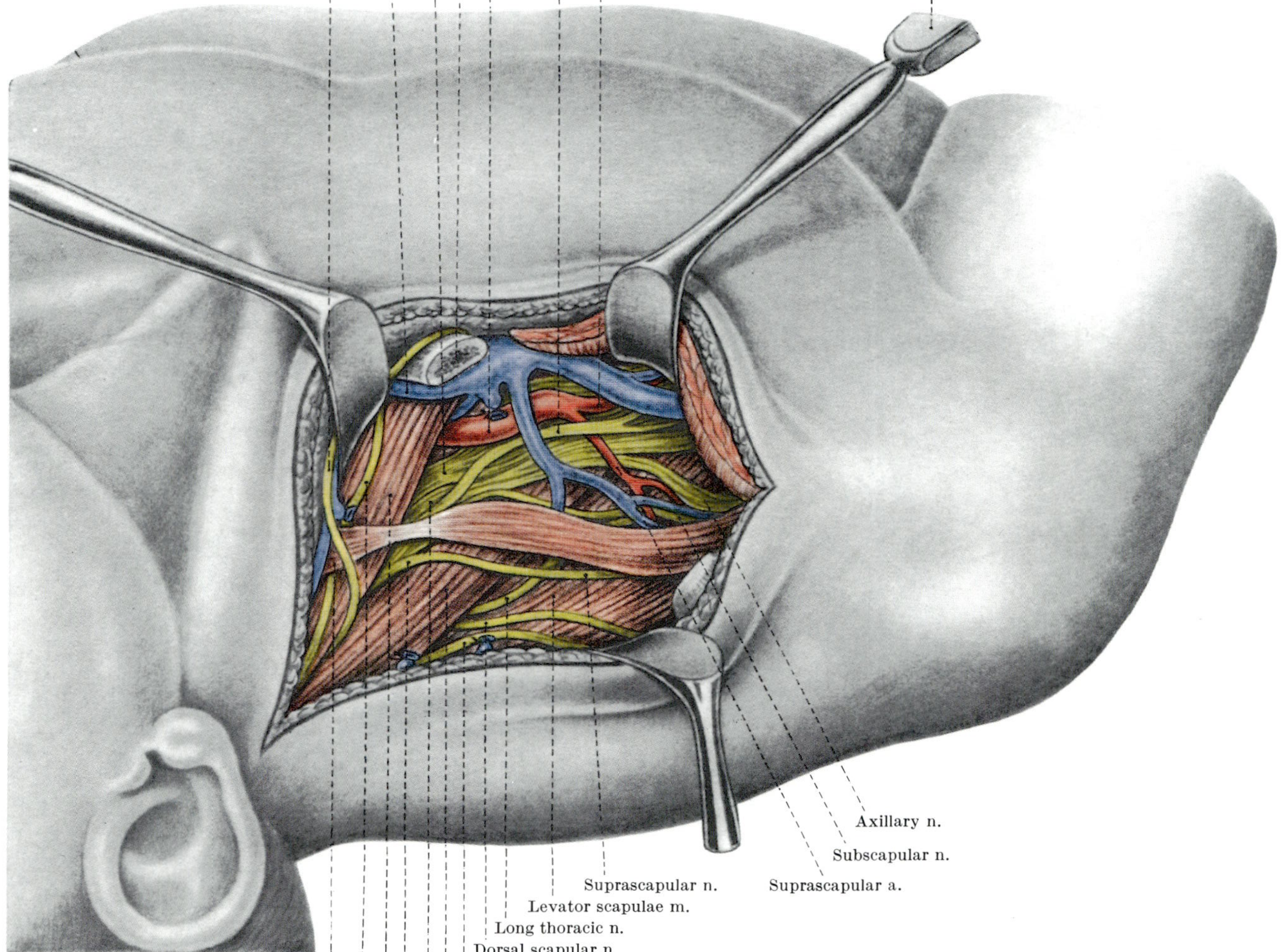

Fig. 179. Exploration of the brachial plexus: Transclavicular approach.

Observe: 1. With this approach all the trunks of the brachial plexus are exposed. 2. The lower trunk is deep to the subclavian artery. 3. Lateral to the first rib, which is palpable, the trunks lie above and behind the first part of the axillary artery where they separate into anterior and posterior divisions. 4. The posterior divisions join to become the *posterior cord* which gives origin to the axillary and radial nerves. 5. The *lateral cord* is formed by the anterior divisions of the upper and middle trunks along the lateral side of the axillary artery. It gives rise to the musculocutaneous nerve (not seen here) and the lateral portion of the median nerve. 6. The *medial cord* is a continuation of the anterior division of the lower trunk and lies along the medial border of the axillary artery. The ulnar nerve and the medial portion of the median nerve arise from this cord.

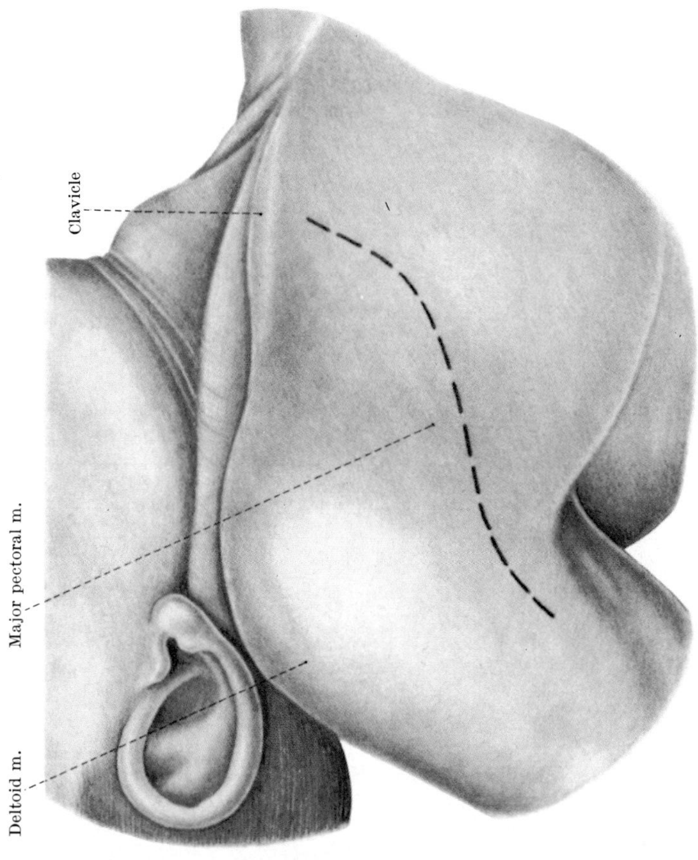

Fig. 180. Exploration of the brachial plexus: Infraclavicular incision.

Observe: 1. The skin incision begins below midportion of the clavicle and extends laterally towards the insertion of the pectoralis major muscle. 2. The arm is abducted to 90°.

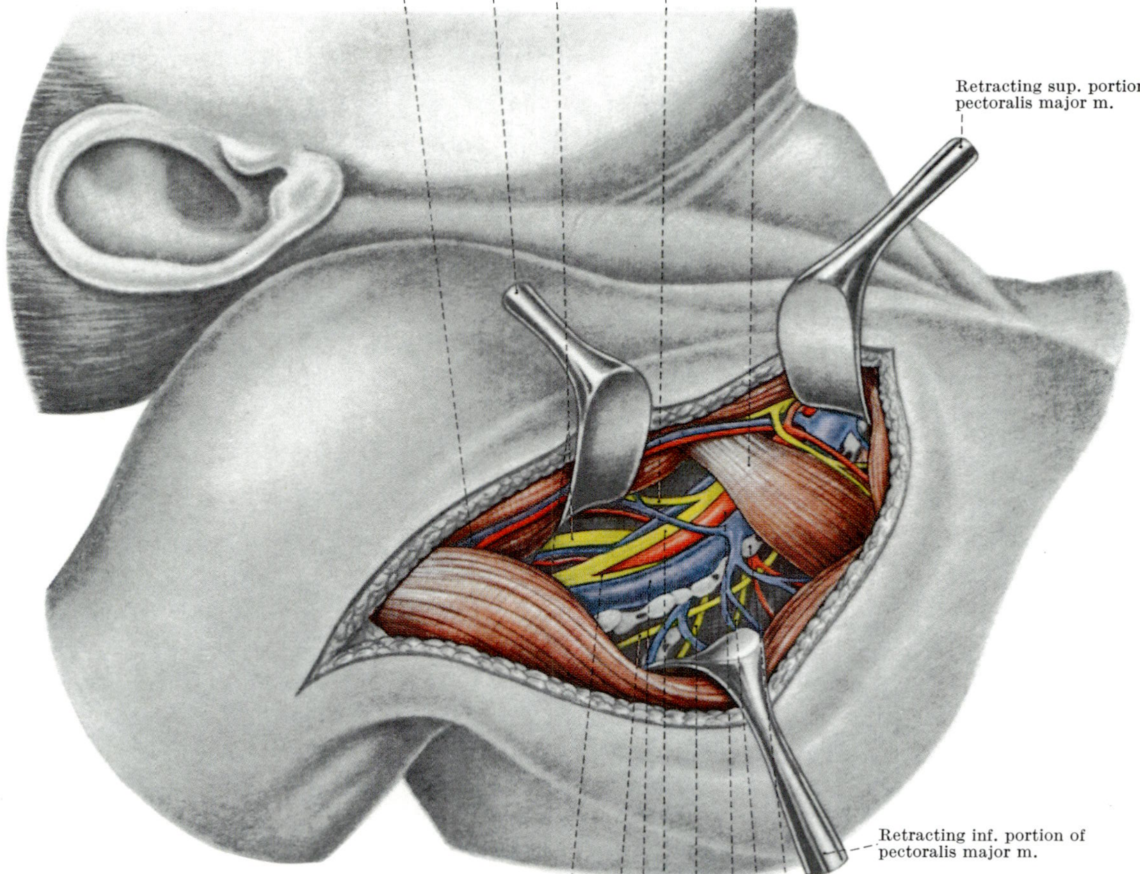

Fig. 181. Exploration of the brachial plexus: Infraclavicular approach.

Observe: 1. The pectoralis major muscle is separated in the direction of the fibers. 2. The brachial plexus runs perpendicular to the pectoralis muscles. 3. The thin fascia covering the neurovascular bundle is opened. 4. The axillary artery lies above and behind the axillary vein.

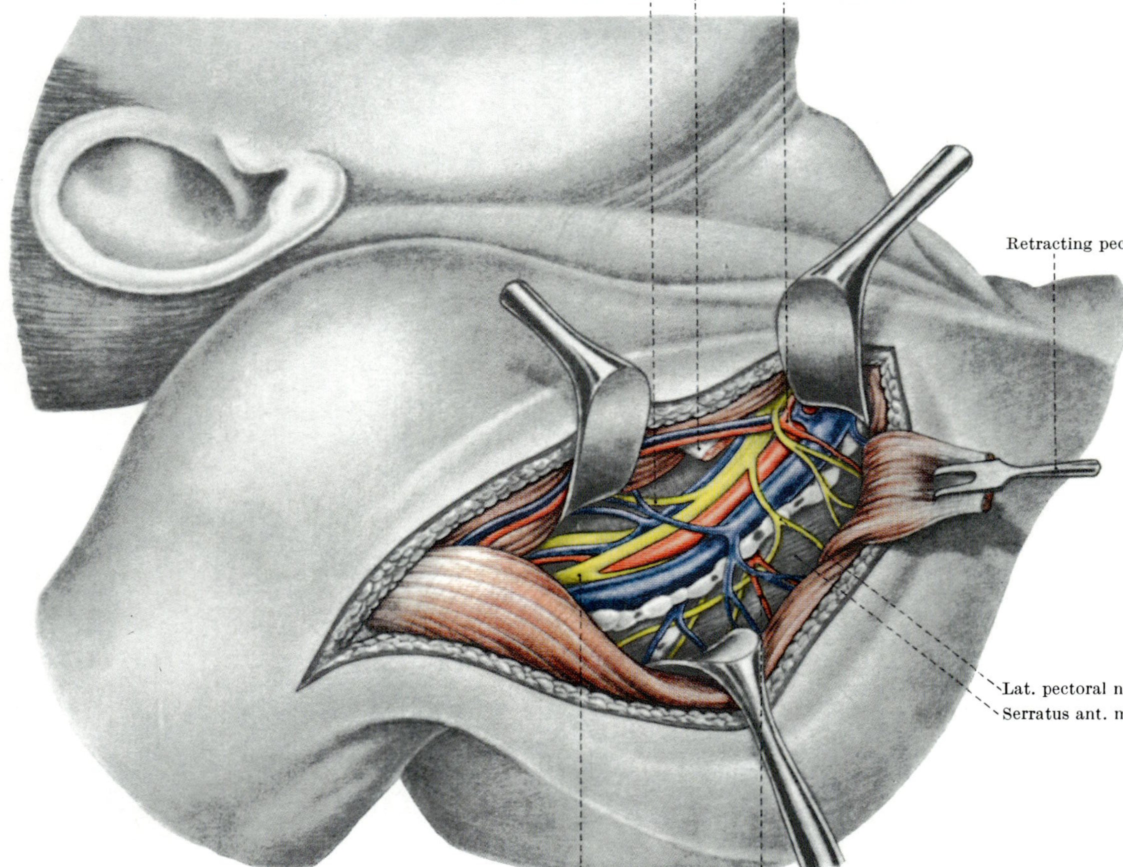

Fig. 182. Exploration of the brachial plexus: Infraclavicular approach.

Observe: 1. The pectoralis minor muscle has been transected at its tendinous insertion to aid in exposure. 2. The thoraco-acromial artery lies beneath the pectoralis minor muscle and may be ligated if it cannot be retracted medially. 3. The musculocutaneous nerve arises from the medial cord and passes into the coraco-brachialis muscle. 4. The medial and lateral cords are seen uniting to form the median nerve.

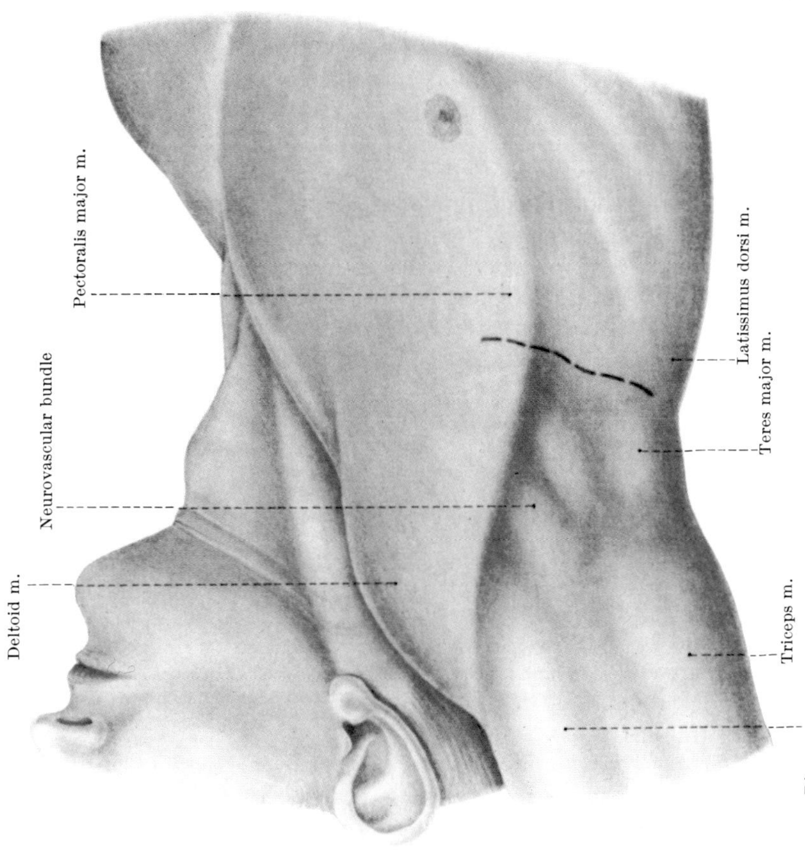

Fig. 183. Exploration of the brachial plexus: Axillary incision for lower brachial plexus. *Observe:* 1. Transverse incision follows axillary skin crease. 2. The arm is abducted 135°.

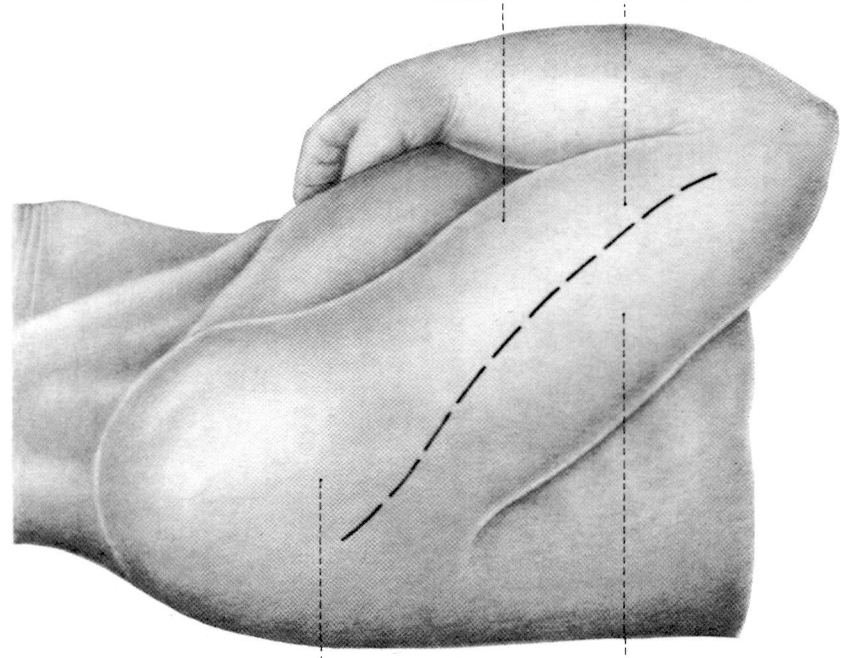

Fig. 185. Exposure of the radial and axillary nerves in the arm: Incision.

Observe: 1. The position of the arm on the thorax. 2. The incision is made from the posterior margin of the deltoid muscle to just above the medial epicondyle at the elbow. 3. Compare with transaxillary exposure Fig. 184.

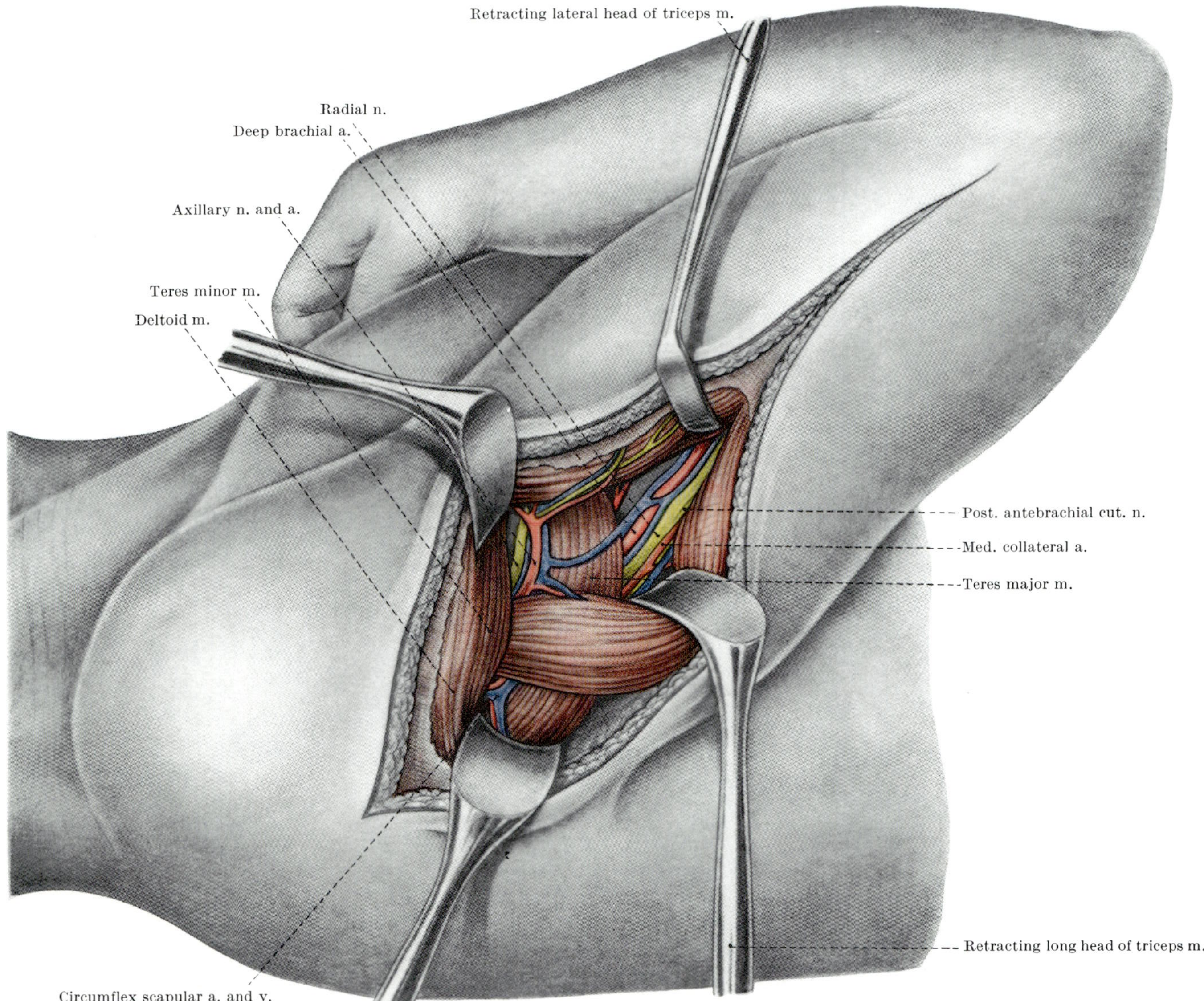

Fig. 186. Exposure of the radial and axillary nerves in the arm.

Observe: 1. The radial nerve is exposed between the long and lateral heads of the triceps muscle. It passes behind the lateral head of the triceps muscle where it is intimately related to the humerus. 2. The axillary nerve follows the upper surface of the teres major muscle toward its insertion on the humerus.

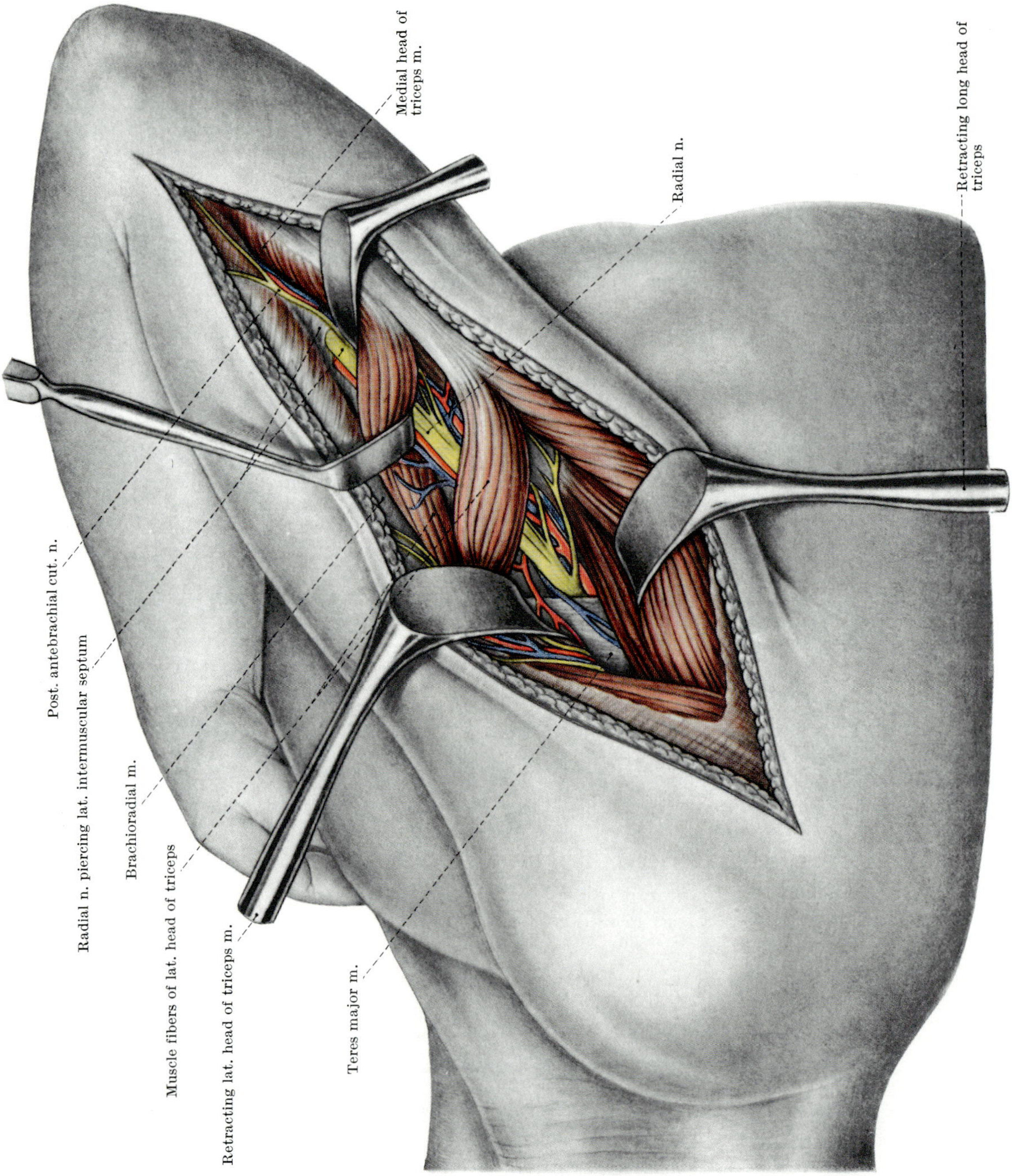

Fig. 187. Exposure of the radial and axillary nerves in the arm.

Observe: The radial nerve can be exposed distally in the arm between the triceps and brachioradialis muscles where it pierces the lateral intramuscular septum to enter the anterior compartment of the arm.

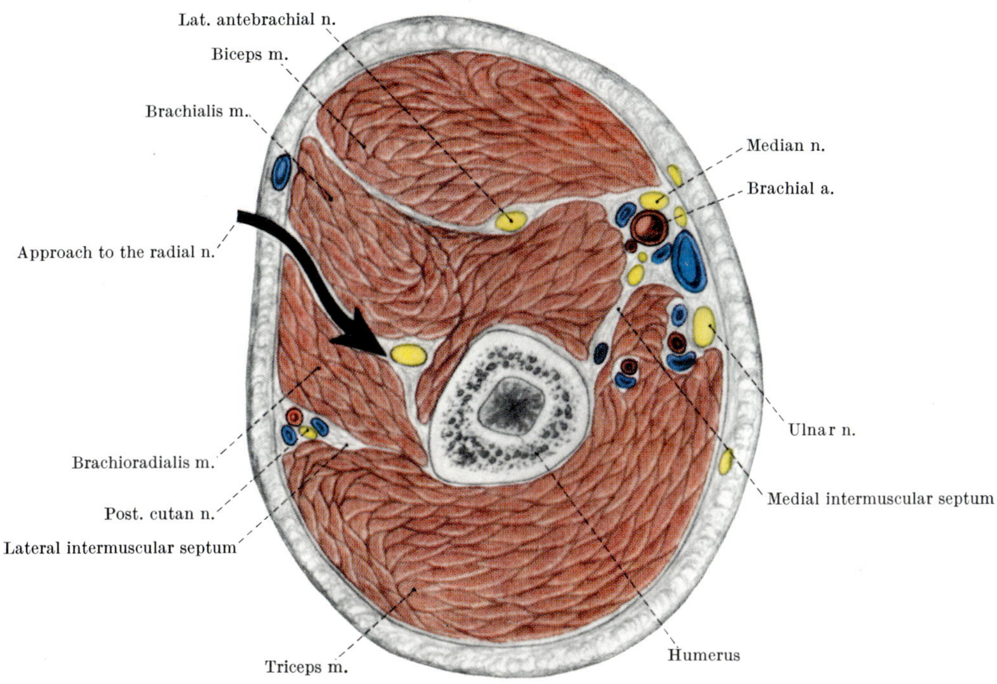

Fig. 188. Exposure of the radial nerve in the arm: Transverse section of the distal third of the arm.

Observe: The operative approach to the radial nerve at this level is between the brachialis and the brachioradialis muscles (corresponding to the operative exposure seen in Fig. 190).

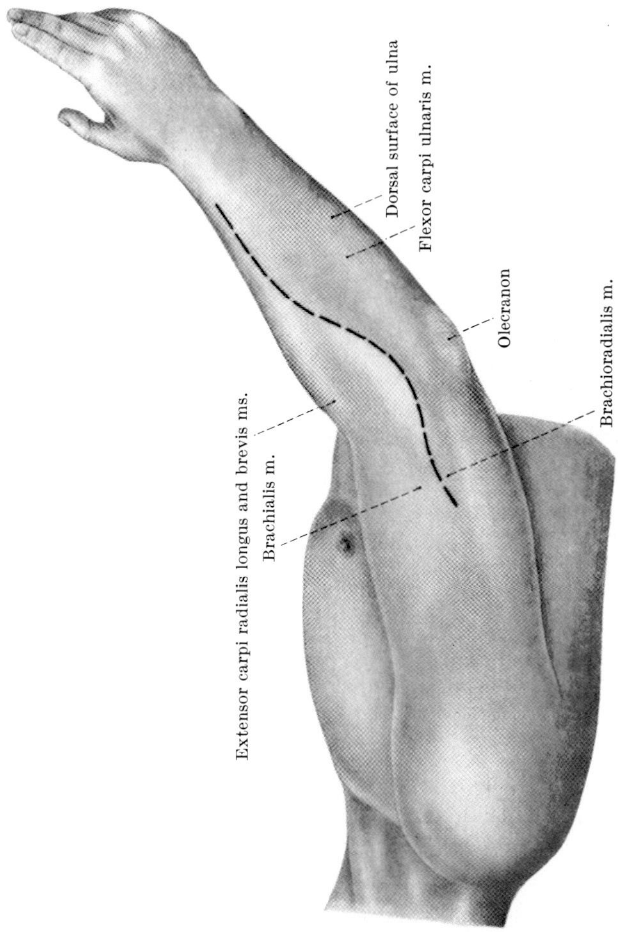

Fig. 189. Exposure of the radial nerve in the lower arm and forearm: Incision.

Observe: 1. The arm is extended and externally rotated as compared to Fig. 185. 2. The skin incision is made from over the groove between the brachialis and brachioradialis muscle to over the extensor carpi radialis muscle.

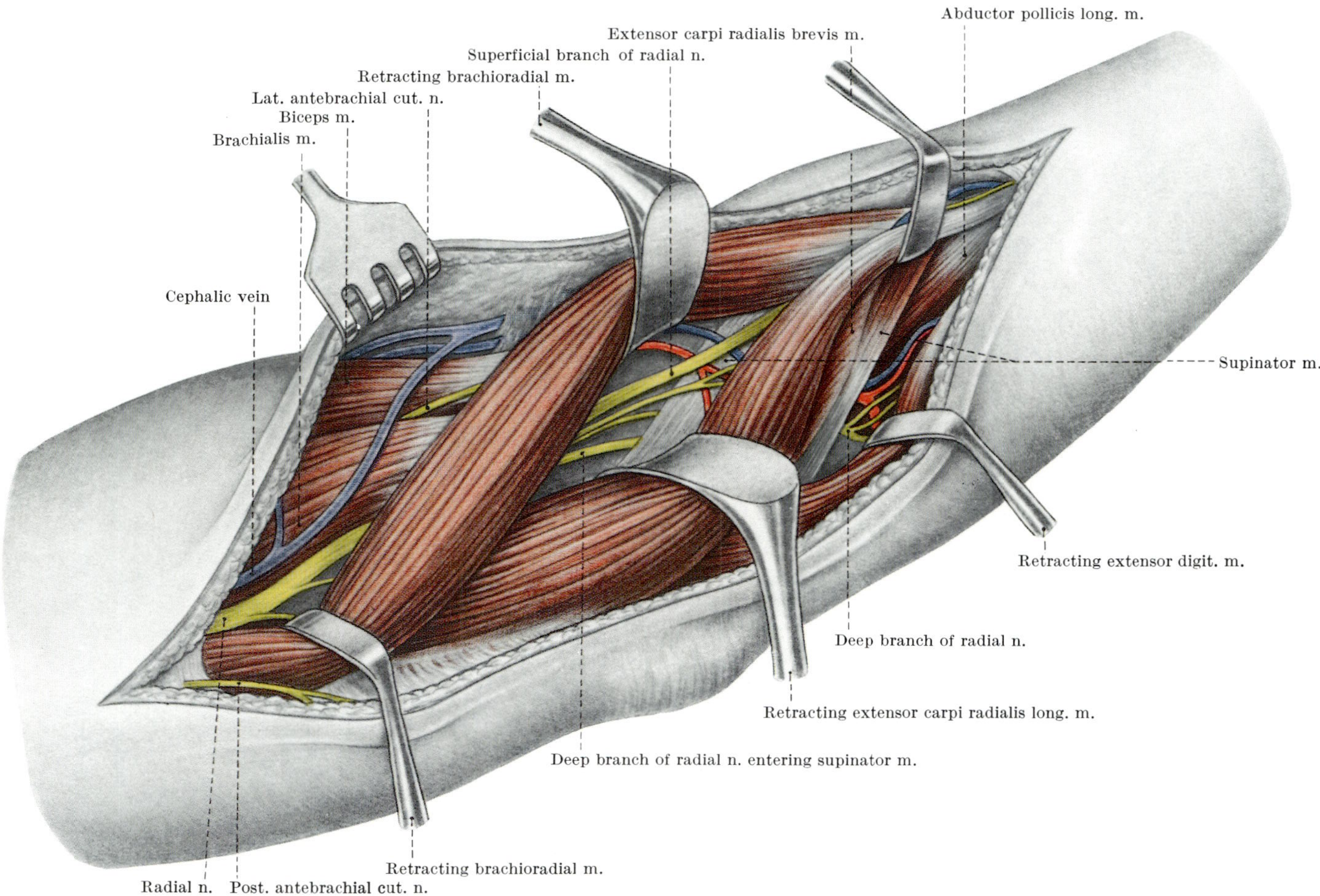

Fig. 190. Exposure of the radial nerve in the lower arm and forearm.

Observe: 1. Prior to entering the groove between the brachialis and brachioradialis muscles the radial nerve is relatively superficial. 2. The radial nerve divides into the deep and superficial branches as it crosses the capsule of the elbow joint. 3. The deep branch enters the supinator muscle and winds around the lateral aspect of the radius. 4. The superficial branch passes along the extensor carpi radialis muscle to become superficial in the distal third of the forearm.

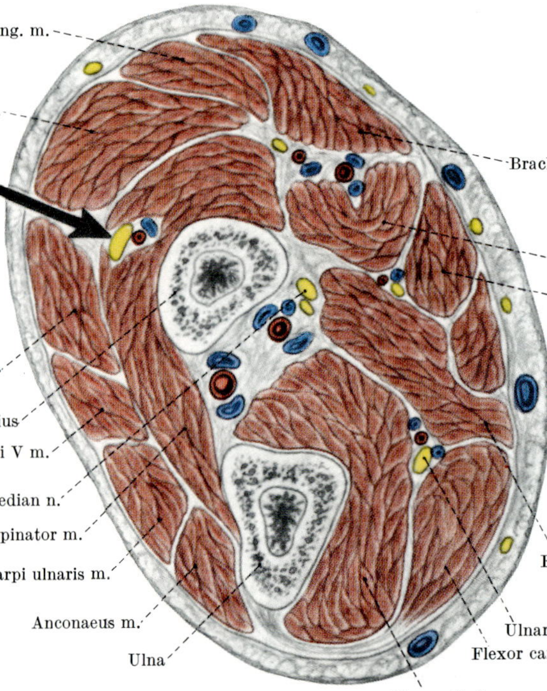

Fig. 191. Exposure of the deep branch of the radial nerve in the forearm: Transverse section of the proximal third of the forearm.

Observe: The operative approach to the deep branch (posterior interosseus nerve) at this level is between the extensor carpi radialis brevis and extensor digitorum muscles.

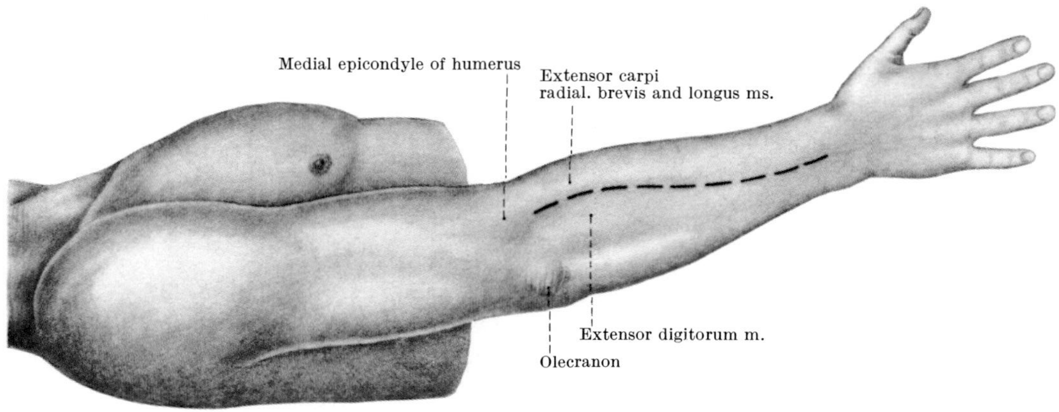

Fig. 192. Exposure of deep branch of the radial nerve in the forearm: Incision.

Observe: The skin incision is made from just in front of the lateral epicondyle of the humerus and extends distally in the groove between the extensor carpi radialis and extensor digitorum muscles.

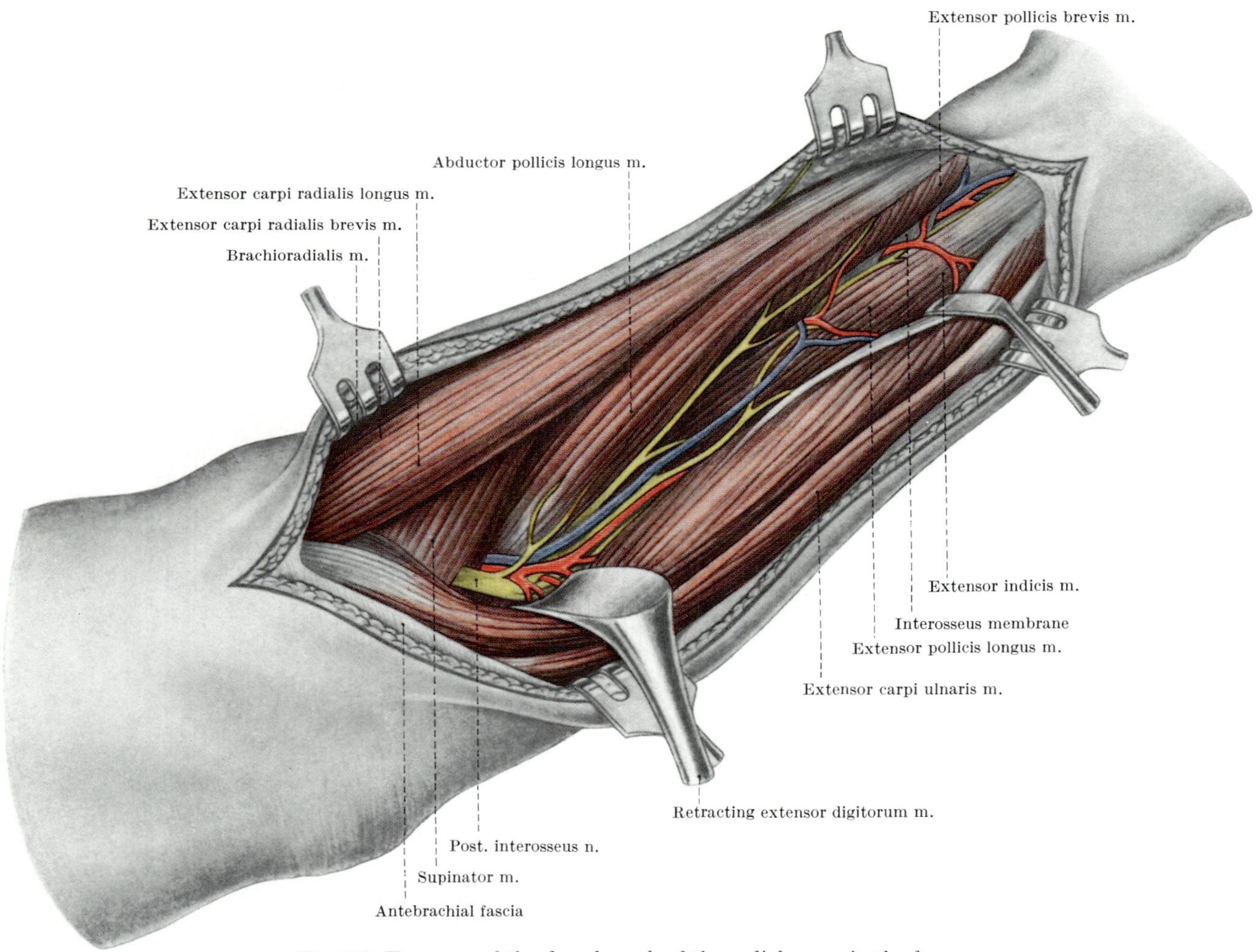

Fig. 193. Exposure of the deep branch of the radial nerve in the forearm.

Observe: 1. The deep branch (posterior interosseus nerve) is exposed as it emerges from the supinator muscle by dissecting between the extensor carpi radialis brevis and the extensor digitorum muscles. 2. To visualize the deep branch as it enters the supinator muscle, dissection is carried down between the brachioradialis and extensor carpi radialis longus muscles (compare Fig. 190). This may be necessary if the distal posterior interosseus nerve cannot be identified because of transection or scar tissue.

5. Median Nerve. Because the medial nerve is the most important nerve of the upper extremity, its importance has been emphasized by using it as an example in discussing nerve grafting (Figs. 169—171) and mobilization of peripheral nerves (Figs. 173 and 174). In dealing with median nerve lesions, remember that without it the hand is useless.

In exposure of the median nerve in the upper arm, the patient is placed on the operating table in the supine position with the arm abducted to 90 degrees and externally rotated so that the upper extremity lies straight (Fig. 194). An incision is made from the axilla to just above the medial epicondyle in the median bicipital groove directly over the neurovascular bundle. In the antecubital fossa the incision is made transversely along a skin flexion crease to the margin of the brachioradialis muscle. To expose the median nerve in the forearm, the incision is carried diagonally across the ventral surface from the medial border of the brachioradialis muscle at the elbow to the ulnar side of the wrist. The skin incision at the wrist follows a transverse skin flexion crease and then extends into the palm along the flexor crease at the base of the thenar eminence. These incisions may be used individually or in combination for exposure of the median nerve.

To expose the median nerve in the arm an incision is made in the skin over the medial bicipital groove. Having retracted the skin margins, the neurovascular bundle is easily palpable. The deep fascia is incised longitudinally over the coracobrachialis muscle. Retracting this muscle laterally will allow exposure of the nerves and brachial artery (Fig. 194); however, in retracting the coracobrachialis muscle one must always be cognizant of the course of the musculocutaneous nerve (Figs. 182 and 184). The median nerve from its origin in the axilla to the antecubital fossa has an intimate relationship with the axillary and brachial arteries. In the axilla, the nerve lies at the anterolateral aspect of the artery. The median nerve then diagonally crosses the artery in its course through the arm to assume a position medial to the artery at the elbow (Fig. 196). The ulnar nerve lies just medial to the artery and median nerve in the upper arm as far as the insertion of the coracobrachialis where it pierces the posterior layer of the intermuscular septum and passes posteriomedially toward the medial epicondyle. Also in close proximity to the median nerve in the upper arm are the medial brachial cutaneous and medial antebrachial cutaneous nerves. These nerves lie medial to the median nerve as far as the level of the insertion of the coracobrachialis muscle where they pierce the deep fascia to become subcutaneous. Having reviewed the close relationship of all these structures within the neurovascular bundle, it is easy to understand why missile wounds so often result in injury to more than one structure.

In exposing the median nerve at the elbow, a *Z*-shaped incision is made beginning five to seven cm. above the medial epicondyle and then following a flexion crease transversely across the antecubital fossa to the margin of the brachioradialis muscle where it is continued distally along the medial margin of this muscle (Figs. 195 and 197). Taking care to preserve the medial and lateral antebrachial cutaneous nerves, the skin margins are undermined and widely retracted (Fig. 198). The fascia is incised longitudinally and the lacertus fibrosus (bicipital aponeurosis) is transected as shown in Figs. 199 and 200. Thus, the median nerve and brachial artery are exposed on the brachialis muscle as they pass into the antecubital fossa medial to the bicipital tendon. Branches of the nerve to the pronator teres muscle must be carefully identified and protected. Having crossed the antecubital fossa the nerve disappears between the two heads of the pronator teres muscle which is a possible site for entrapment of this nerve (Honeymoon paralysis). Just above the upper margin of this muscle the brachial artery divides into the radial and ulnar arteries.

Exposure of the median nerve in the forearm requires a longitudinal incision along the volar aspect of the forearm (Fig. 195). The nerve after passing between the two heads of the pronator teres muscle proceeds under the tendinous arch of the flexor digitorum superficialis muscle and descends through the middle of the forearm adherent to the fascia on the underside of this muscle. Dissection is carried out between the pronator teres and the flexor carpi radialis muscles (Fig. 201) and the fibers of the flexor digitorum superficialis muscle are separated to expose the nerve immediately beneath it. Small short muscular branches to this muscle must be kept in mind when mobilizing the median nerve in the forearm (Figs. 173, 174 and 201). A great deal of additional mobility of the nerve can be attained by division of the pronator teres muscle (Fig. 173) allowing superficial transposition of the nerve.

The median nerve at the wrist is most often exposed in the treatment of the carpal tunnel syndrome. A transverse skin incision over a flexion crease of the wrist is made under local anesthesia (Fig. 202). The thin superficial fascia is divided to expose the transverse carpal ligaments (flexor retinaculum). The ligament is incised parallel to the median nerve and perpendicular to the fibers of the ligament (Fig. 203). It is of utmost importance that the ligament is transected in its entire width (Fig. 205). The median nerve is superficial to the flexor tendons in the carpal tunnel. An external neurolysis is not indicated in the treatment of the carpal tunnel syndrome since the entrapment is relieved by section of the transverse carpal ligament. Therefore, it is not necessary to dissect out the nerve as long as the incision of the ligament is done on the ulnar half of the wrist.

Surgical exposure of the median nerve in the palm is performed through an *S*-shaped incision illustrated in Figs. 195 and 204. The superficial fascia and the transverse carpal ligament are opened permitting wide retraction of the skin flaps (Fig. 205). At the distal border of the transverse carpal ligament a large branch leaves the radial side of the median nerve and curves sharply into the muscles of the thenar eminence. This is the motor branch of the median nerve (recurrent thenar branch), and it represents the only hazard to exposure of th median nerve in the hand. Having given off its motor branch, the median nerve then divides into three common palmar digital nerves (Fig. 206). The ulnar nerve may be exposed by this same incision. In dissection at the ulnar side of the wrist it is crucial to remember that, although the ulnar nerve is deep to the volar carpal ligament and the palmaris brevis muscle, it is superficial to the transverse carpal ligament.

The median and ulnar nerves at the wrist and hand are exposed using a slightly different skin incision in Figs. 207 and 208.

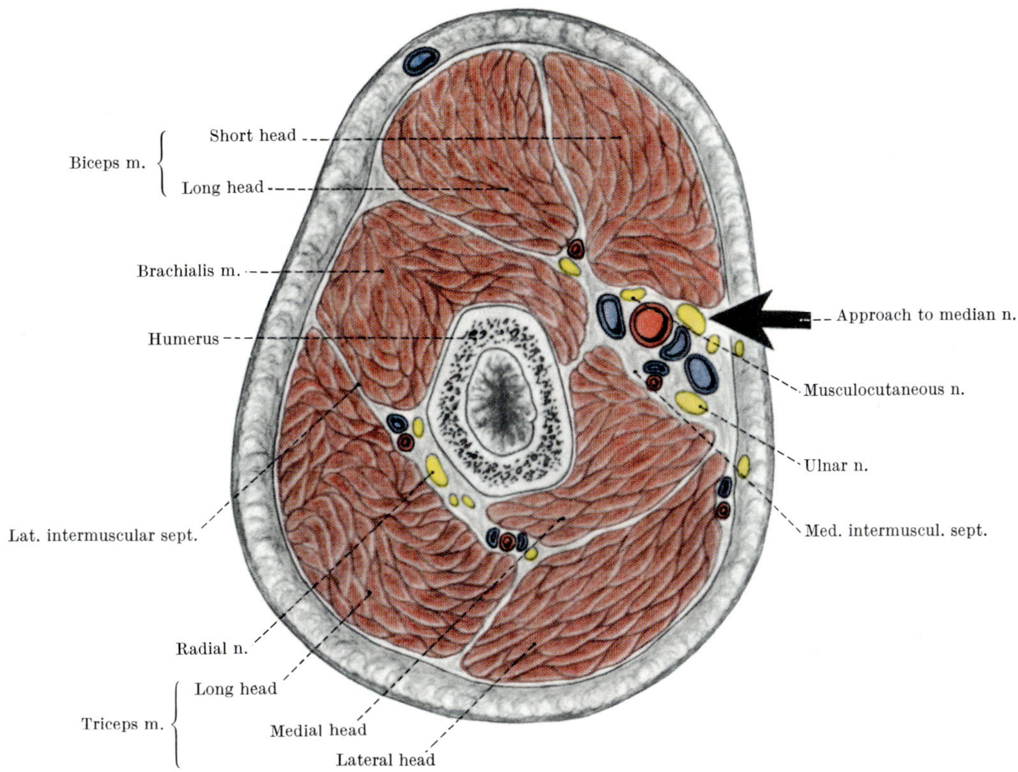

Fig. 194. Exposure of the median and ulnar nerves in the arm: Transverse section of the upper third of the arm.

Observe: The operative exposure is between the biceps and triceps muscles.

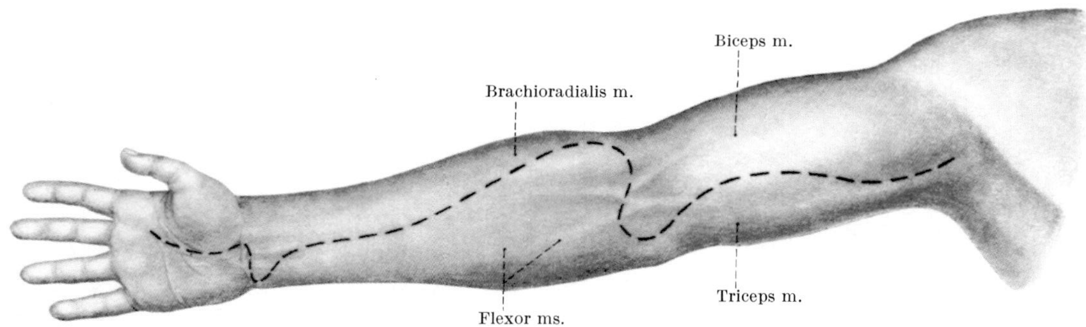

Fig. 195. Exposure of the median nerve: Incision.

Observe: 1. In the arm the median nerve is exposed by an incision over the neurovascular bundle between the biceps and triceps muscles. This same incision is used to expose the ulnar nerve in the arm. 2. In the antecubital fossa a transverse incision is made following a normal skin crease to the medial border of the brachioradialis muscle. 3. In the forearm the incision is made along the medial border of the brachioradialis muscle. The incision is gradually slanted toward the medial side of the forearm so that at the wrist it approaches the pisiform bone. This incision is also applicable for exposure of the ulnar nerve in the distal forearm. 4. At the wrist the incision is made transversely following a flexion crease (see Fig. 202). 5. The incision in the hand is made through the flexion crease at the base of the thenar eminence.

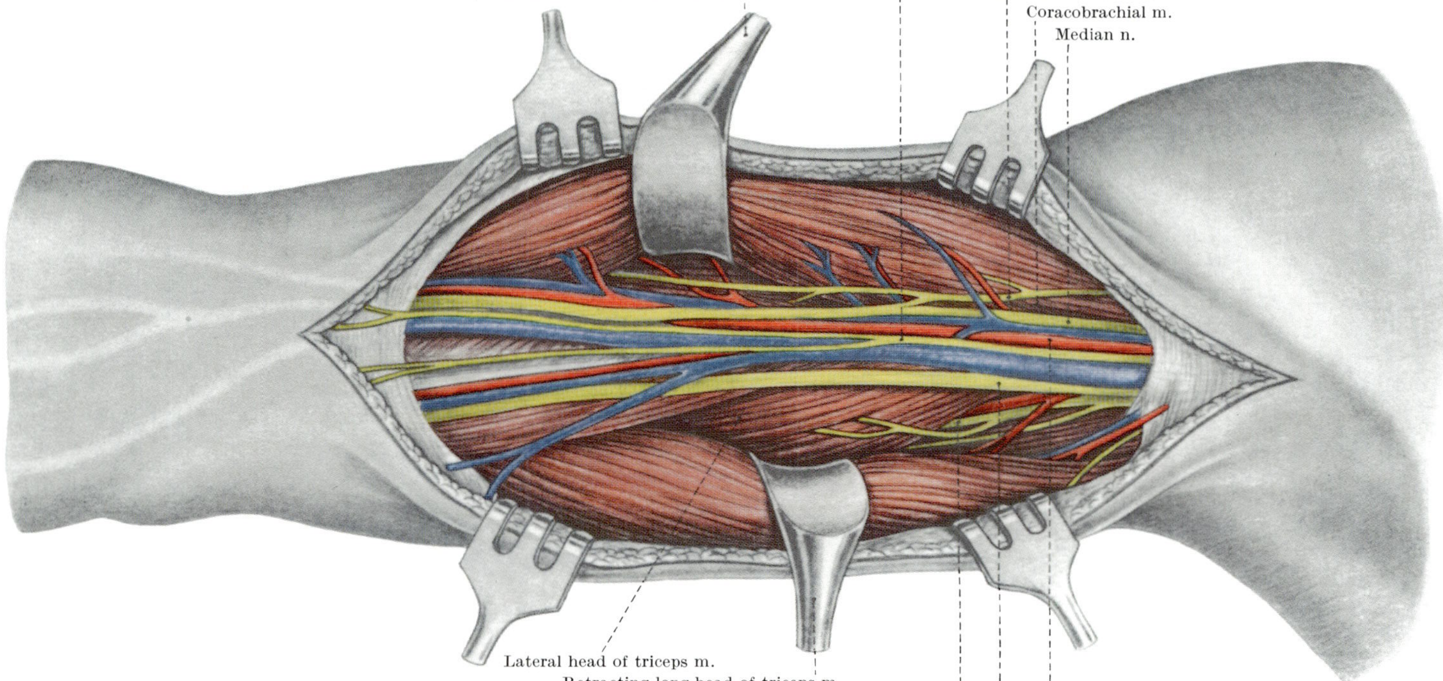

Fig. 196. Exposure of the median and ulnar nerves in the arm.

Observe: 1. The median nerve has an intimate relationship to the brachial artery. Proximally it lies lateral to the artery but it crosses the artery anteriorly to assume a medial position at the elbow. 2. The long and lateral heads of the triceps muscle are separated to reveal the radial nerve just before it disappears around the humerus. 3. The musculocutaneous nerve having penetrated the coracobrachialis muscle appears here between that muscle and the biceps muscle.

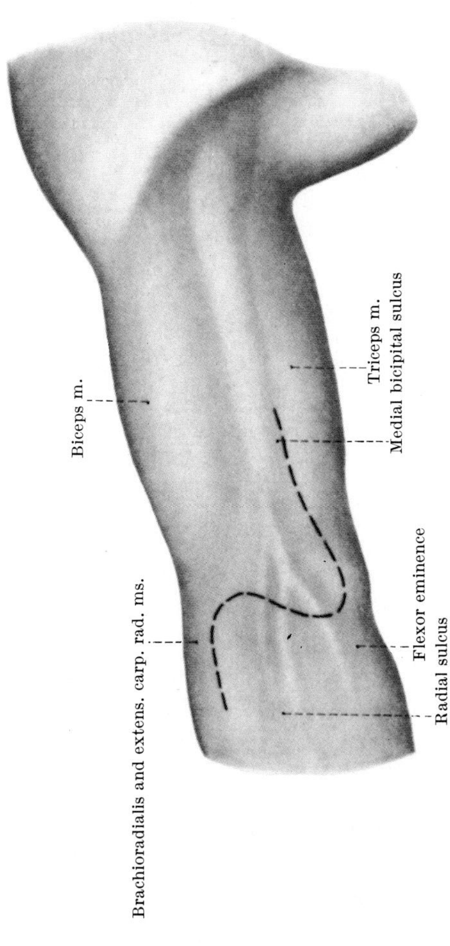

Fig. 197. Exposure of the median nerve at the elbow: Incision.

Observe: 1. The arm is abducted to 90° and the elbow joint is fully extended.
2. A *Z*-shaped incision is made to avoid crossing a flexion crease.

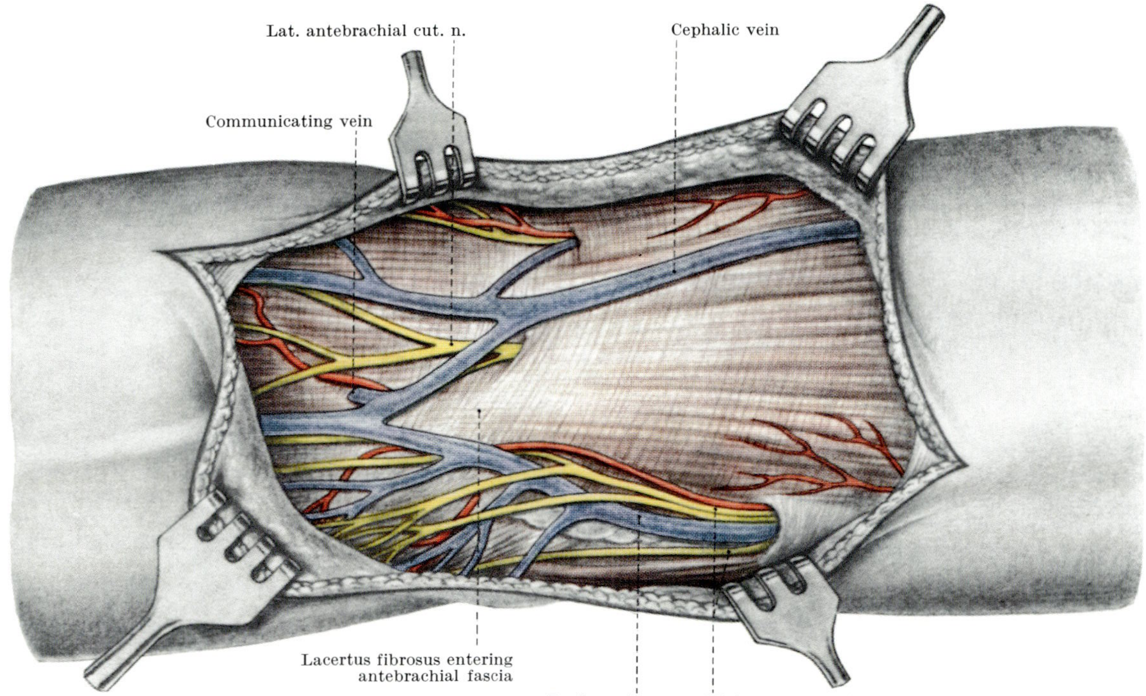

Fig. 198. Exposure of the median nerve at the elbow.

Observe: 1. Subcutaneous dissection provides a wide exposure of the antecubital fascia. 2. The medial and lateral antebrachial cutaneous nerves are identified and protected.

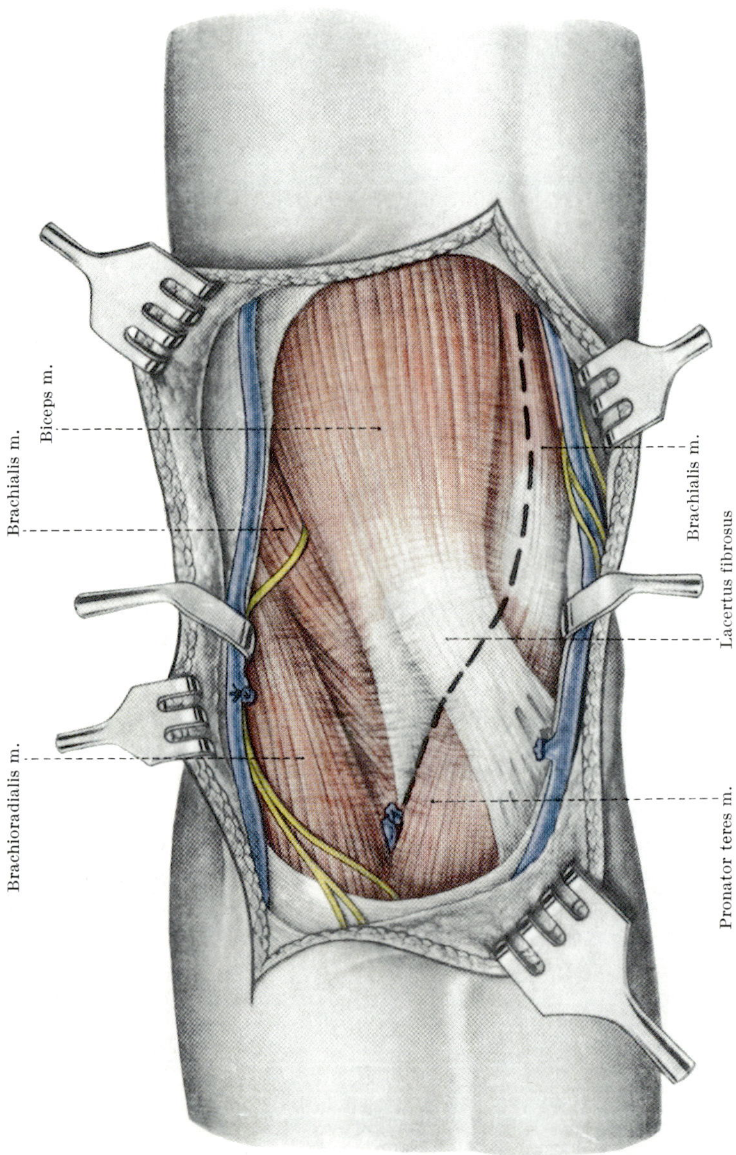

Fig. 199. Exposure of the median nerve at the elbow.

Observe: 1. The antecubital fascia has been incised and retracted. 2. Dotted line marks the course of the median nerve and brachial artery.

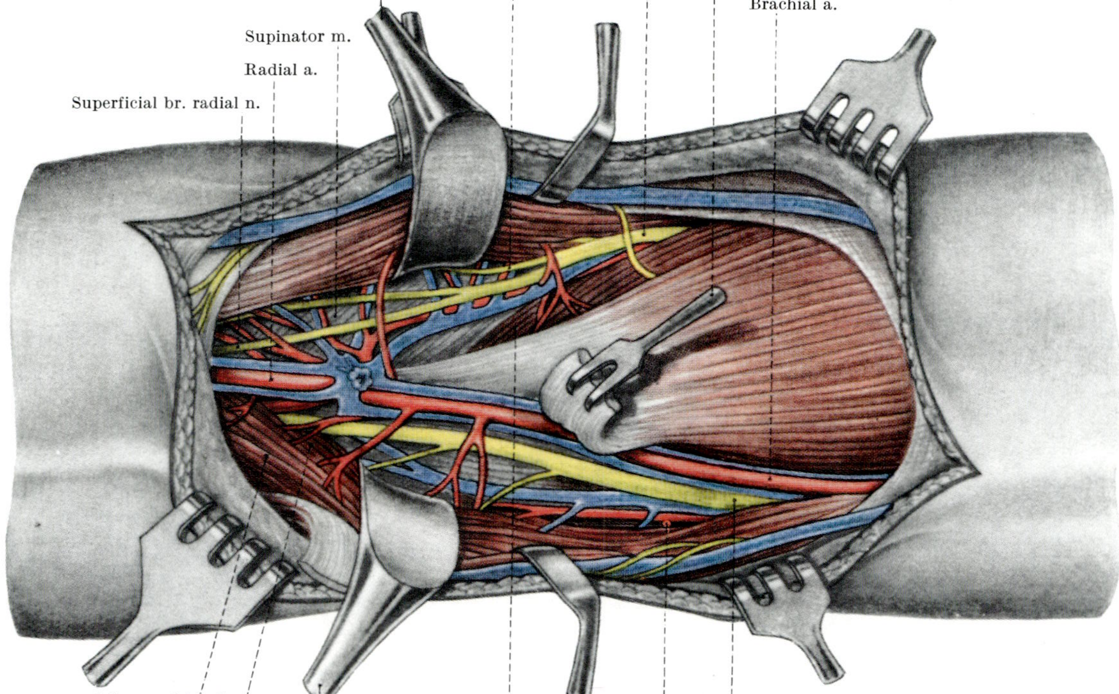

Fig. 200. Exposure of the median nerve at the elbow.

Observe: 1. The lacertus fibrosus has been transected. 2. The median nerve is separated from the humerus only by the brachialis muscle. 3. The median nerve passes between the two heads of the pronator teres muscle as it proceeds into the forearm. 4. The radial nerve is also seen in this exposure. It perforates the supinator muscle and divides into the deep and superficial branches (compare Figs. 190, 191 and 193).

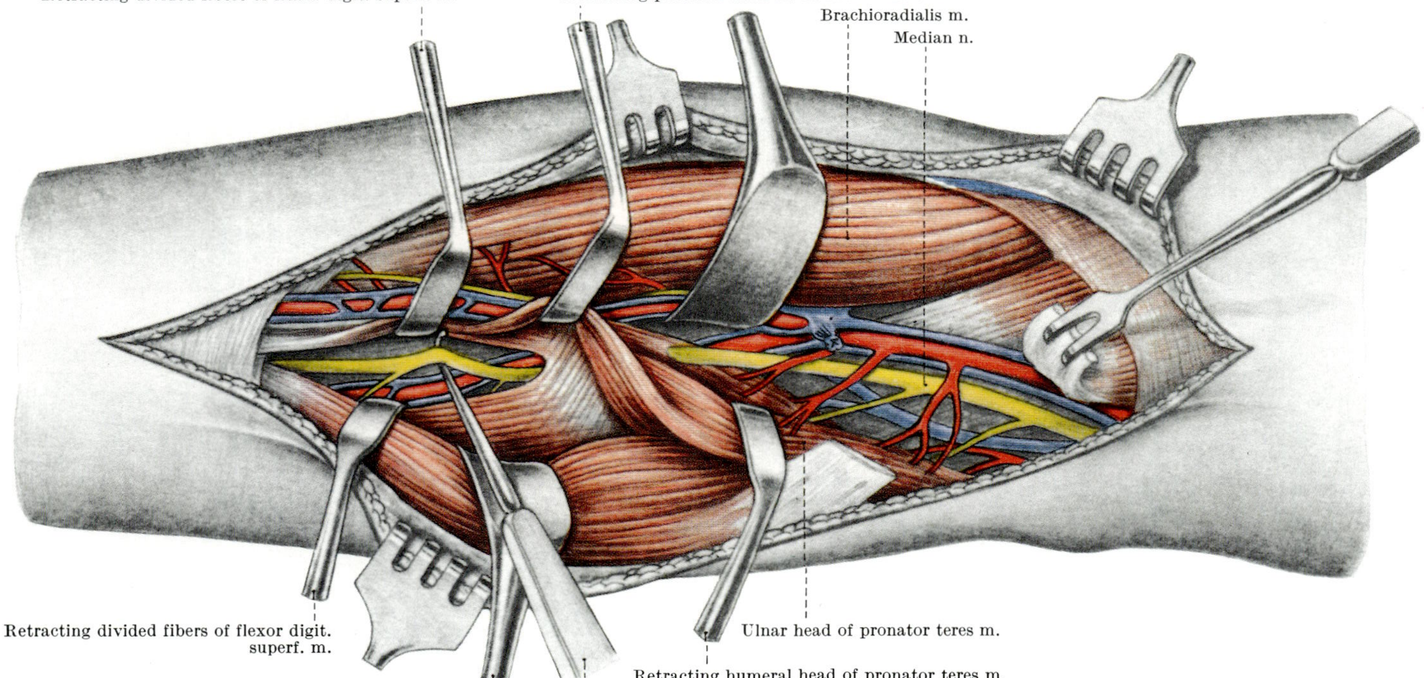

Fig. 201. Exposure of median nerve in the forearm.

Observe: 1. After passing between the two heads of the pronator teres muscle the median nerve assumes an intimate relationship with the deep surface of the flexor digitorum superficialis muscle (compare Figs. 173 and 174). 2. Branches to the pronator teres muscle must be identified and protected. 3. Separation of the pronator teres muscle from the flexor carpi radialis muscle inferiorly gives additional exposure of the median nerve.

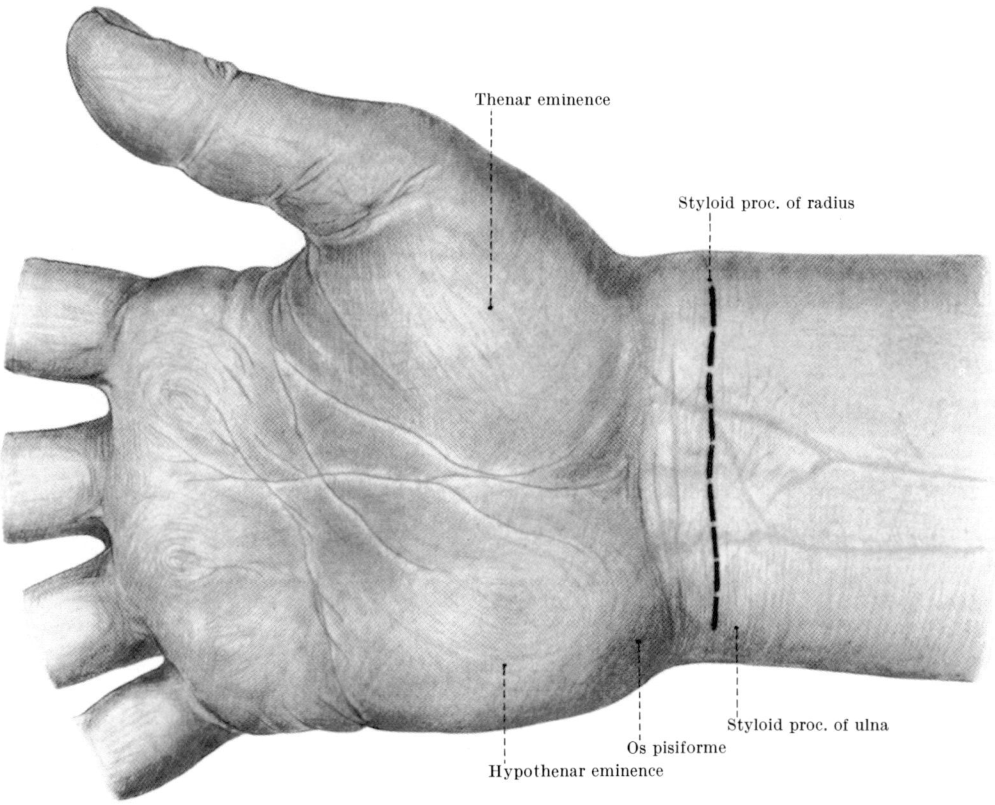

Fig. 202. Exposure of the median and ulnar nerves at the wrist: Incision.

Observe: A transverse incision is made in a flexion skin crease.

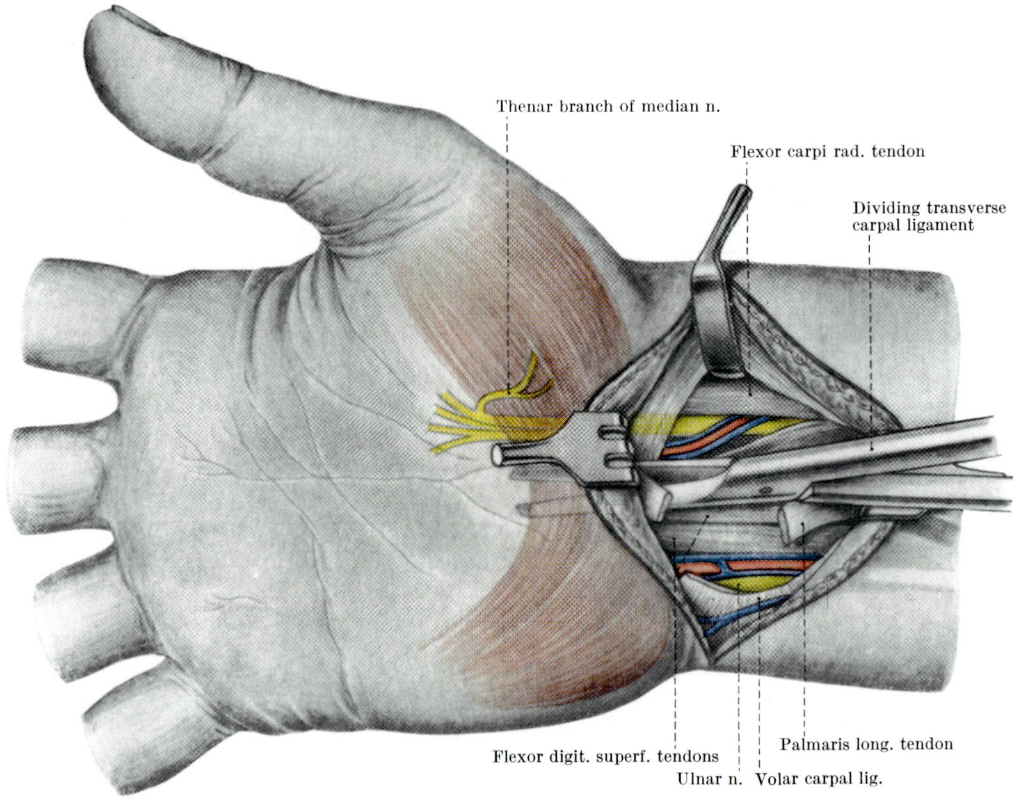

Fig. 203. Exposure of the median and ulnar nerves at the wrist.

Observe: 1. The transverse carpal ligament is divided medial to the median nerve to protect the recurrent branch as well as the two sensory branches to the thumb (see Fig. 205). 2. If mobilization of the median nerve is required the incision shown in Fig. 204 is used.

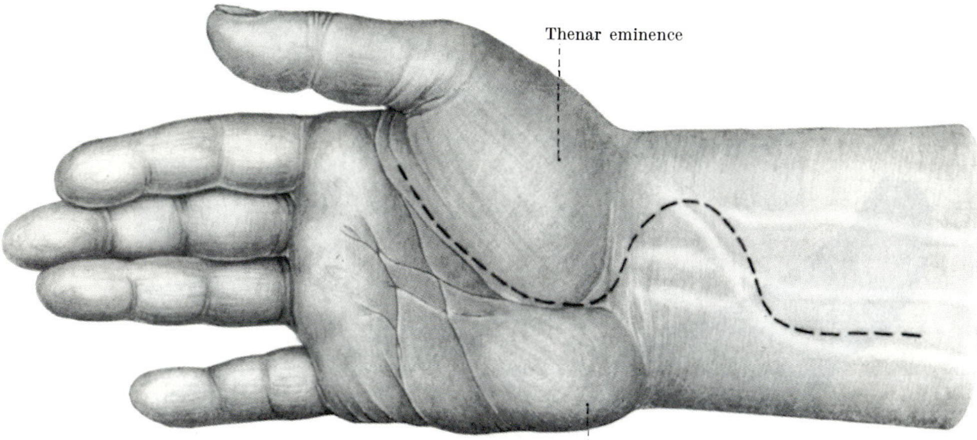

Fig. 204. Exposure of the median nerve from forearm to palm: Incision.

Observe: A curvilinear incision is used to prevent crossing flexor creases. The palmar extension follows the skin crease at the base of the thenar eminence.

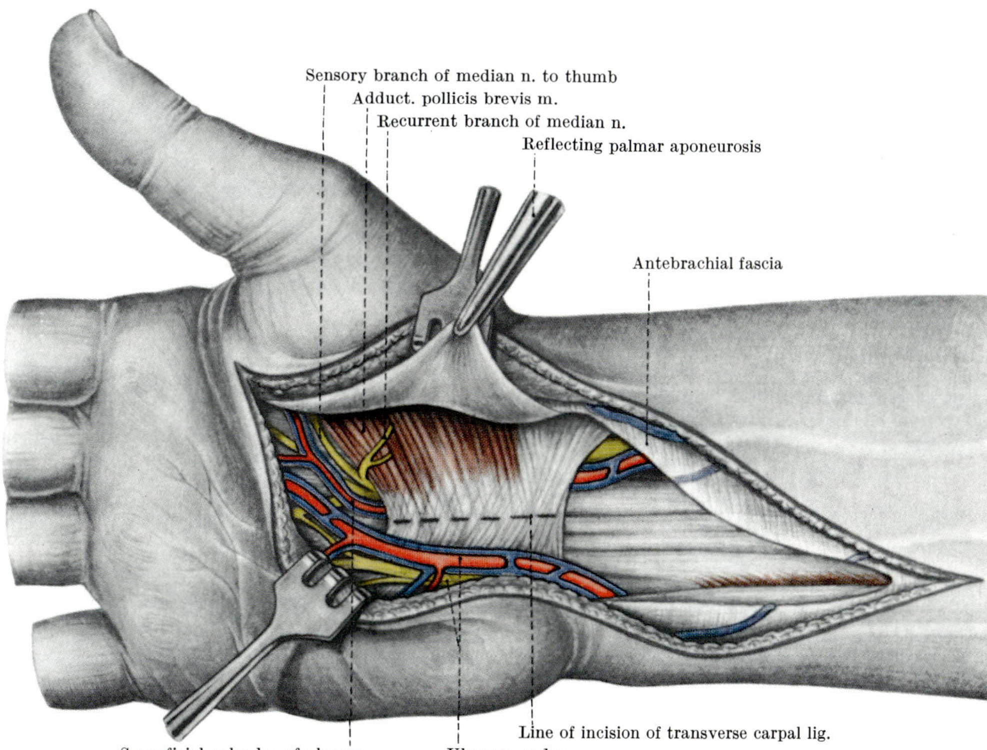

Fig. 205. Exposure of the median nerve from forearm to palm.

Observe: 1. The superficial position of the recurrent branch at the inner margin of the adductor pollicis brevis muscle. 2. The width of the transverse carpal ligament.

6. Ulnar Nerve. Exposure of the ulnar nerve as it arises from the medial cord of the brachial plexus is gained by the previously described transaxillary approach (Figs. 183 and 184).

The operative approach to the ulnar nerve in the arm has also been discussed in the section on the median nerve (Figs. 195 and 196) since these nerves share a common fascial compartment in the upper arm. It must be remembered, however, that the ulnar nerve leaves the neurovascular bundle at the level of the insertion of the coracobrachialis muscle passing posteriorly to lie on the medial head of the triceps muscle on its way toward the medial epicondyle. Having left the neurovascular bundle the nerve is covered only by the deep fascia. The ulnar nerve has no branches in the arm until just above the medial epicondyle where several fine articular branches leave the nerve. The nerve then passes the back of the elbow between the olecranon and the medial epicondyle of the humerus. The ulnar nerve in the arm is accompanied by the superior ulnar collateral branch of the brachial artery, the ulnar collateral branch of the radial nerve and the ulnar collateral veins. Preserving this vascular accompaniment is usually the only difficulty in the dissection of the ulnar nerve in the arm.

Anterior transposition of the ulnar nerve at the elbow is a very common neurosurgical exercise. This operation is done either for a tardy ulnar palsy or to gain additional length in performing a neurorrhaphy. The arm is positioned in extension and is externally rotated (Fig. 209). An incision is made from the medial bicipital groove ten cm. above the medial epicondyle to the lateral surface of the flexor carpi ulnaris muscle of the forearm in a lazy *S*-shaped curve. An incision behind the medial epicondyle should be avoided since this is a common pressure point. The deep fascia is initially opened proximally and the nerve identified. The deep fascia is then incised following the course of the nerve over the entire length of the skin incision (Fig. 210). The secret to a successful transposition of the ulnar nerve lies in the management of the dissection at the two extremes of the wound. Dissection proximally must be carried as high as the insertion of the coracobrachialis muscle where the ulnar nerve leaves the neurovascular bundle to be certain that the nerve is transposed anteriorly and not angulated over the firm intermuscular septum. Distally the nerve must be mobilized between the two heads of the flexor carpi ulnaris muscle (Fig. 211). The fibrous arch between these two parts of the muscle must be completely divided so that when the nerve is anteriorly transposed no angulation will occur. Having completed these two crucial steps the remaining mobilization of the nerve is simply done. Muscular branches to the flexor carpi ulnaris muscle should be preserved, and stripping of these branches from the parent nerve easily provides enough mobility so that the nerve can be transposed without any tension. A few sutures in the antecubital fascia over the nerve will secure its new position anterior to the medial epicondyle.

The forearm incision for exposure of the ulnar nerve is made along the flexor carpi ulnaris muscle (Fig. 209). The course of the ulnar nerve in the forearm can be traced by drawing a straight line between the medial epicondyle of the humerus and the lateral edge of the pisiform bone at the wrist. The deep fascia is incised along the lateral border of the flexor carpi ulnaris muscle, and this muscle is bluntly dissected from the flexor digitorum superficialis muscle laterally and the flexor digitorum profundus muscle below. The nerve is exposed lying on the anterior surface of the flexor digitorum muscle (Figs. 212 and 213). At the mid forearm level the nerve is joined by the ulnar artery which assumes a position on the lateral side of the nerve. Fig. 212 also illustrates muscular branches of the nerve which supply the flexor carpi ulnaris and the ulnar portion of the flexor digitorum profundus muscles and the dorsal cutaneous branch which leaves the nerve in the distal third of the forearm to supply sensation to the ulnar side of the back of the hand. In the distal third of the forearm the ulnar nerve emerges at the radial side of the flexor carpi ulnaris tendon and is covered only by the antebrachial fascia. This superficial position of the nerve at the wrist makes it vulnerable to injury, particularly by laceration.

To expose the ulnar nerve at the wrist a curvalinear incision is made beginning at the base of the hypothenar compartment, curving medially at the wrist to avoid cutting across flexion creases and then continuing into the forearm along the radial side of the flexor carpi ulnaris tendon (Fig. 214). The ulnar nerve is identified proximally just beneath the antebrachial fascia and dissection then proceeds distally. The volar carpal ligament (palmar carpal ligament) and the palmaris brevis muscle are incised as the ulnar nerve is followed in its course past the radial side of the pisiform bone (Fig. 215). Once again it must be emphasized that the ulnar nerve is superficial to the transverse carpal ligament (flexor retinaculum) as it crosses the wrist to enter the palm. Along the radial aspect of the pisiform bone the ulnar nerve divides into its terminal branches to the hand, the superficial and deep branches.

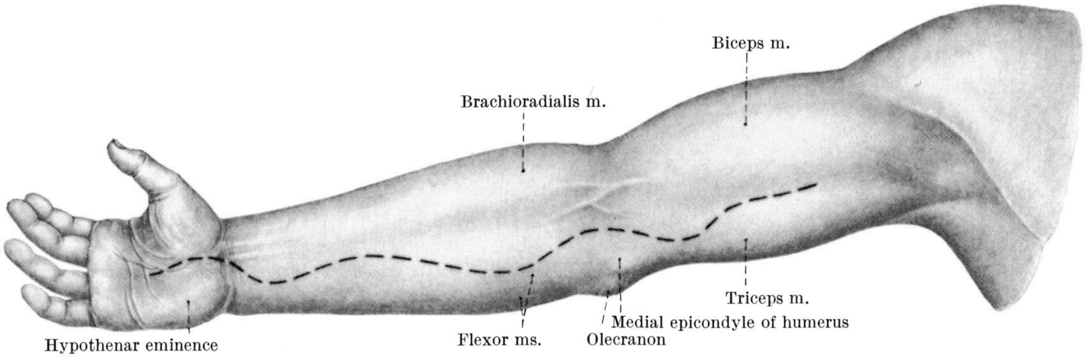

Fig. 209. Exposure of the ulnar nerve: Incision.

Observe: 1. In the arm the ulnar nerve is exposed using the same incision as for the median nerve (see Fig. 195). 2. At the elbow the incision is made ventral to the medial epicondyle of the humerus. 3. At the wrist a medial detour is made to avoid crossing the flexion creases before swinging into the crease between the thenar and hypothenar eminences.

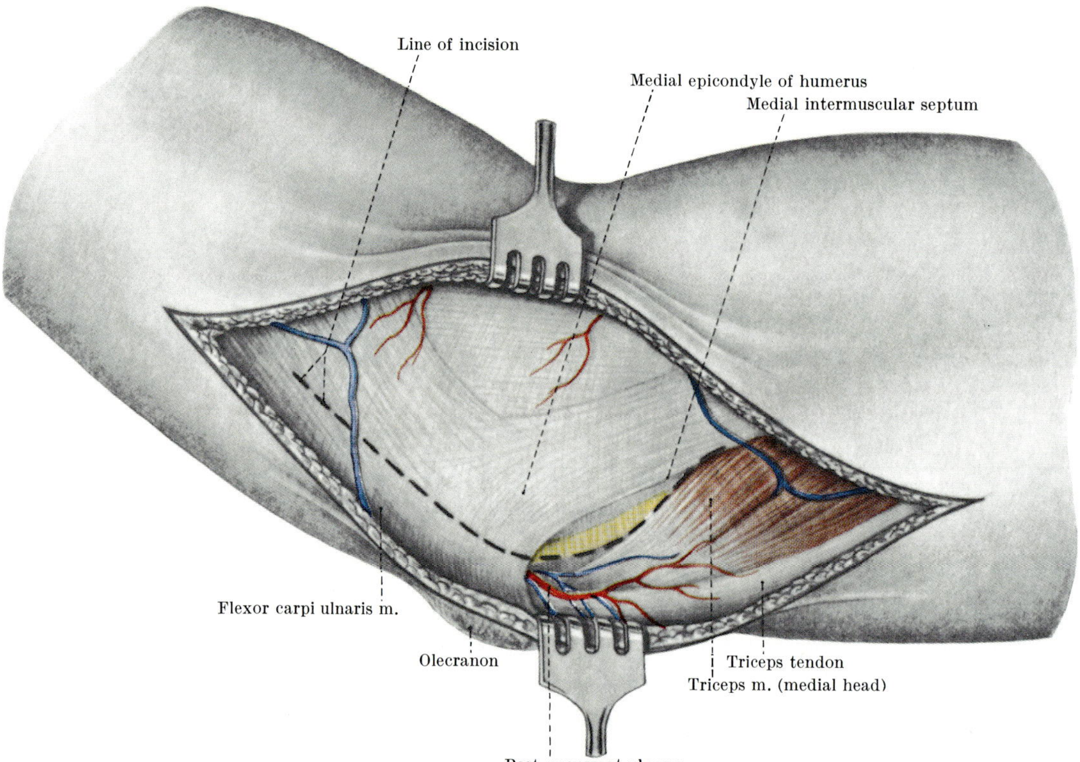

Fig. 210. Exposure of the ulnar nerve at the elbow: Transposition of the ulnar nerve.
Observe: The fascia is incised directly over the course of the ulnar nerve.

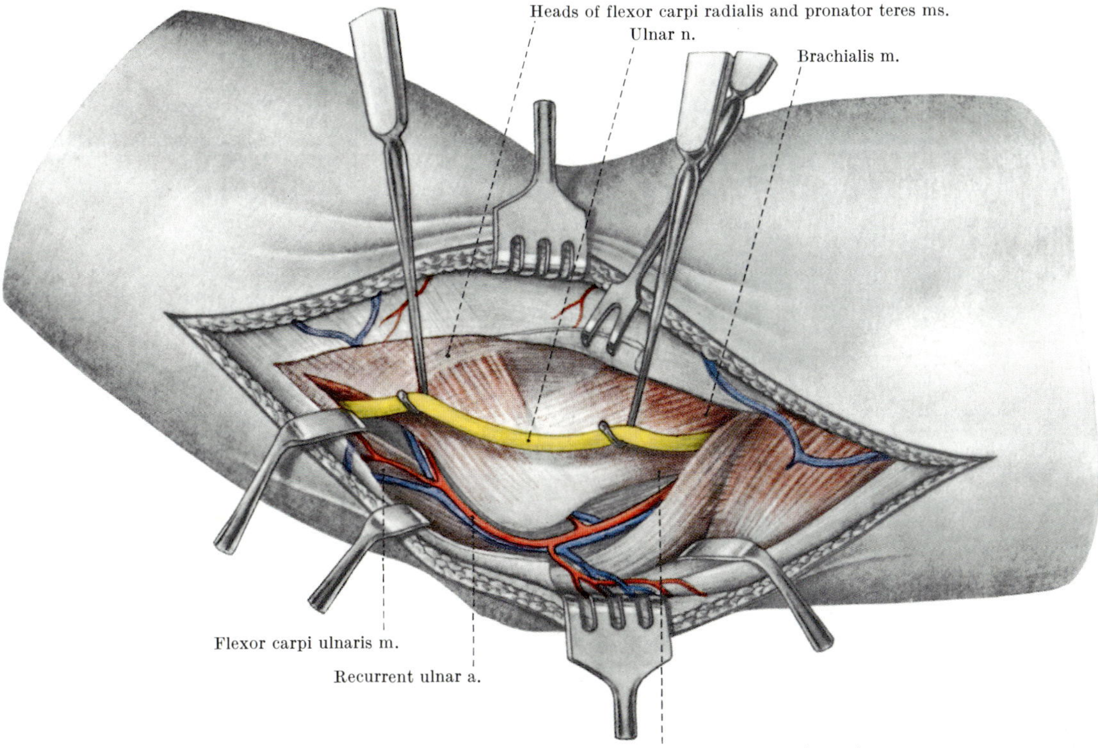

Fig. 211. Exposure of the ulnar nerve at the elbow: Transposition of the ulnar nerve.

Observe: 1. Proximal dissection must be to the level of the insertion of the coracobrachialis muscle. Incision of the intermuscular septum is a key step in preventing angulation of the nerve. 2. Distal mobilization must include division of the fibrous arch between the two heads of the flexor carpi ulnaris muscle.

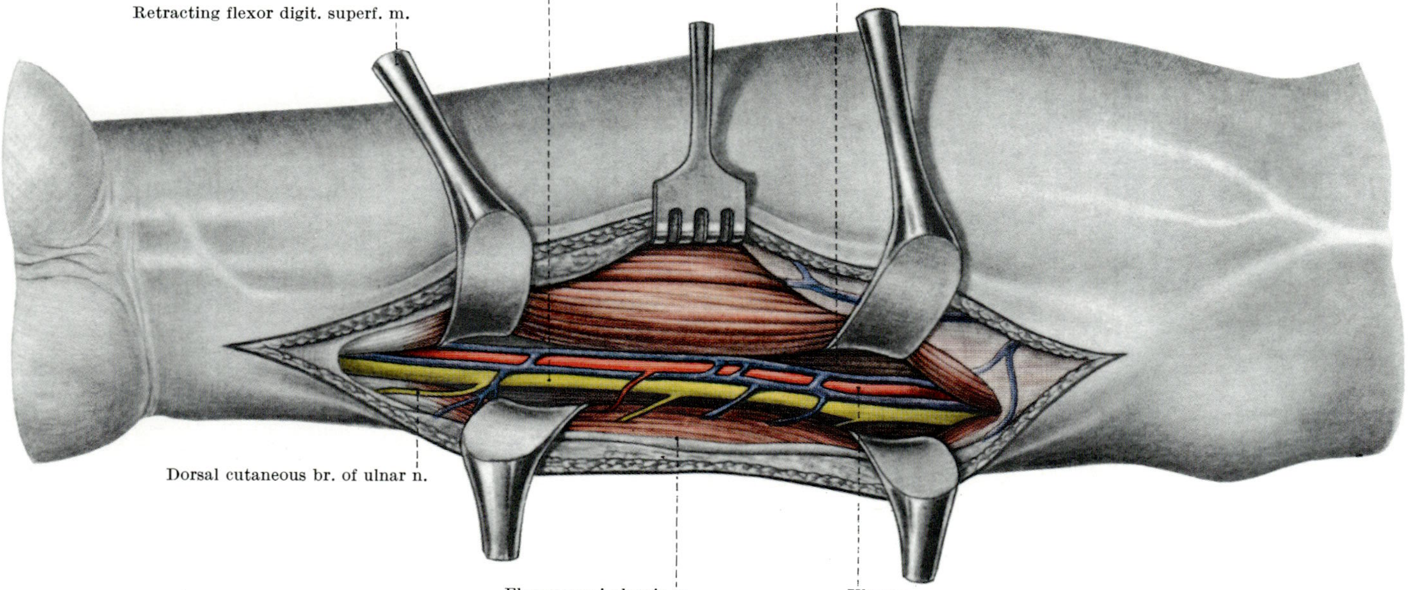

Fig. 212. Exposure of the ulnar nerve in the forearm.

Observe: 1. The deep fascia is incised between the flexor carpi ulnaris and the flexor digitorum superficialis muscles. 2. The ulnar artery lies on the radial side of the nerve and supplies many short nutrient branches to the nerve. 3. The dorsal cutaneous branch of the ulnar nerve originates in the distal third of the forearm.

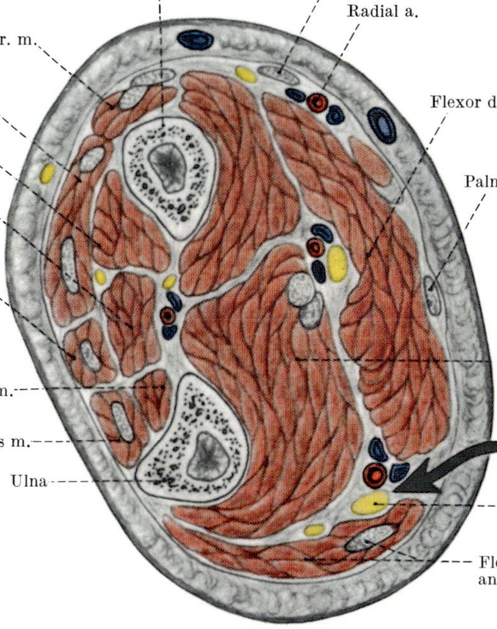

Fig. 213. Exposure of the ulnar nerve in the forearm: Transverse section through the middle third of the forearm.

Observe: The operative exposure is between the flexor carpi ulnaris and flexor digitorum superficialis muscles.

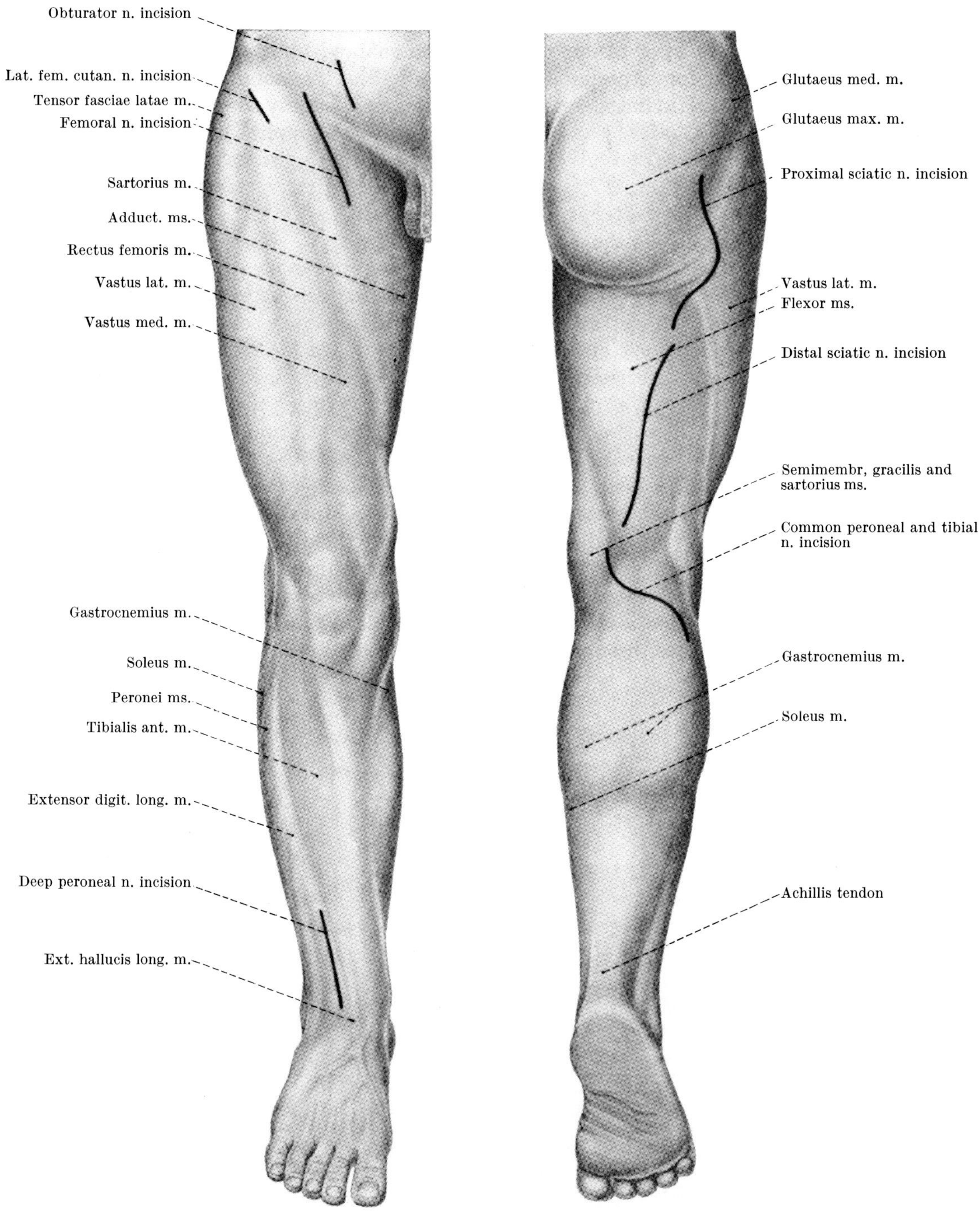

Fig. 216. Exposure of peripheral nerves in the lower extremity: Incisions.

Observe: Each incision will be discussed in more detail later but notice that all incisions are made in such a way that maximum exposure will be obtained with the most favorable cosmetic result.

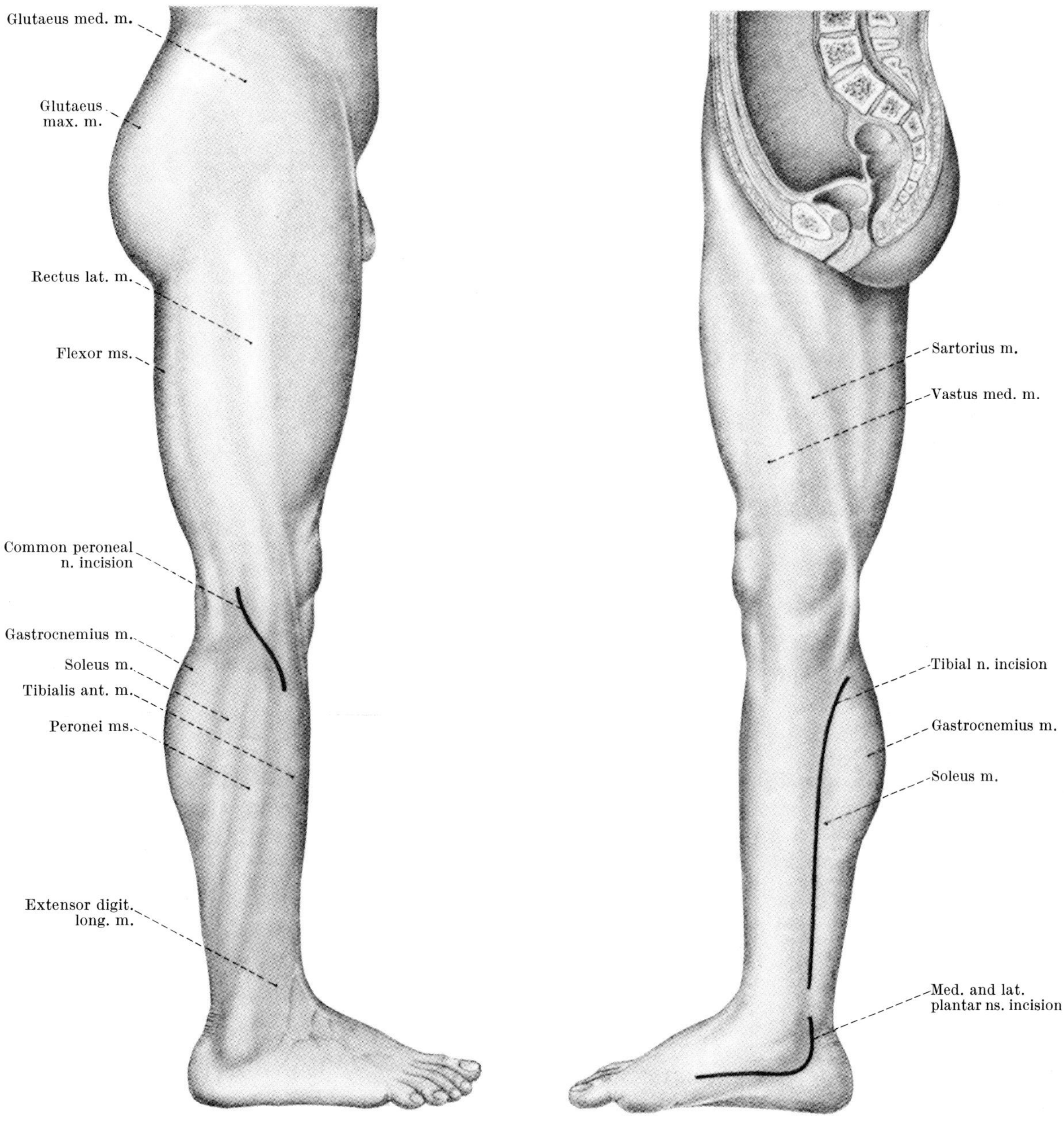

Fig. 217. Exposure of peripheral nerves in the lower extremity: Incisions.

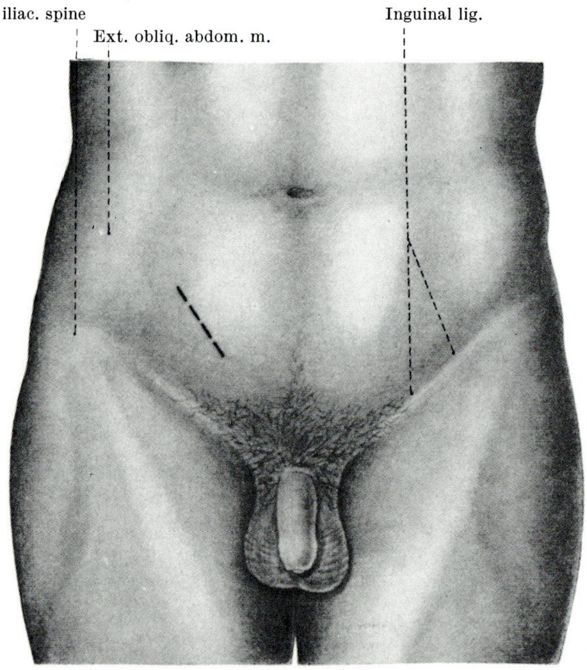

Fig. 218. Exposure of the obturator nerve: Incision for transabdominal extraperitoneal approach.

Observe: The incision is made 4 cm. above and parallel to the inguinal ligament.

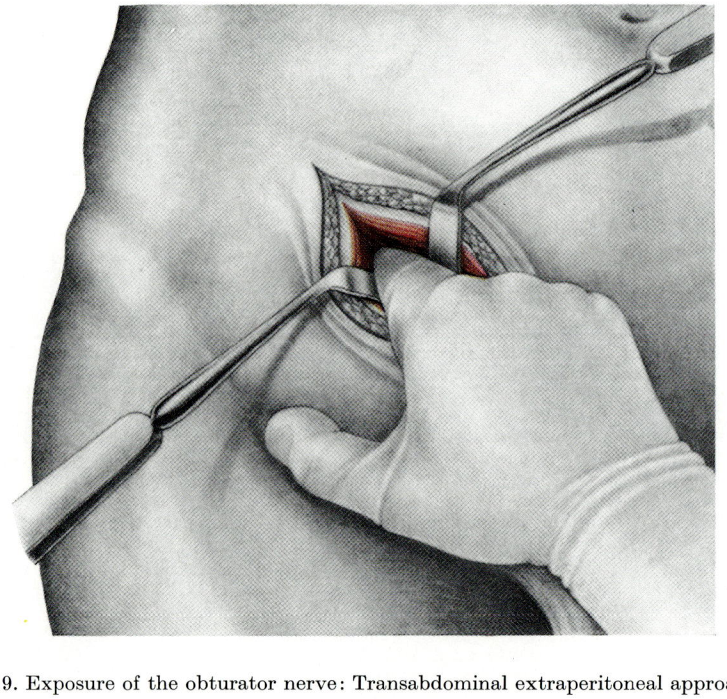

Fig. 219. Exposure of the obturator nerve: Transabdominal extraperitoneal approach.

Observe: 1. A muscle splitting incision is used. 2. Having visualized the peritoneum, the index finger dissects it from the abdominal wall.

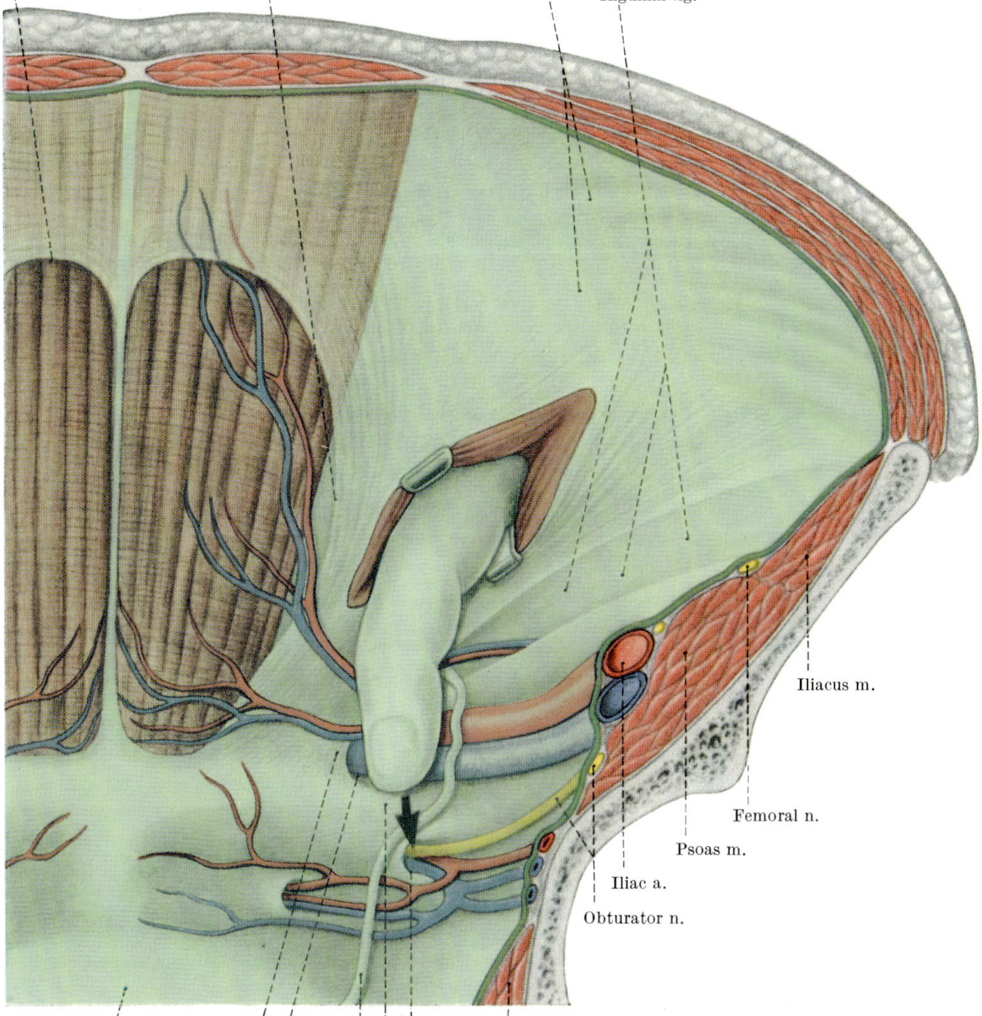

Fig. 220. Exposure of the obturator nerve: Transabdominal extraperitoneal approach as seen from the inside.

Observe: 1. The index finger in the preperitoneal space covers the deep inguinal ring and the femoral canal. 2. The superior ramus of the pubis is being palpated. The obturator nerve is intimately related to this structure as it passes out the obturator canal. 3. This same approach is used to expose the femoral nerve in the pelvis.

8. Lateral Femoral Cutaneous Nerve. Meralgia paresthetica is a syndrome consisting of paresthesias, pain and sensory loss over the anterolateral surface of the thigh. This affliction of the lateral femoral cutaneous nerve is often caused by entrapment of the nerve at the level of the inguinal ligament. The lateral femoral cutaneous nerve arises from the posterior branches of the second and third lumbar nerves along the lateral border of the psoas muscle. It crosses the iliacus muscle and passes into the thigh immediately beneath the lateral extent of the inguinal ligament at the anterior superior spine of the ilium. Once again it must be emphasized that more proximal lesions of the nerve must be distinguished before treatment is undertaken. Lesions of the ilium, cecum or sigmoid colon may compress the nerve at the level of the psoas muscle. A herniated intervertebral disc at L_{1-2} or L_{2-3} will occasionally cause symptoms indistinguishable from meralgia paresthetica. Therefore, prior to surgical treatment of this syndrome, a nerve block using local anesthetics is indicated. The needle is inserted one finger breadth medial to and below the anterior superior iliac spine. Ten cc. of a one percent solution are sufficient. Most unsuccessful attempts are the result of inserting the anesthetic too deeply.

The operative exposure of the lateral femoral cutaneous nerve is made under local anesthesia. A three cm. incision immediately beneath the lateral extent of the inguinal ligament (Fig. 221) is carried down to the fascia lata which is incised in the same direction (Fig. 223). By retracting the fascia lata the nerve can be identified by blunt dissection as it passes just medial to the anterior superior iliac spine (Fig. 224). Actually the nerve passes through a triangle in most instances which has as its borders the inguinal ligament anterosuperiorly, the bone laterally and the attachment of the iliacus fascia to the inguinal ligament inferiorly. Having exposed the nerve it can be pulled downward and transected (Fig. 224) or transposed medially by incising the shelving border of the inguinal ligament (Fig. 225). This latter procedure gives the nerve a more direct course, as can be appreciated from Fig. 222, and removes the nerve from its bony boundary by the ilium.

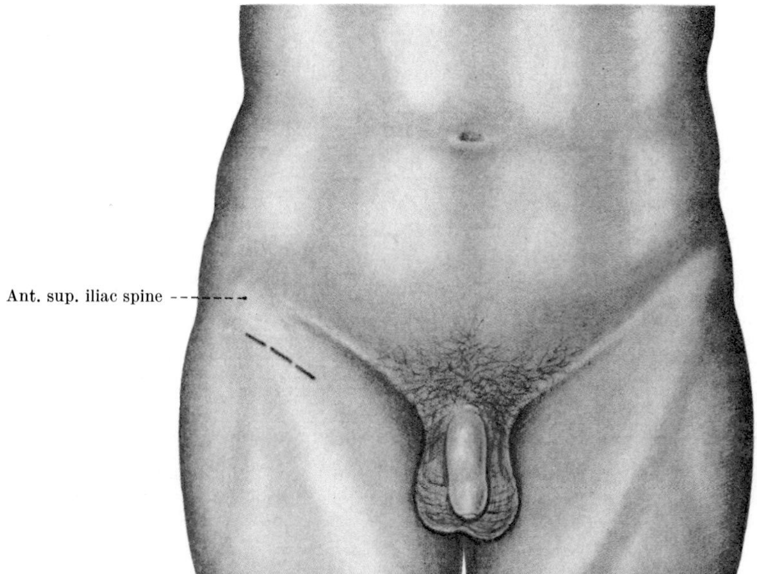

Fig. 221. Exposure of the lateral femoral cutaneous nerve: Incision.

Observe: The incision is made 3 cm. below the anterior superior spine of the ilium and parallel to the inguinal ligament.

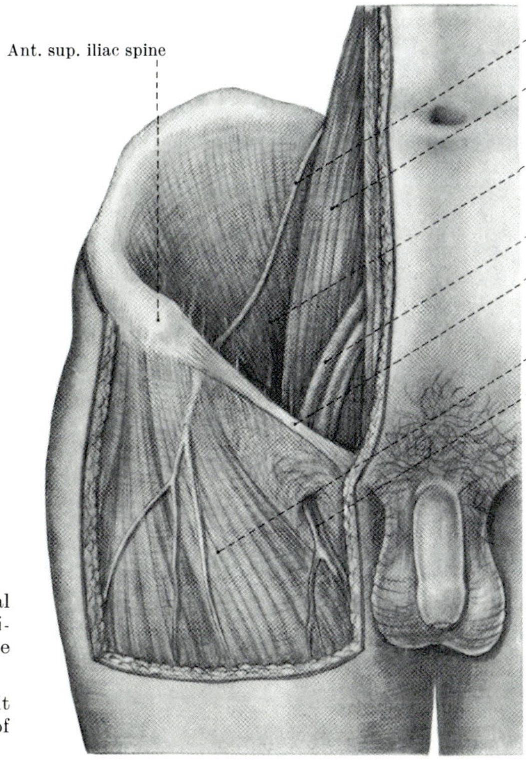

Fig. 222. Exposure of the lateral femoral cutaneous nerve: Anatomical view to demonstrate the course of this nerve.

Observe: The nerve angulates as it leaves the pelvis at the origin of the inguinal ligament.

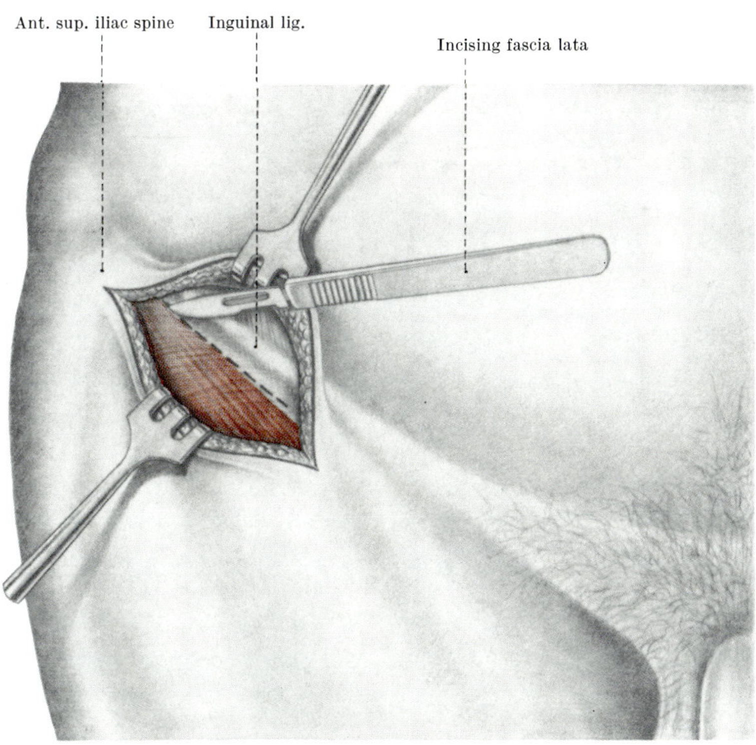

Fig. 223. Exposure of the lateral femoral cutaneous nerve.

Observe: The fascia lata is incised parallel to the inguinal ligament.

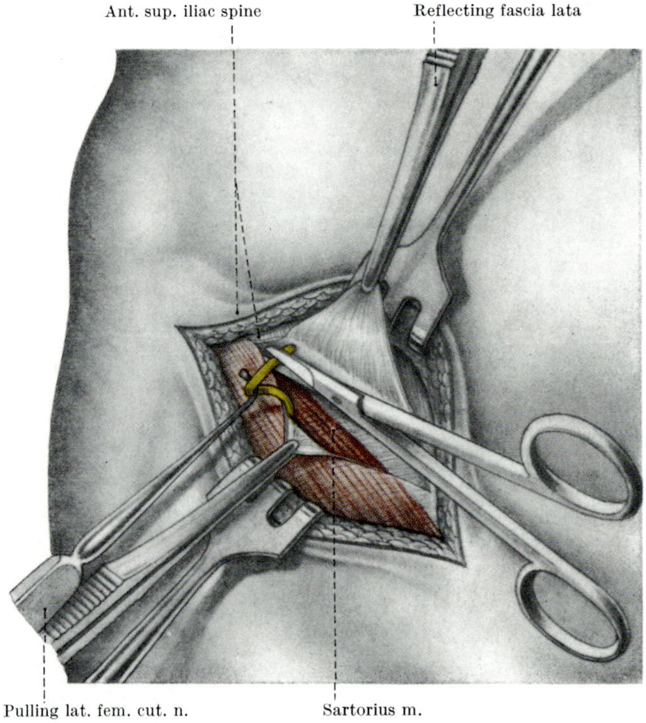

Fig. 224. Exposure of the lateral femoral cutaneous nerve: Transection of the nerve.

Observe: 1. The nerve is identified as it passes through a triangle formed by the anterior superior iliac spine and the two origins of the inguinal ligament. 2. Traction is applied to the nerve prior to transection.

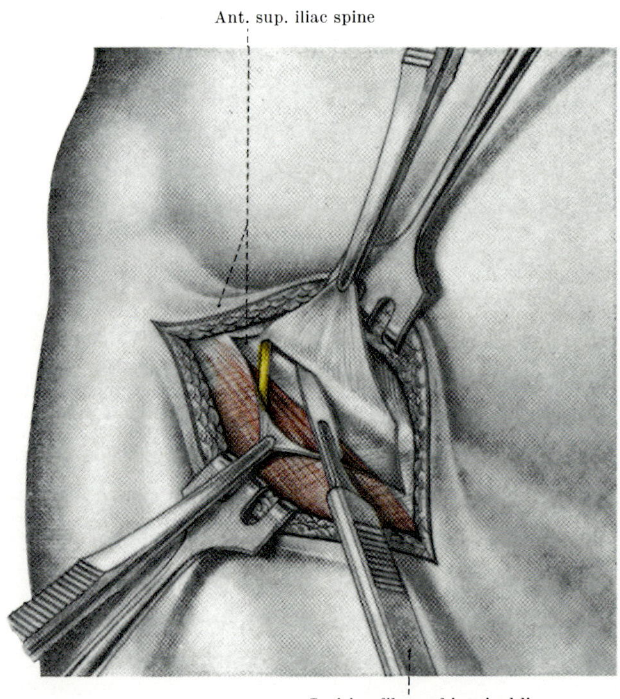

Fig. 225. Exposure of the lateral femoral cutaneous nerve: Transposition.

Observe: By transecting the attachment of the inguinal ligament to the iliacus fascia the nerve can easily be transposed several centimeters medially on the iliopsoas muscle.

9. Femoral Nerve. The femoral nerve, formed by the posterior divisions of the second, third and fourth lumbar nerves, is the largest branch of the lumbar plexus. Passing inferiorly in a groove formed by the adjacent psoas and iliacus muscles, it is joined by the external iliac artery (Fig. 220). Together they pass beneath the inguinal ligament into the femoral triangle. At this level the external iliac artery becomes the femoral artery, and it is separated from the laterally situated femoral nerve by psoas muscle fibers and the iliacus fascia (Fig. 228).

The surgical approach to the lumbar plexus and proximal femoral nerve is identical to that used for lumbar sympathectomy (see p. 241).

In the pelvis the femoral nerve is exposed by the transabdominal retroperitoneal approach described for the obturator nerve (Figs. 219 and 220).

The femoral nerve in the thigh is approached through a vertical incision which is made beginning at the mid portion of the inguinal ligament and continued inferiorly along the medial border of the sartorius muscle (Fig. 226). Camper's fascia is incised and retracted widely. A *T*-shaped incision is made into the fascia lata and the falciform margin of the fossa ovalis as shown in Fig. 227. The fascia lata incision is parallel to the medial margin of the sartorius muscle. On retracting the incised fascia, the femoral artery and vein and deep inguinal lymph nodes become visible. Fig. 228 illustrates these structures without showing the femoral sheath. The artery is then gently retracted medially and a vertical incision is made into the iliacus fascia (deep layer of the fascia lata) to expose the femoral nerve in its groove between the iliacus and psoas muscles (Fig. 228). Three to five cm. below the inguinal ligament the nerve divides into terminal muscular, articular and sensory branches.

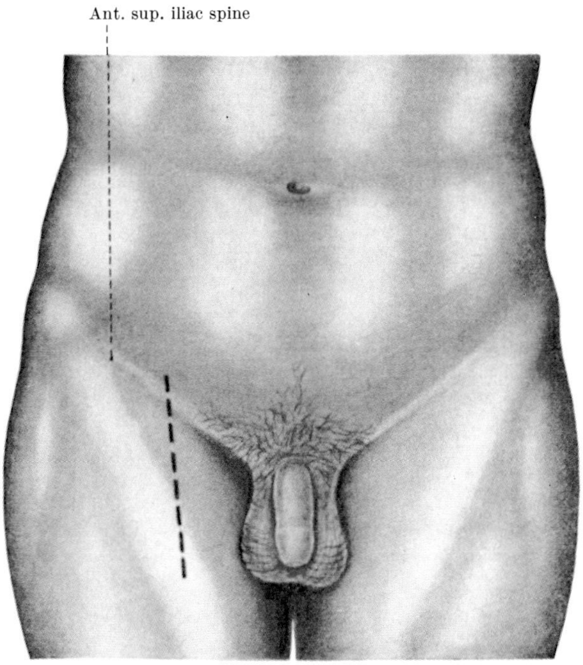

Fig. 226. Exposure of the femoral nerve: Incision.

Observe: The incision is made from the mid portion of the inguinal ligament downward following the medial border of the sartorius muscle.

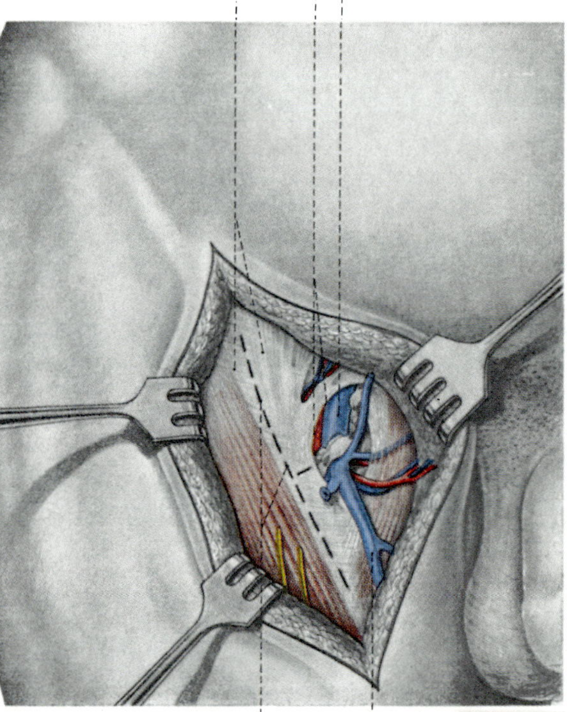

Fig. 227. Exposure of the femoral nerve.

Observe: 1. Camper's fascia has been incised and retracted. 2. A *T*-shaped fascial incision of the falciform margin of the fossa ovalis and the fascia lata is made parallel to the sartorius muscle.

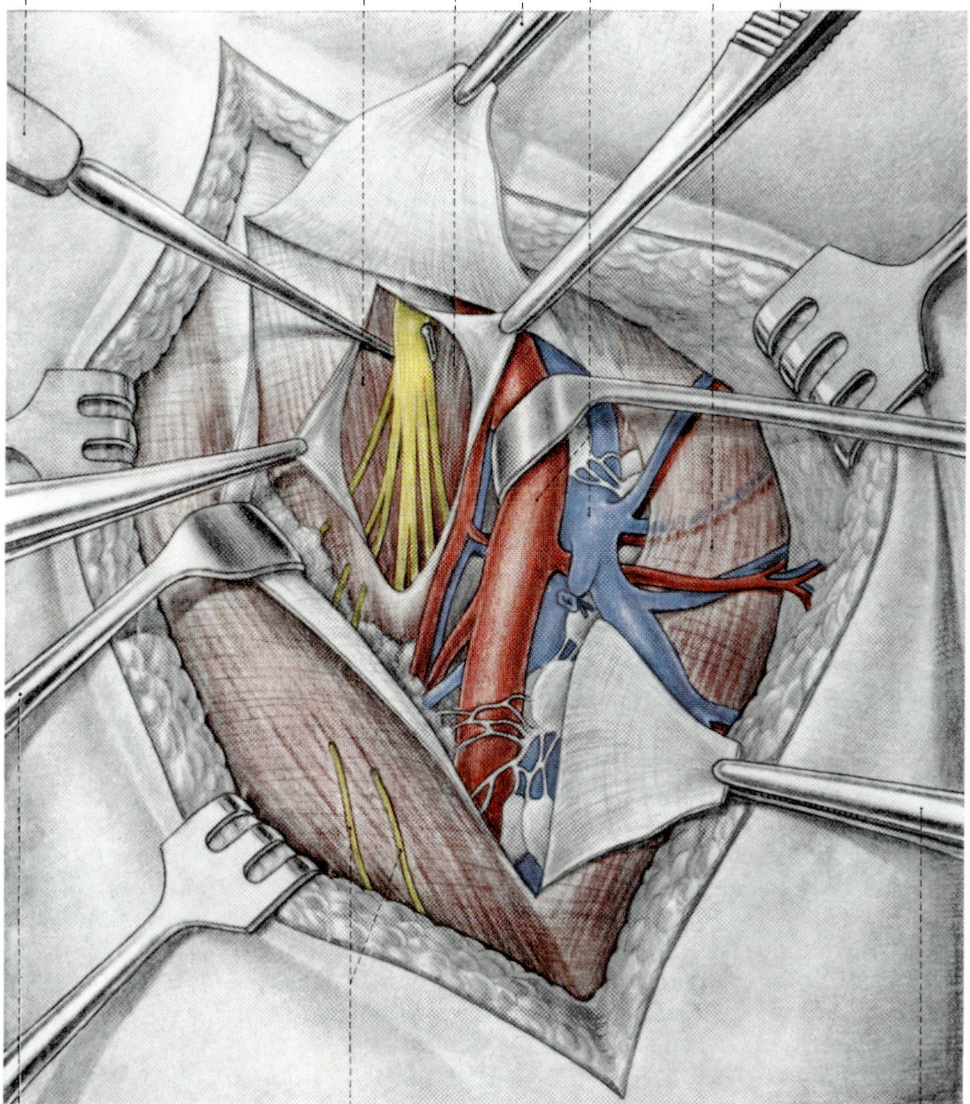

Fig. 228. Exposure of the femoral nerve.

Observe: The iliacus fascia (deep leaf of the fascia lata) must be incised to expose the femoral nerve in the groove between the psoas and iliacus muscle.

10. Sciatic Nerve. The sciatic nerve is actually two nerves contained within a common connective tissue sheath — the common peroneal and the tibial nerves. This large mass of nerve fibers arises from spinal cord segments L_4 to S_3. The tibial division is formed from the anterior division of the entire series of nerve roots, and the common peroneal is formed from the posterior branches of nerves L_4 through S_2. Occasionally the separate identity of the two nerves is clear throughout the thigh. The tibial division is the medial part of the sciatic nerve; the common peroneal is lateral in the nerve. The sciatic nerve leaves the pelvis through the lower part of the greater sciatic foramen and extends straight down the thigh until its two parts bifurcate at the level of the distal one-third of the femur.

The sciatic nerve roots are exposed to possible traumatic injury as they pass over the ala of the sacrum in direct contact with it. Since the common peroneal nerve arises from the posterior divisions of the rootlets, it is not surprising that trauma in this area results in a selective injury to this nerve. The sciatic nerve roots are separated from the hollow of the sacrum only by the piriformis muscle. For this reason it must be emphasized that a complete rectal examination should be performed on any patient who has symptoms suggesting sciatic nerve pathology.

Operative treatment of sciatic nerve lesions in the gluteal region usually yield disappointing results. This, as has been shown by SUNDERLAND [1], is due to the large number of small fascicles which are separated by large amounts of epineural connective tissue and due to the relatively long distance from target organs of many of the fascicles. Even though the prognosis is not good, lesions at this level should have the benefit of surgical exploration. Because of the long delay in spontaneous recovery functional following axonotemesis or neuronotemesis, early exploration of these injuries is indicated.

The exposure of the sciatic notch is performed with the patient prone by making a curvalinear incision from above the greater trochanter to the insertion of the gluteus maximus muscle at the mid thigh (Fig. 229). After opening the fascia, the gluteus maximum muscle is transected close to its insertion into the iliotibial band of the fascia lata (Fig. 230). The gluteus maximus is then hinged medially to expose the sciatic nerve beneath the piriformis muscle as it leaves the pelvis (Fig. 231). The surgeon should be aware that anatomical variations in the relationship to the nerve to the piriformis muscle are not uncommon. The piriformis muscle occasionally passes between the two divisions of the nerve. Rarely the entire sciatic nerve will pass over the piriformis muscle. These anatomic variants may constrict the nerve with resulting sciatic nerve irritative symptoms. The surgeon must be aware that important vascular contributions are made to the sciatic nerve at the level of the notch from the inferior gluteal artery and lower in the thigh from many perforating branches of the deep femoral artery.

In the thigh, the sciatic nerve is exposed through a vertical midline incision which is curved laterally at the gluteal fold and medially at the popliteal fossa (Fig. 232). The fascia must be carefully opened and gently retracted to avoid injury to the posterior femoral cutaneous nerve which is located immediately beneath the fascia. The cleft between the semitendinosis and biceps femoris muscles is opened to expose the sciatic nerve deep within this groove (Fig. 233). In this dissection, care must be taken to avoid injuring small muscular branches to the hamstring muscles. To overcome a gap in the sciatic nerve, additional length may be obtained by extending the thigh at the hip and flexing the leg at the knee. As previously mentioned, the leg must not be flexed greater than 90 degrees at the knee, and after the cast is removed the leg must be very gradually straightened. The common peroneal nerve is especially sensitive to stretch injury because, as SUNDERLAND points out, it has more small fascicles and less adipose tissue in the epineurium than the tibial nerve. An additional difference in these two nerve components is that the common peroneal nerve has an angular course and is fixed not only at the

[1] SUNDERLAND, S., RAY, L. J.: The intraneural topography of the sciatic nerve and its popliteal division in man. Brain **71**, 242 (1948).

fibular head but also at the sciatic notch. Many excellent surgical repairs of this nerve have resulted in no functional recovery because of post operative stretch injuries.

The sciatic nerve usually bifurcates at the lower one-third of the thigh as it enters the popliteal space; however, occasionally the separate identity of the tibial and common peroneal nerves is maintained throughout the thigh. At the popliteal space these nerves separate, and the common peroneal nerve follows the tendon of the biceps femoris muscle to wind around the head of the fibula, whereas, the tibial nerve continues the straight course of the sciatic nerve vertically through the popliteal space.

To expose the bifurcation of the sciatic nerve as well as the common peroneal and tibial nerves within the popliteal fossa, a *Z*-shaped incision is made (Fig. 234). The horizontal limb of the incision crosses the popliteal space transversely along a flexion crease. The proximal extension is made upward parallel to the hamstring tendons. The distal limb curves downward along the fibula. Fig. 235 illustrates the fascial exposure after retracting the skin margins. The popliteal fascia is incised vertically taking care once again to preserve the posterior femoral cutaneous nerve. The biceps femoris muscle is separated from the semitendinosus and semimembranosus tendons at the superior extent of the incision. The common peroneal nerve is identified as it follows along the medial margin of the biceps femoris muscle (Fig. 236) and followed distally to the neck of the fibula. This dissection is carried out on the lateral surface of the nerve to avoid injury to the lateral sural nerve which leaves its medial aspect within the popliteal space and to muscular and articular branches which leave at the level of the head of the fibula. The tibial nerve is identified in the midline lateral as well as posterior to the popliteal artery and vein. In dissection of the tibial nerve in the popliteal space, articular, muscular and the medial sural branches must be preserved. Within the popliteal space both the common peroneal and tibial nerves receive nutrient arteries from the popliteal artery — the tibial nerve, which is closely approximated to the artery, by small perforating vessels and the common peroneal nerve from more laterally placed genicular and muscular branches.

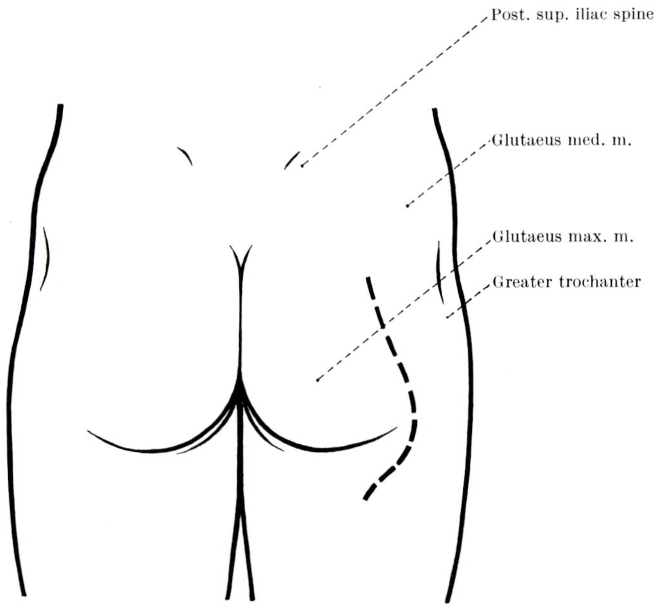

Fig. 229. Exposure of the sciatic nerve at the sciatic notch: Incision.

Observe: The incision is made from above the level of the greater trochanter medially to the below the insertion of the gluteaus maximus muscle at the mid thigh.

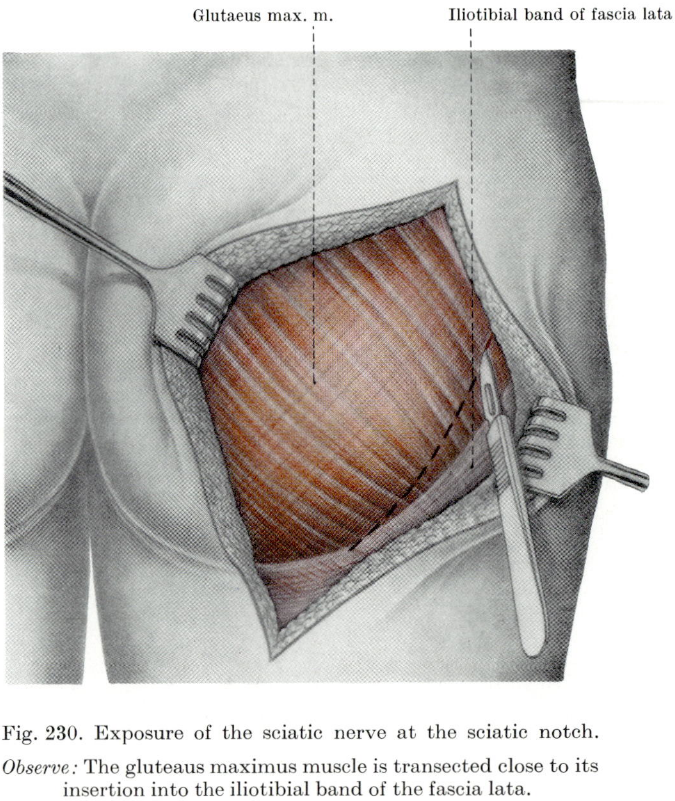

Fig. 230. Exposure of the sciatic nerve at the sciatic notch.

Observe: The gluteaus maximus muscle is transected close to its insertion into the iliotibial band of the fascia lata.

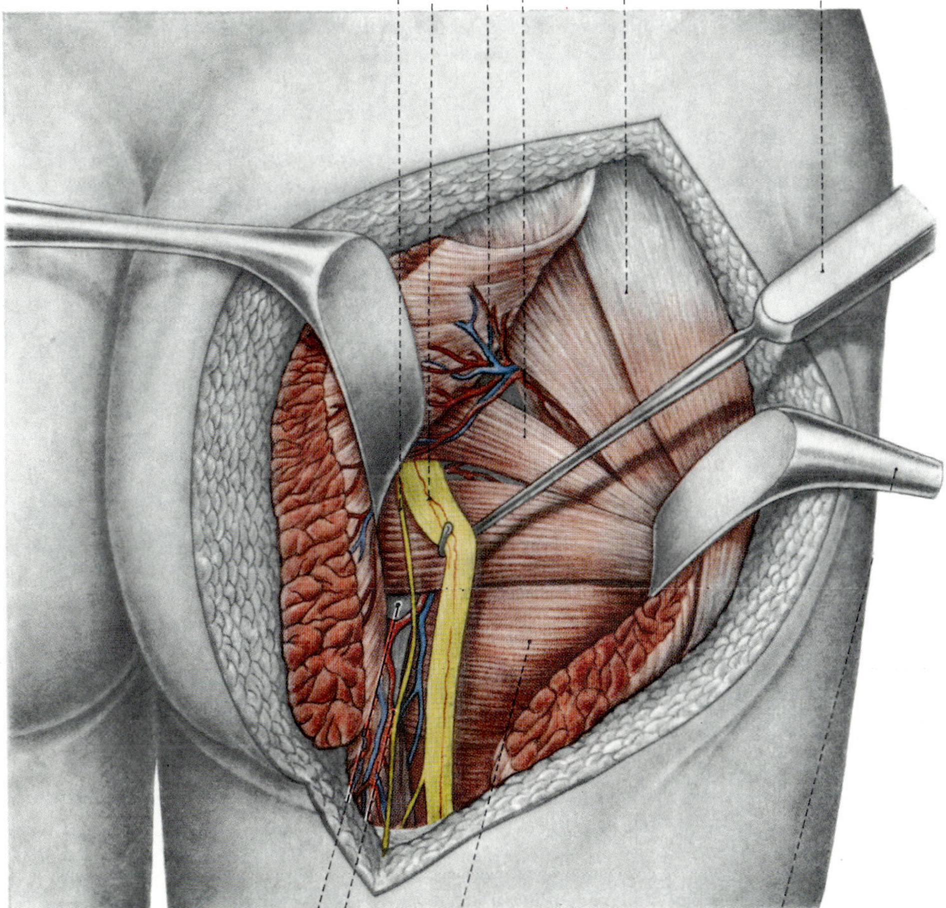

Fig. 231. Exposure of the sciatic nerve at the sciatic notch.

Observe: 1. An important arterial supply to the nerve is from the inferior gluteal and medial circumflex femoral arteries. 2. The ischial tuberosity separates the greater and lesser sciatic notches.

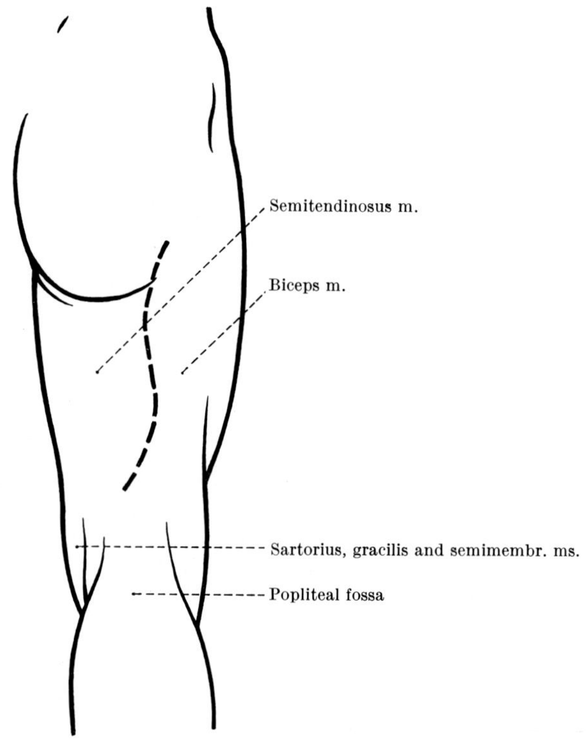

Fig. 232. Exposure of the sciatic nerve in the thigh: Incision.

Observe: Superiorly the incision curves laterally at the gluteal fold and inferiorly it deviates medially as the popliteal fossa is approached (see Fig. 234).

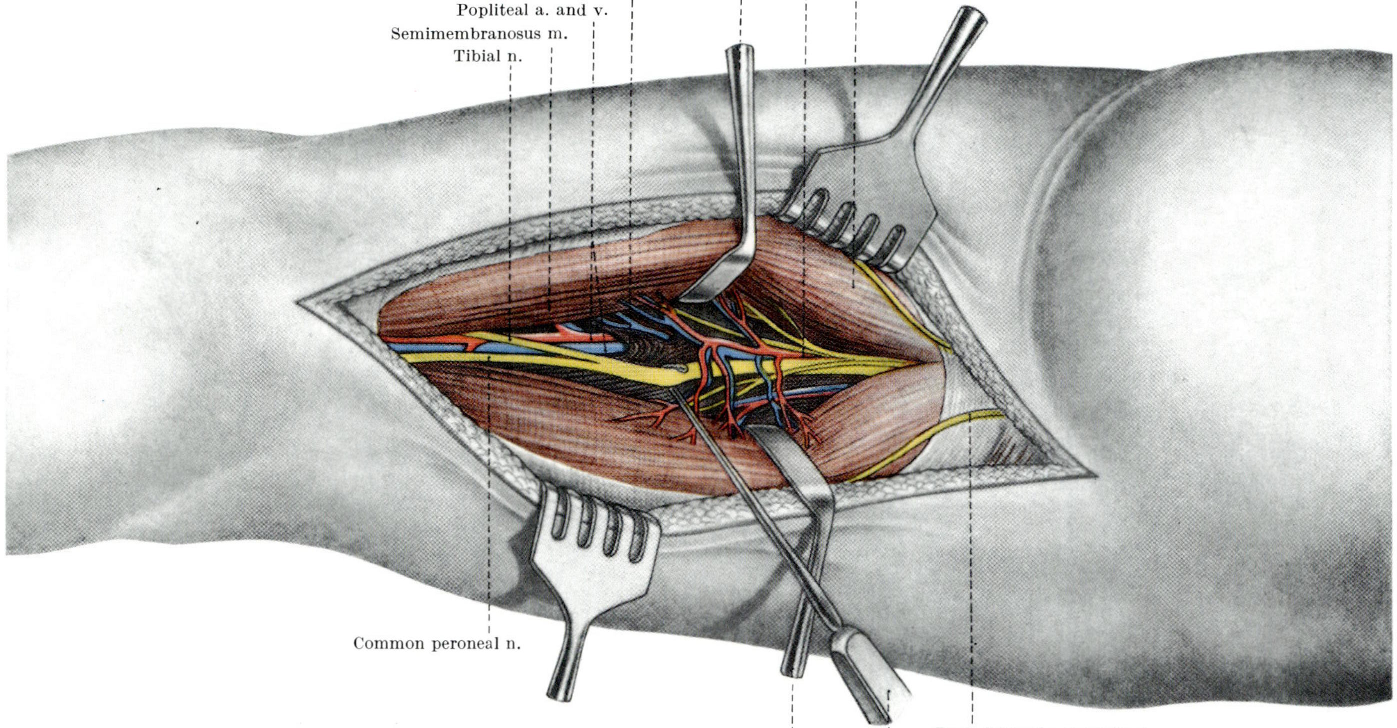

Fig. 233. Exposure of the sciatic nerve in the thigh.

Observe: 1. In opening the fascia the posterior femoral cutaneous nerve has been preserved. 2. The dissection is between the biceps femoris and semitendinosus muscles and the muscular branches to these muscles must be preserved. 3. At the level of the adductor hiatus the nerve is close to the femur.

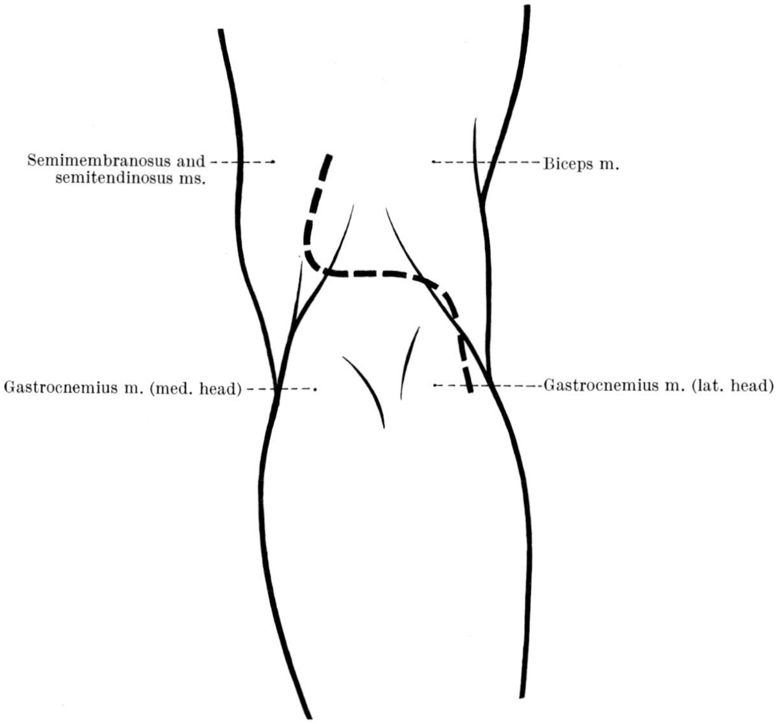

Fig. 234. Exposure of the tibial and common peroneal nerves at the popliteal fossa: Incision.

Observe: Z-shaped incision allows for healing without contracture.

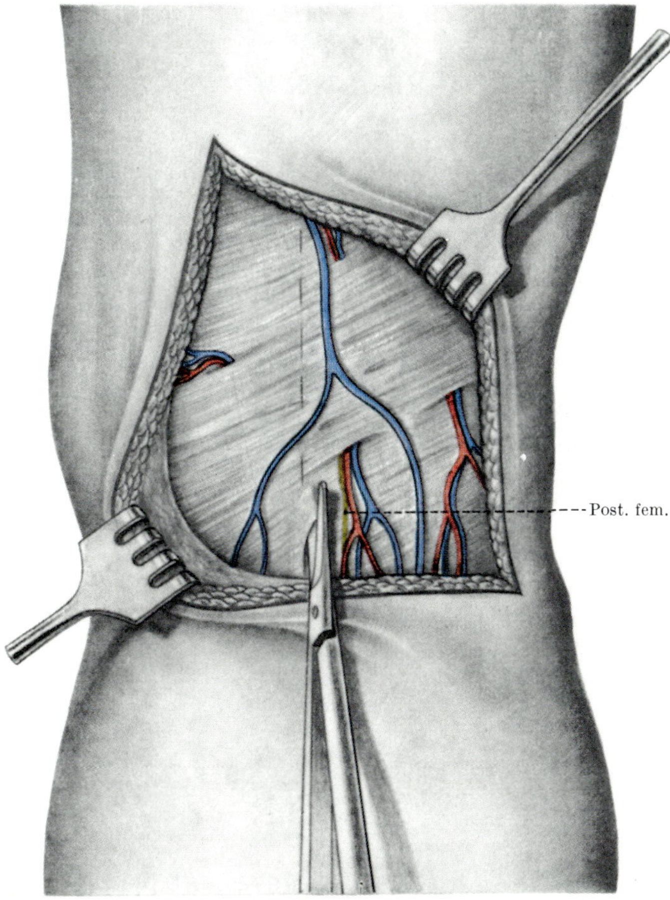

Incising popliteal fascia

Fig. 235. Exposure of the tibial and common peroneal nerves at the popliteal fossa.

Observe: The posterior femoral cutaneous nerve is identified and preserved.

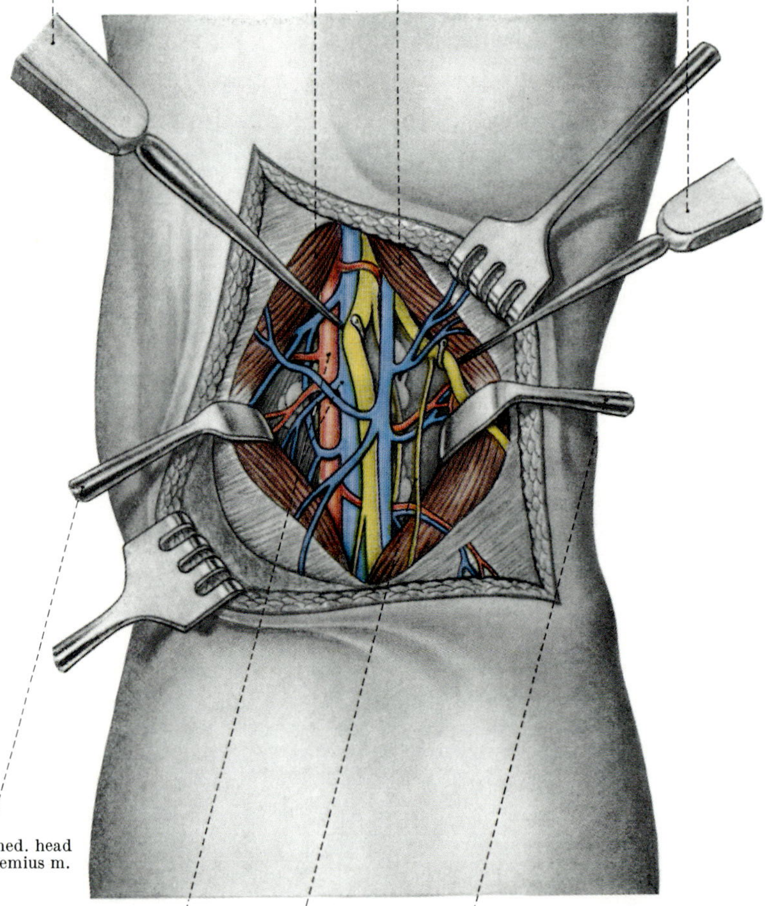

Fig. 236. Exposure of the tibial and common peroneal nerves at the popliteal fossa.

Observe: 1. The common peroneal nerve follows the tendon of the biceps femoris muscle along the lateral margin of the popliteal space. It gives origin to the lateral sural cutaneous nerve as it crosses the lateral head of the gastrocnemius muscle. 2. The tibial nerve proceeds inferiorly directly in the midline at the lateral side of the popliteal vein.

11. Common Peroneal Nerve. Having followed the biceps femoris tendon through the popliteal space to the back of the head of the fibula, the common peroneal nerve enters the leg by turning forward around the neck of the fibula beneath the uppermost fibers of the peroneus longus muscle, where it divides into its superficial and deep branches. The anatomical relationship of this nerve in this area cannot be overemphasized because this site requires the most frequent surgical exposure of a peripheral nerve in the lower extremity. The vulnerability of the common peroneal nerve to stretch injury has already been emphasized. Its superficial position while held against a bony structure makes it a frequent victim of direct trauma. Not only is the nerve easily compressed in this area but its nutrient vessels may also be compromised leading to ischemic damage to the nerve.

To expose the common peroneal nerve at the fibular head requires a complete knowledge of the anatomy of the popliteal space (see section on *Sciatic Nerve*, p. 215) since the nerve often has to be exposed as far proximally as the sciatic bifurcation. The surgical incision demonstrated in Fig. 237 represents an inferior extension of the popliteal fossa incision shown in Fig. 234, and these two incisions often must be used together. After incising the fascia the nerve is identified at the level of the fibular head. The nerve is followed distally as it penetrates the peroneus longus muscle, then passes between the superficial and deep heads of this muscle and, at this point, divides into its superficial and deep branches (Fig. 238). The superficial head of the muscle may have to be partially reflected to expose the bifurcation of the nerve. The common peroneal nerve is securely fixed during its course below the head of the fibula even before entering the peroneus longus muscle by the deep fascia which attaches to the fibula. This means that additional length cannot be gained in this nerve by mobilization distally. Gaps in the common peroneal nerve must be made up by proximal mobilization of the nerve and flexion of the knee joint.

12. Deep Peroneal Nerve. The deep peroneal nerve continues the forward and downward course of the common peroneal nerve, passing through the upper part of the origin of the extensor digitorum longus muscle to the lateral border of the tibialis muscle. At this point in the anterior compartment of the leg, it takes up a position along the lateral aspect of the anterior tibial artery and descends with it to the ankle.

In addition to direct injuries, this nerve, particularly in the military situation, is not infrequently involved in an ischemic nerve lesion — the "anterior tibial syndrome". This syndrome is characterized by severe pain, swelling and discoloration over the anterior compartment of the leg after strenuous activity. Neurologically there is a foot drop and loss of sensation over the first interdigital space. The treatment of this condition is to enlarge the osseo-fascial compartment and relieve obstructed circulation by surgical incision.

The skin incision for the operative exposure of the deep peroneal nerve is shown in Fig. 239. The incision is made parallel to the palpable tibialis anterior muscle. Having incised the crural fascia, dissection is carried between the tibialis anterior and the extensor hallucis longus tendons to expose the deep peroneal nerve lateral to the anterior tibial artery and vein (Fig. 240).

13. Tibial Nerve. The anatomy and surgical exposure of the tibial nerve within the popliteal fossa have been described with the sciatic nerve (see p. 215). Leaving the popliteal area, the nerve passes under the tendinous arch of the soleus muscle and descends immediately beneath the transverse intermuscular septum where it overlies the tibialis posterior muscle as it proceeds toward the medial malleolus.

The tibial nerve in the leg is exposed by an incision along the medial border of the gastrocnemius and soleus muscles (Fig. 241). A posterior midline muscle-splitting incision is contraindicated. The fan-like arrangement of the muscles prevents separation of the fibers without extensive destruction of muscle tissue. The crural fascia is incised parallel to the skin incision. The medial border of the gastrocnemius muscle is retracted to reveal the popliteus and soleus muscles. It is necessary to go through some fibers of the soleus muscle medially to expose the transverse intermuscular septum. This fascial layer is then opened vertically to expose the tibial nerve and the tibial artery on its medial border (Fig. 242). To obtain additional proximal exposure the soleus muscle may be mobilized from the popliteus muscle. However, it must be remembered that the popliteus muscle while crossing over the soleus muscle passes under the tibial nerve.

Exposure of the distal tibial nerve at the ankle may be indicated for laceration, painful neuroma or external compression of the nerve. Entrapment of this nerve causes a painful condition analogous to the carpal tunnel syndrome. It is revealed by incision of the retinaculum over the tibial nerve. The skin incision follows the course of the flexor digitorum longus tendon posterior to the medial malleolus and curves anteriorly over the medial surface of the navicular bone (Fig. 243). This incision must stay well above the sole of the foot. The fascia and flexor retinaculum are incised parallel to the skin incision (Fig. 244) to expose the tibial nerve and posterior tibial vessels. The nerve and vessels enter the foot by passing deep to the origin of the abductor hallucis muscle and, under that muscle, divide into medial plantar and lateral plantar nerves and vessels. By retracting the flexor digitorum longus tendon dorsally and the abductor hallucis and flexor digitorum brevis muscles plantarward, these structures are easily seen and can be dissected well into the sole of the foot (Fig. 245). Following repair of the tibial nerve at the ankle, sensory return has been quite rewarding, but reinnervation of intrinsic foot muscles is a rare event.

Fig. 237. Exposure of the common peroneal nerve: Incision.

Observe: This skin incision can be used as an inferior extension of the popliteal fossa incision shown in Fig. 234.

Fig. 238. Exposure of the common peroneal nerve.

Observe: The common peroneal nerve crosses the fibers of the gastrocnemius and soleus muscles arising from the head of the fibula. It then passes between the two heads of the peroneus longus muscle where it divides.

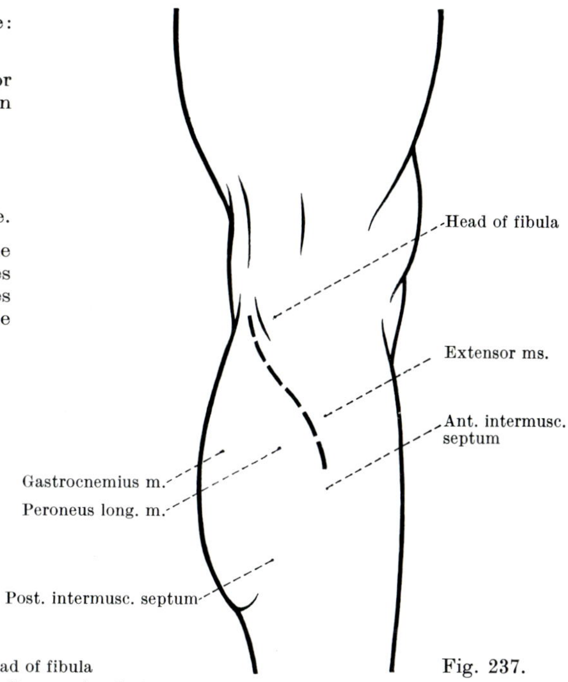

Fig. 237.

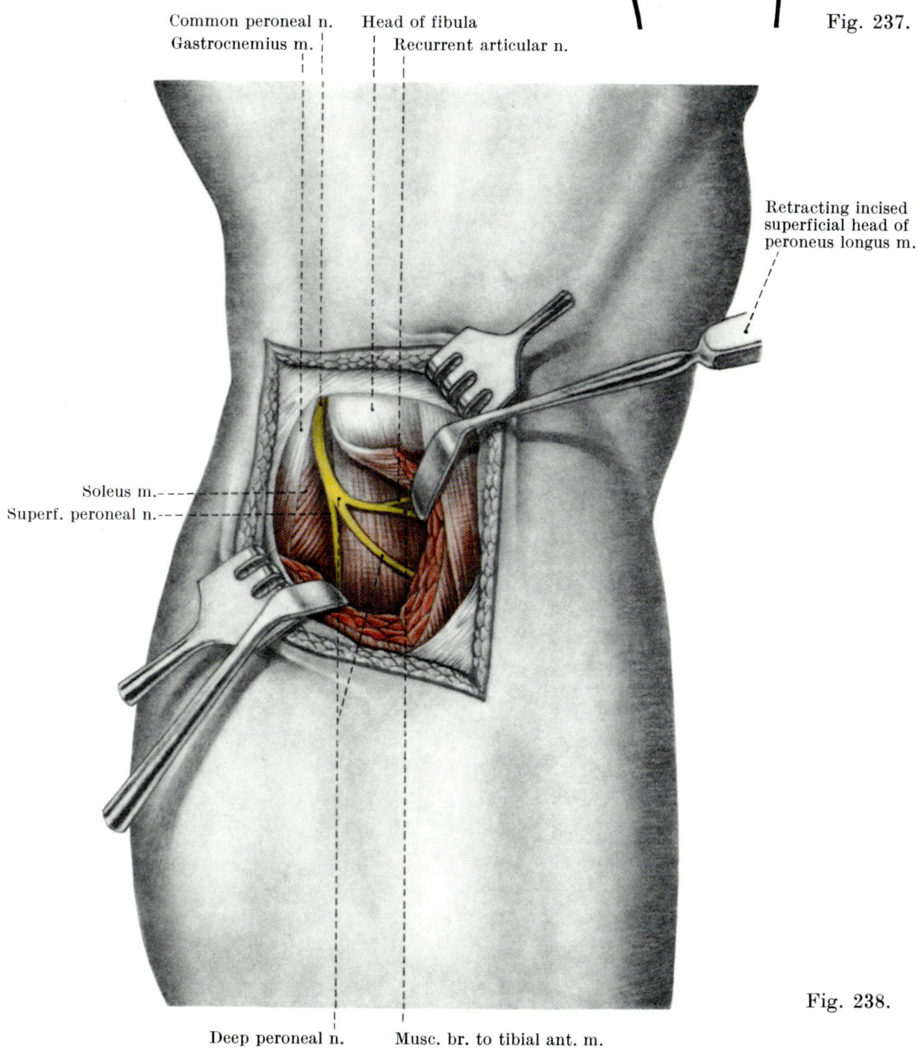

Fig. 238.

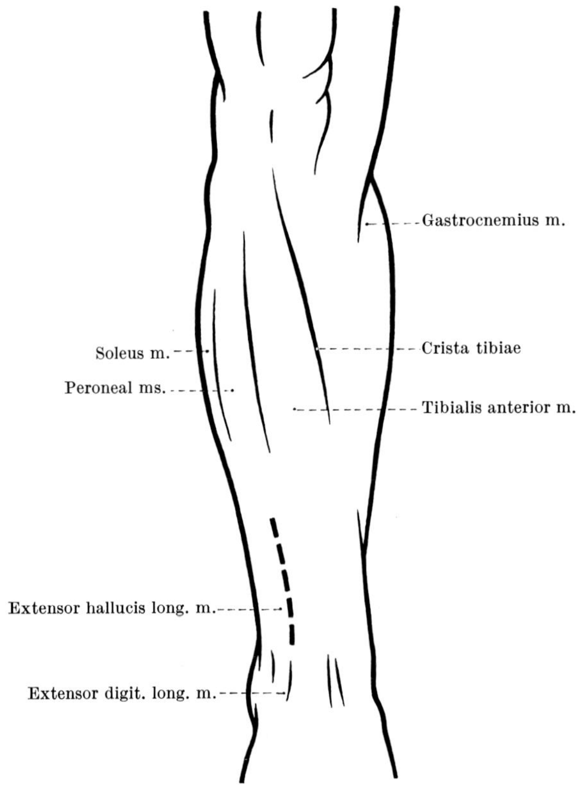

Fig. 239. Exposure of the deep peroneal nerve in the leg: Incision.

Observe: 1. The skin incision is made between the anterior tibial and extensor hallucis longus muscles. 2. This incision is used for the anterior tibial syndrome.

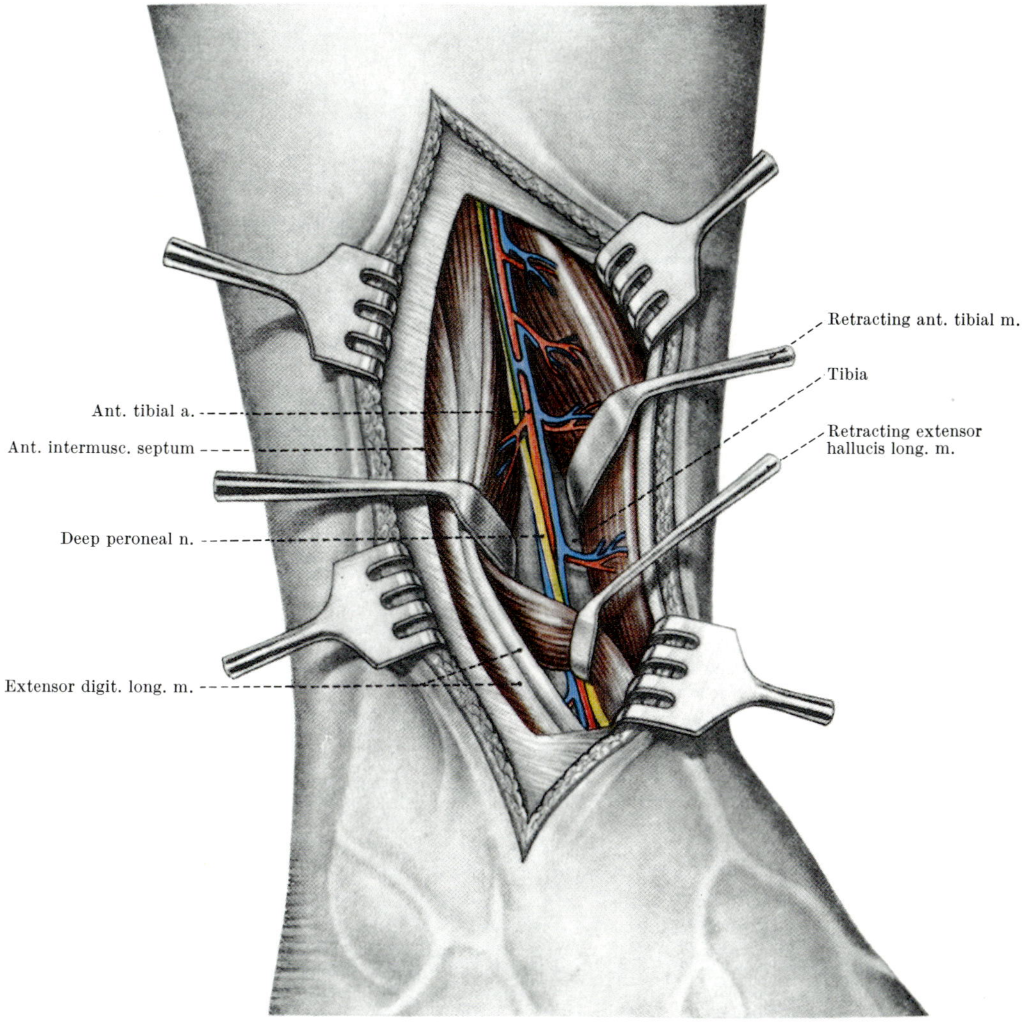

Fig. 240. Exposure of the deep peroneal nerve in the leg.

Observe: 1. The relationship of the deep peroneal nerve to the lateral surface of the tibia and the overlying extensor hallucis longus muscle. 2. The intimate relationship between nerve and artery. Nutrient branches must be preserved.

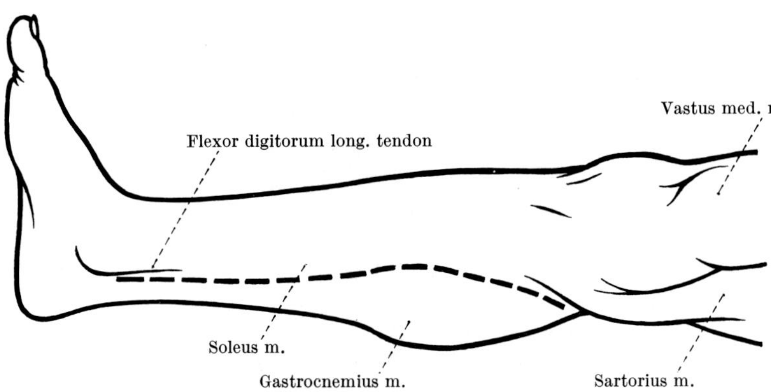

Fig. 241. Exposure of the tibial nerve in the leg: Incision.

Observe: 1. The skin incision is made along the medial border of the gastrocnemius and soleus muscles. 2. A posterior incision is contraindicated because the fan-like arrangement of the muscles prevent muscle splitting without destruction of the muscle tissue.

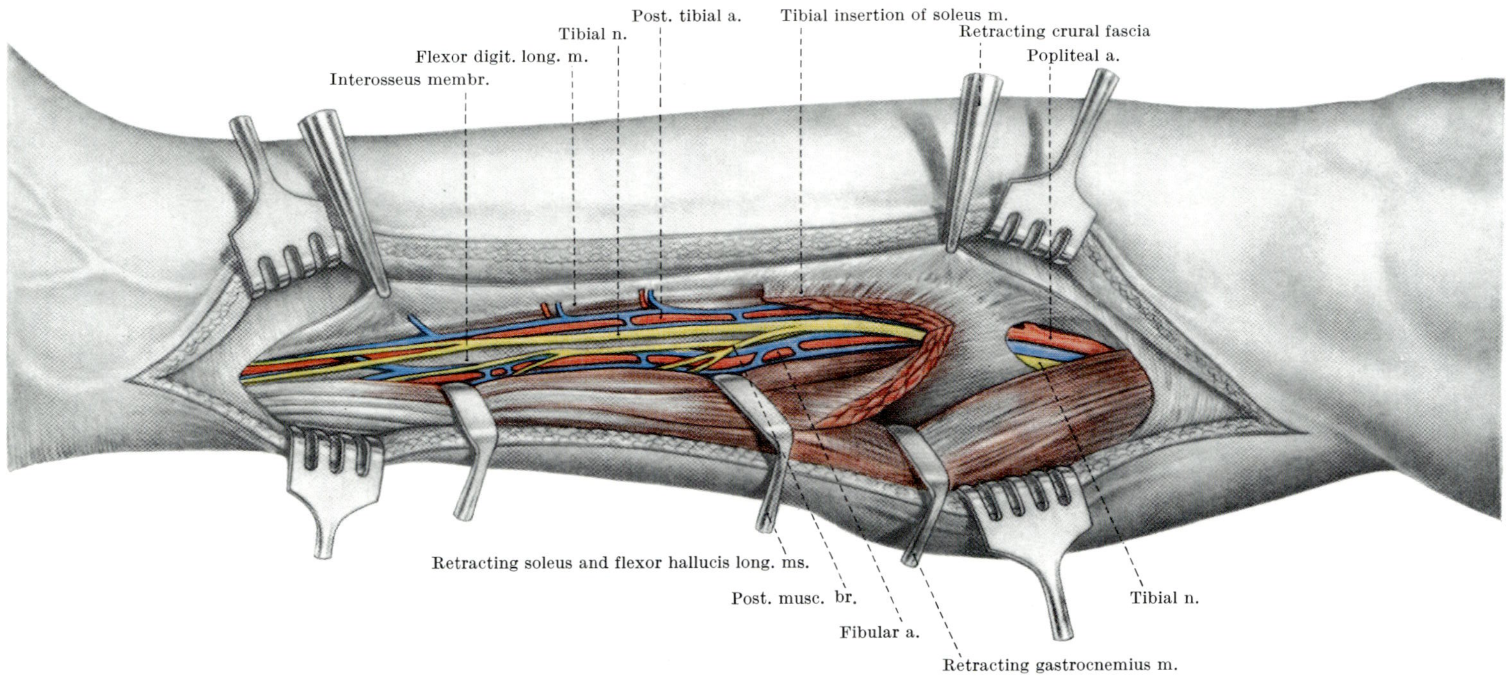

Fig. 242. Exposure of the tibial nerve in the leg.

Observe: 1. Dissection is between the soleus and flexor digitorum longus muscles. 2. The flexor digitorum longus muscle is freed at its origin from the interosseus membrane.

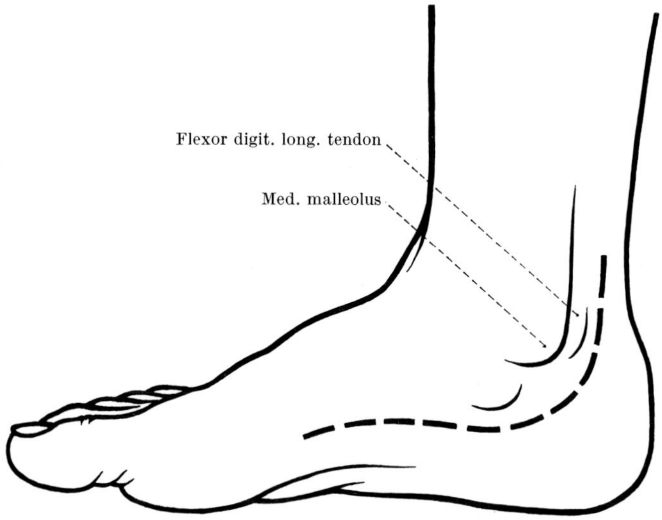

Fig. 243. Exposure of the medial and lateral plantar nerves: Incision.

Observe: 1. The skin incision is made along the flexor digitorum longus tendon and is curved anteriorly along the medial surface of the navicular bone. 2. The incision stays well above the sole of the foot.

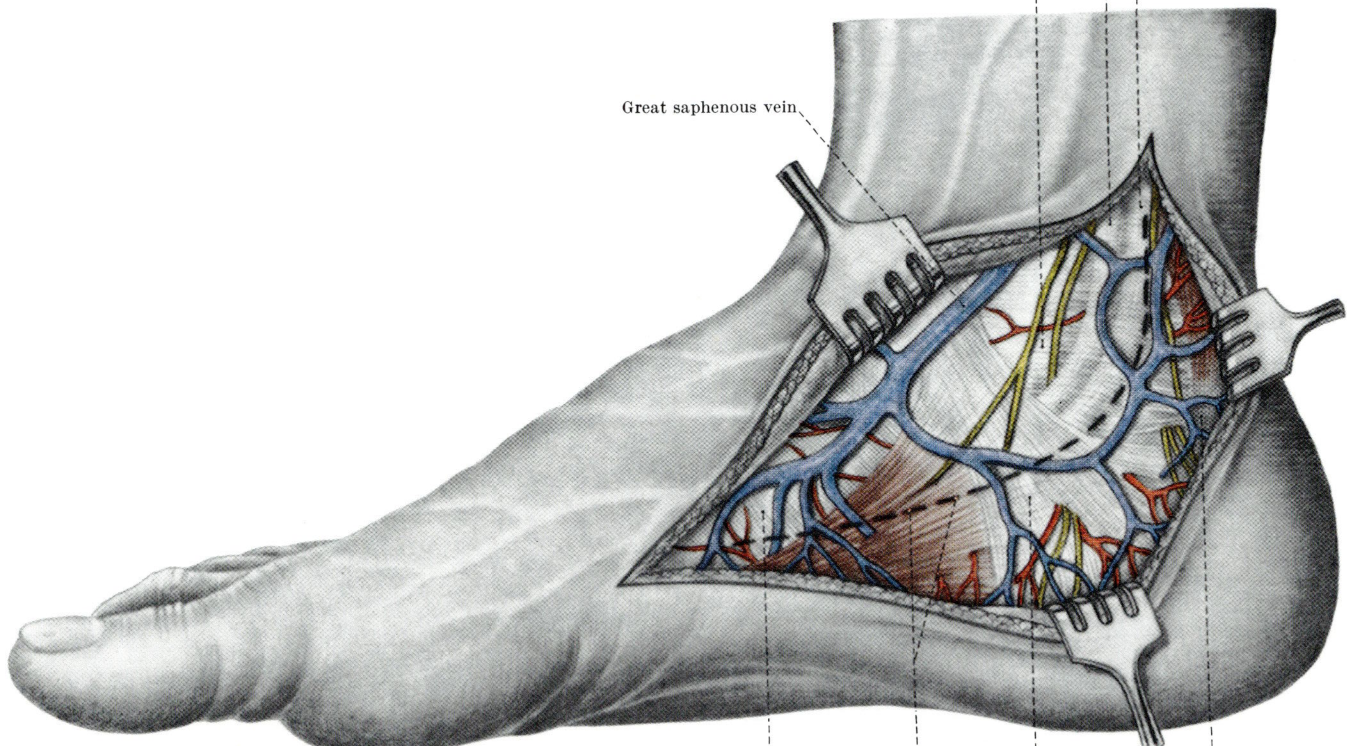

Fig. 244. Exposure of the medial and lateral plantar nerves.

Observe: The incision of the flexor retinaculum is made in the same direction as the skin incision.

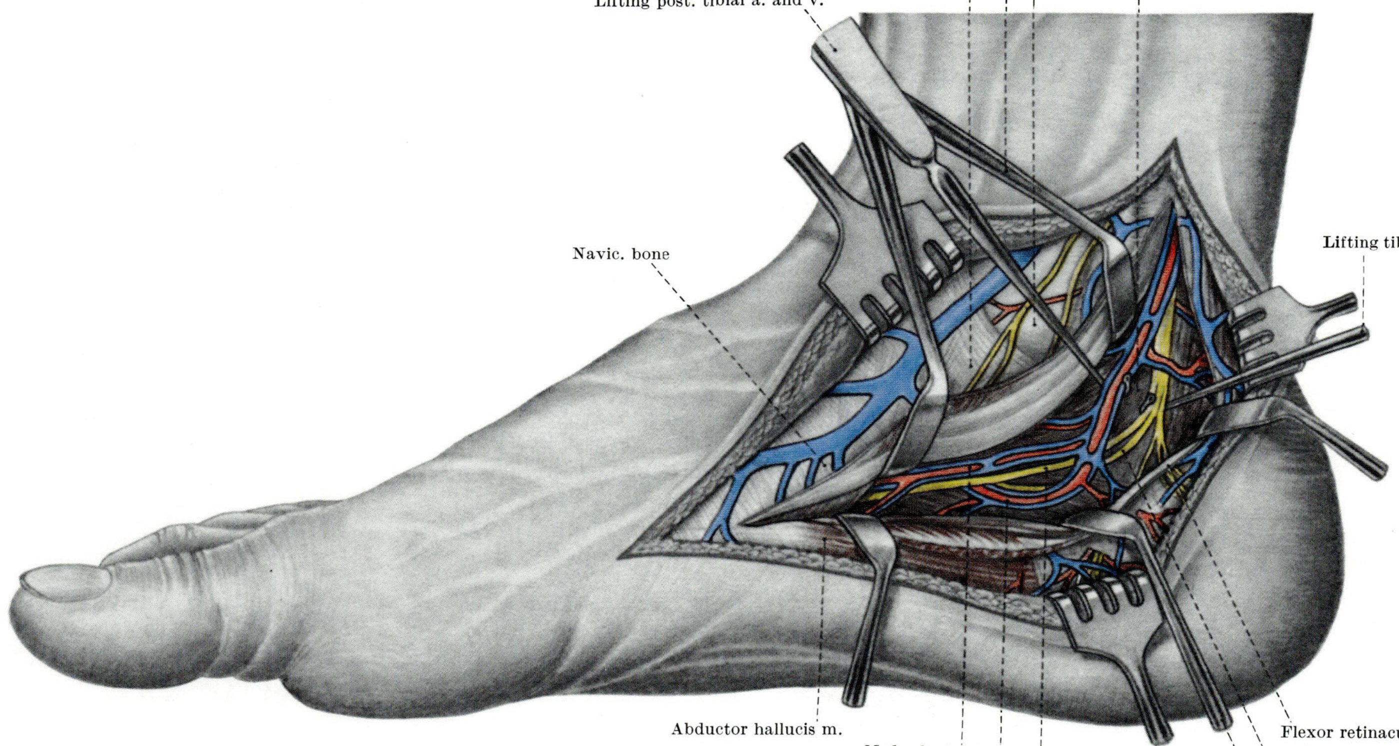

Fig. 245. Exposure of the medial and lateral plantar nerves.

Observe: 1. Having incised and retracted the flexor retinaculum, the tibial nerve is identified behind the medial malleolus posterior to the flexor digitorum longus tendon. 2. The medial and lateral plantar arteries lie within the fork of the medial and lateral plantar nerves. 3. The flexor digitorum brevis muscle provides a soft cushion for the vessels and nerves.

Chapter XXII

Hypoglossal-Facial Anastomosis

Paralysis of the facial nerve causes a severe cosmetic deformity. Following intracranial operations in which the facial nerve was found to be irreparably damaged, an early nerve crossing operation should be done to restore tone to the facial muscles as soon as possible. When the status of the nerve lesion intracranially is unknown, several months of clinical observation with electrical testing should be allowed for spontaneous reinnervation to take place.

The hypoglossal-facial anastomosis is preferred to the accessory-facial combination primarily because of the extensive muscular atrophy of the upper trapezius and sternocleidomastoid muscles which seems to bother most patients more than hemiatrophy of the tongue. In addition, if the descendens hypoglossi nerve is anastomosed to the distal hypoglossal nerve, the atrophy may be minimal in some patients. Another advantage, it would appear, is that there are less adaptive readjustment difficulties following use of the hypoglossal nerve.

Following hypoglossal-facial anastomosis, the prognosis for return of tone to the facial muscles is excellent in those patients who have had early surgery. This return of tone is crucial for cosmesis and restores a great deal of the symmetry to the face at rest. The degree to which voluntary control returns is dependent to a large extent on the motivation of the patient.

This operation is performed with the patient in the supine position with the head turned slightly away from the operative side. A six to eight cm. skin incision is made from two cm. above the mastoid process obliquely down the neck to two cm. behind the angle of the jaw (Fig. 246). The platysma muscle is divided along the same line and retracted (Fig. 247). The tendinous insertion of the sternocleidomastoid muscle is incised over the mastoid process as shown in Fig. 247, and using a periosteal elevator the tip of the mastoid process is denuded of all tendinous insertions. The deep fascia is incised along the line of the initial incision (Fig. 248) while taking care to avoid the capsule of the parotid gland which often reaches surprisingly far posteriorly. The tail of the parotid gland with its capsule intact is then gently retracted. The tip of the mastoid process is rongeured away, and any exposed mastoid air cells are closed with bone wax. The posterior belly of the digastric is identified as it leaves its origin at the mastoid notch of the temporal bone and is retracted downward and posteriorly. This allows exposure of the facial nerve as it leaves the stylomastoid foramen. On retracting the posterior belly of the digastric, a small branch of the nerve to this muscle may be recognized as it enters the superomedial aspect of the muscle and traced proximally to the parent nerve trunk. In exposing the facial nerve there is a tendency on the part of inexperienced surgeons to search too deeply for the facial nerve, particularly when the tail of the parotid gland has been elevated since this may also make the facial nerve more superficial. A nerve stimulator may be of aid especially if the facial nerve has been injured at the stylomastoid foramen, and the nerve has to be identified distally. Having identified the nerve, it is divided at the stylomastoid foramen (Fig. 249). Bleeding from the foramen is easily controlled by inserting a short probe and electrocoagulating the small vessels accompanying the nerve.

The simplest method of exposing the hypoglossal nerve is to retract the sternocleidomastoid muscle laterally and expose the carotid sheath at the lower portion of the incision.

The hypoglossal nerve is easily identified as it turns forward at this level, loops around the occipital artery and passes between the internal carotid artery and jugular vein. It is freed upward to the point where it enters the carotid sheath. As the nerve hooks around the occipital artery, it gives off the descendens hypoglossi. The hypoglossal nerve is dissected distally until it enters the submandibular triangle beneath the digastric muscle where it is sharply divided. The descendens hypoglossi is followed down the carotid sheath as far as possible (Fig. 250) and is also divided sharply.

The proximal hypoglossal nerve is then approximated to the distal facial nerve either above or below the posterior belly of the digastric muscle. Because these nerves are small, this anastomosis should be performed using magnifying loops. The technique of nerve suture does not differ from that described in the chapter on peripheral nerves (see p. 151).

To put frosting on the cake, the descendens hypoglossi can be anastomosed to the distal hypoglossal nerve (Fig. 251). This adds only a few minutes to the operating time and may prevent some of the glossal hemiatrophy.

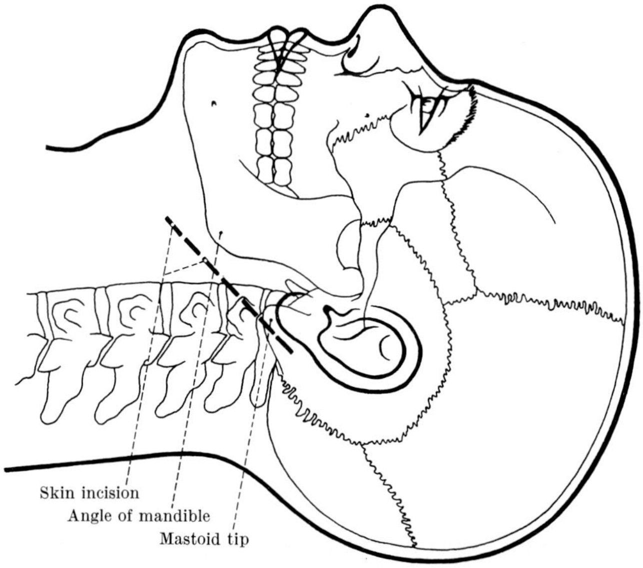

Fig. 246. Hypoglossal-facial anastomosis: Skin incision.

Observe: A 12 cm. oblique incision is made from 2 cm. above the mastoid process to 2 cm. behind the angle of the mandible.

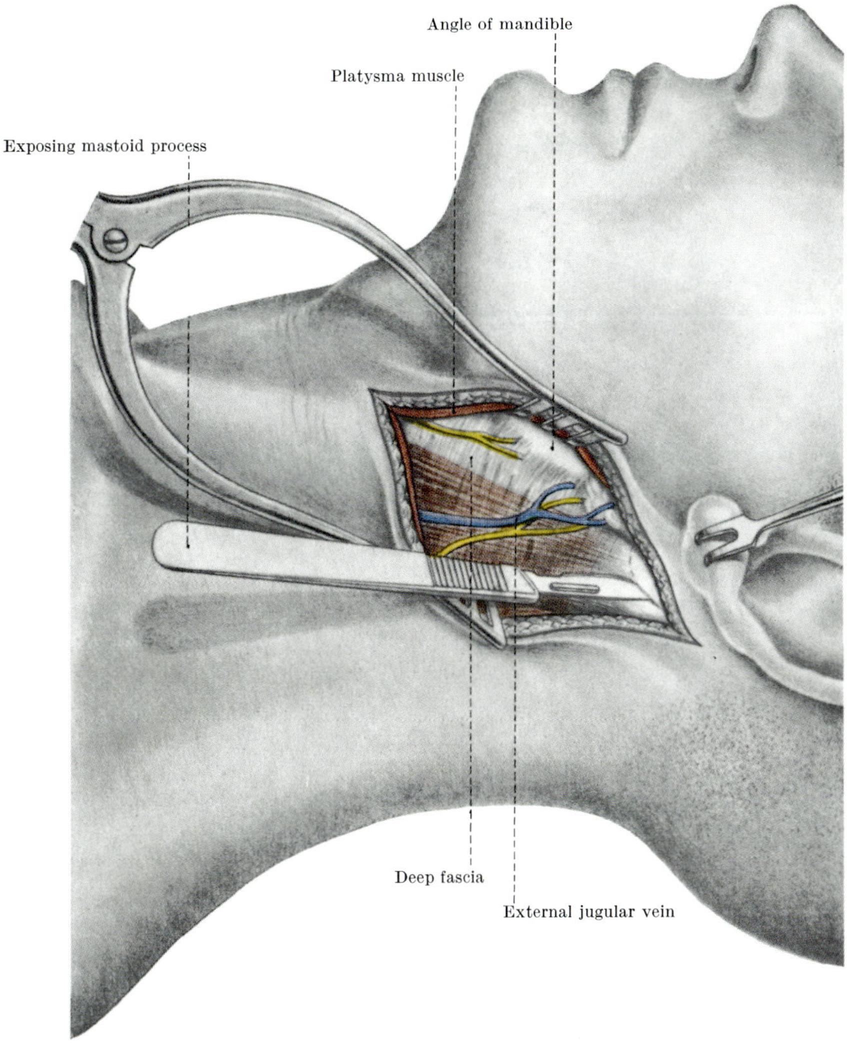

Fig. 247. Hypoglossal-facial anastomosis: Operative exposure after incision and retraction of platysma muscle.

Observe: 1. Incision of tendinous insertion of sternocleidomastoid muscle over the mastoid process. 2. Exposure of deep cervical fascia.

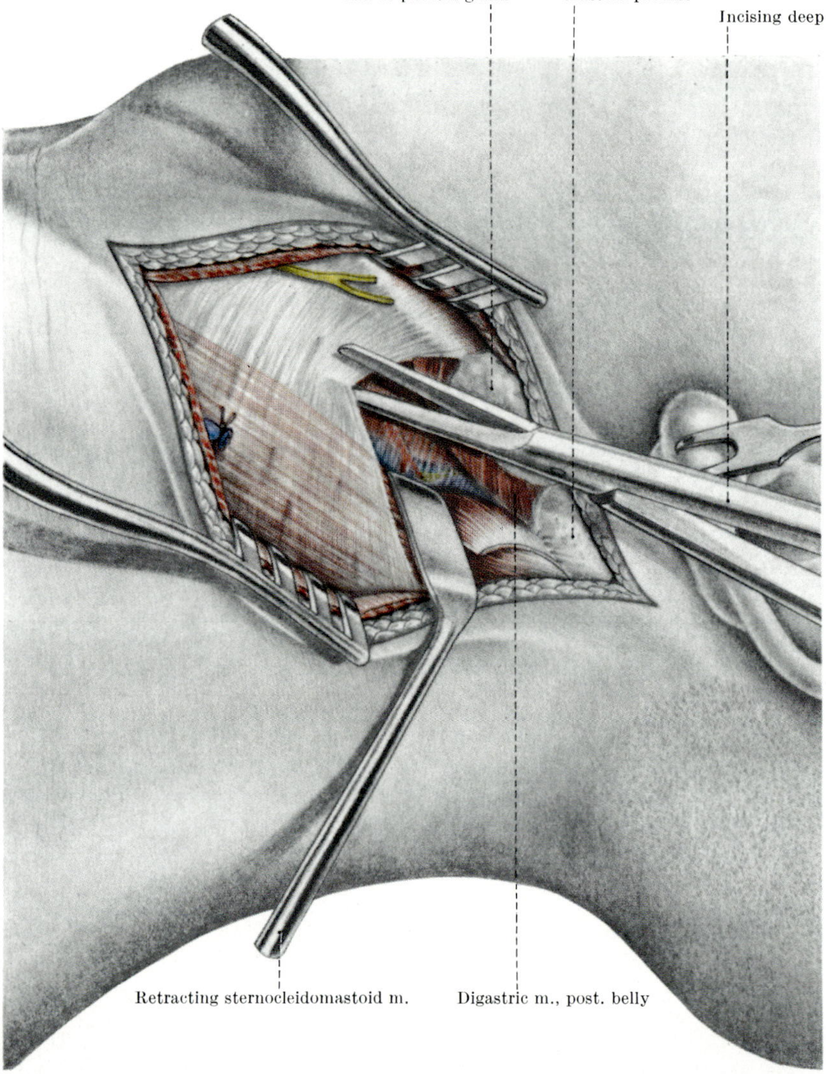

Fig. 248. Hypoglossal-facial anastomosis: Incision of deep fascia parallel to the anterior border of the sternocleidomastoid muscle.

Observe: 1. The tail of the parotid gland is carefully retracted anteriorly. 2. The posterior belly of the digastric muscle is identified at its origin from the mastoid process.

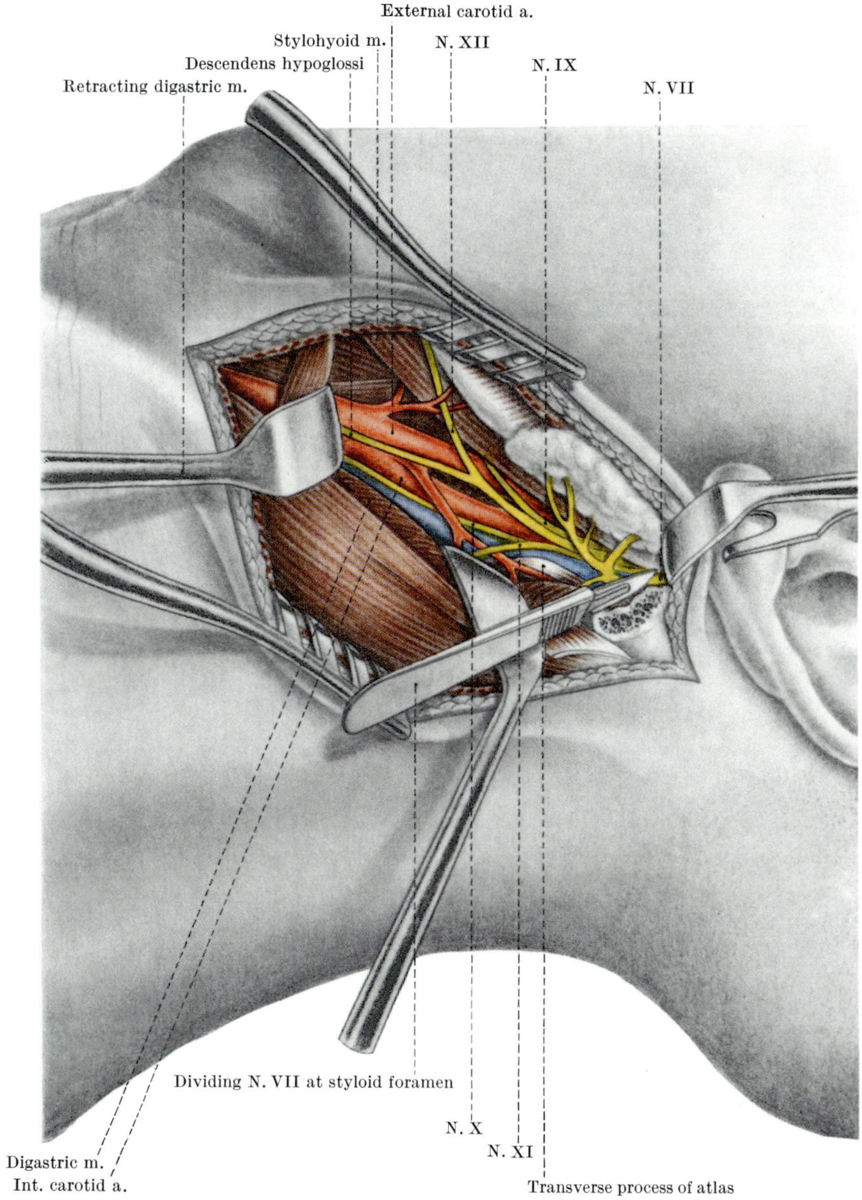

Fig. 249. Hypoglossal-facial anastomosis: Exposure of the facial nerve.

Observe: 1. The tip of the mastoid process is removed to help in exposure of N. VII. 2. All nerves and vascular structures are anterior to the transverse process of the atlas.

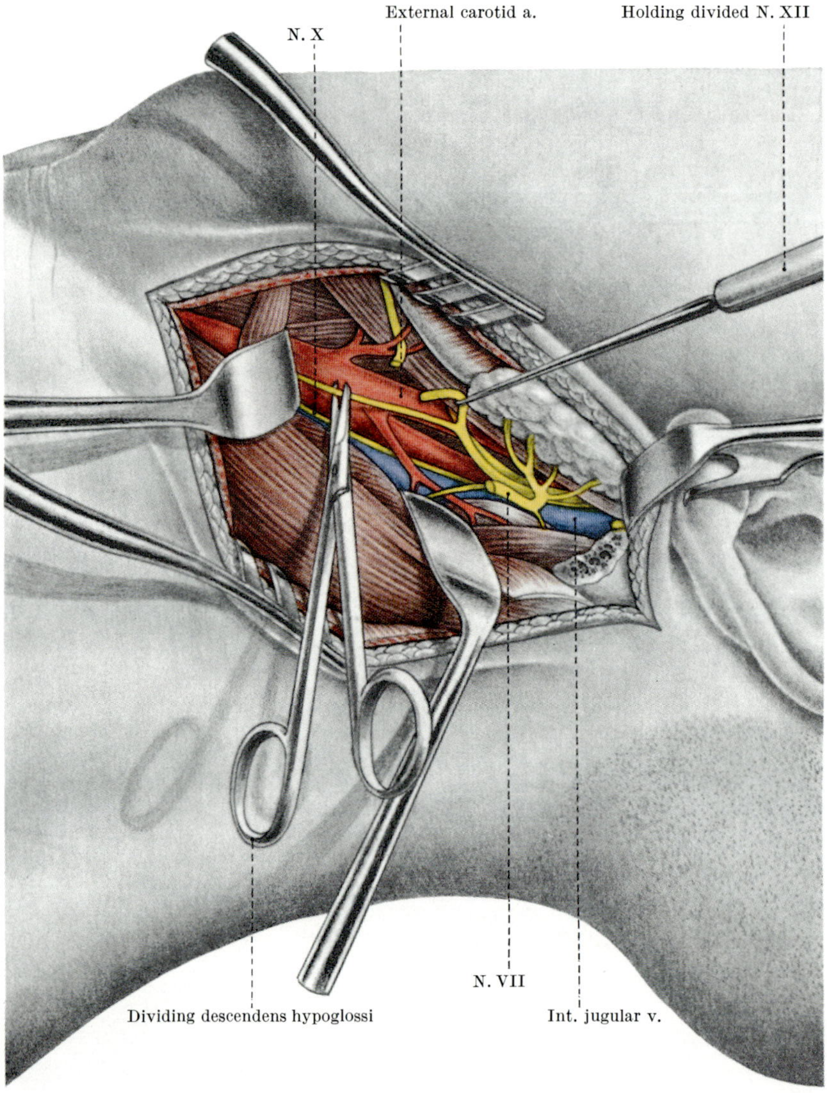

Fig. 250. Hypoglossal-facial anastomosis: Exposure and division of hypoglossal nerve.

Observe: 1. The posterior belly of the digastric muscle is pulled downward to expose the distal portion of the hypoglossal nerve traversing the external carotid artery.

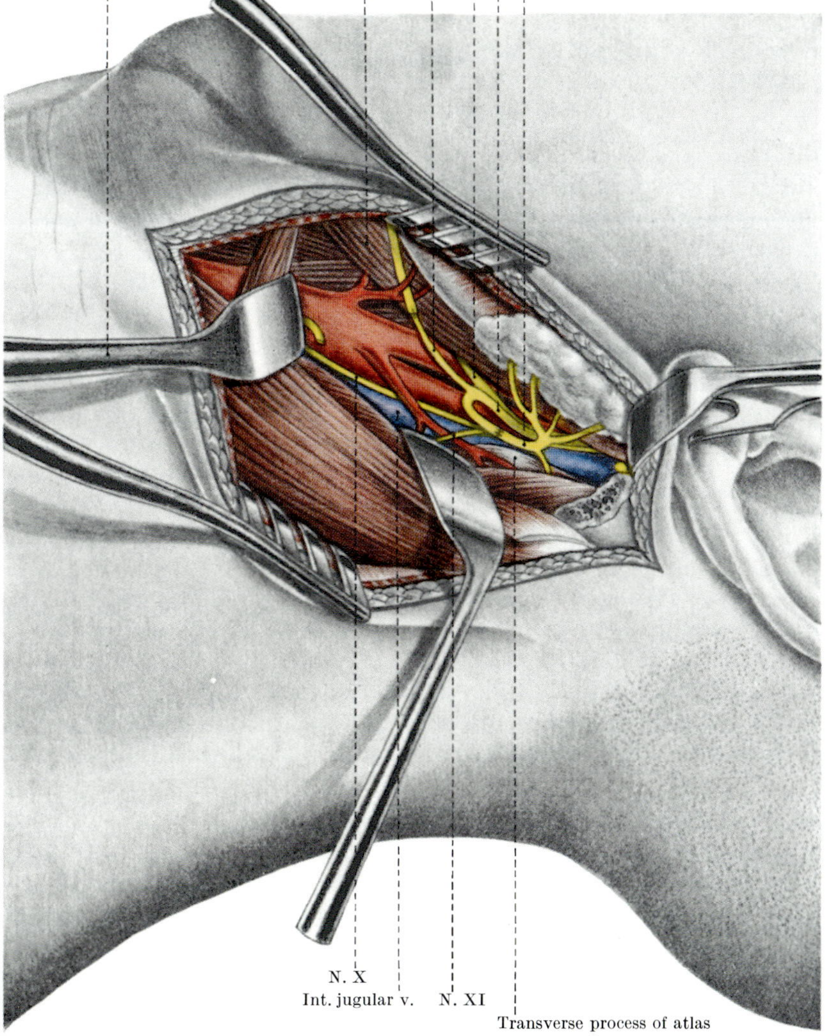

Fig. 251. Hypoglossal-facial anastomosis: Relationship following anastomoses.

Observe: 1. The hypoglossal nerve is brought medial to the digastric muscle and anastomosed with the facial nerve. 2. The descendens hypoglossi is sutured to the distal end of the hypoglossal nerve.

Chapter XXIII

Sympathectomy

A. Low Cervical — Upper Thoracic

The indications for low cervical — upper thoracic sympathectomy include causalgia, Sudeck's post-traumatic dystrophy, post-traumatic neuralgia, hyperhydrosis and vascular disease. Our experience in recent wars has once again taught us the importance of sympathectomy early in the course of the patient's symptoms. To be effective, sympathectomy should be done within three months of the onset of symptoms. The author prefers the anterior cervical approach because of its technical ease and because of the absence of post-operative incisional pain. There is no difficulty in reaching as low as the third thoracic ganglion with this approach.

Under endotracheal anesthesia, the patient is placed in the supine position with the head and chest elevated twenty degrees. This elevation is important since it facilitates the exposure and visualization of the sympathetic chain down into the chest. The head is turned away from the side of the operation (Fig. 252). The skin incision is made parallel to and one fingerbreadth above the clavicle beginning over the clavicular head of the sternocleidomastoid muscle and extending horizontally for 5—7 cm. The platysma muscle is divided. The external jugular vein usually has to be ligated and divided. The clavicular head of the sternocleidomastoid muscle is transected at its insertion to obtain adequate medial exposure. The omohyoid muscle, running obliquely across the wound, is dissected from surrounding adipose tissue and retracted superiorly (Fig. 253). On the left side large lymphatic channels may be identified as they pass in a loop toward the angle between the internal jugular and subclavian veins. The thoracic duct should be protected by a wet cotton pledget. The phrenic nerve is then identified and dissected from the fascia over the anterior scalene muscle (Fig. 253). This nerve may be retracted laterally with the anterior scalene muscle as shown in Fig. 254, or the nerve may be retracted laterally and the muscle transected. If the anterior scalene muscle is well developed, it should be transected. The muscle is elevated by curved hemostats and divided in small increments using a scalpel. The key to finding the stellate ganglion is exposure of the subclavian artery posterior to the anterior scalene muscle. This artery is followed medially to the take-off of the vertebral artery from its superodorsal surface. At this point the vertebral artery is surrounded by fibers from the upper part of the cervico-thoracic sympathetic chain (Fig. 254). The thyrocervical trunk must not be mistakenly identified as the vertebral artery. The thyrocervical trunk is usually short, larger in diameter and arises from the antero-superior surface of the artery. Having identified the sympathetic chain at the origin of the vertebral artery, the fibers are clipped superiorly above the stellate ganglion and transected. The stellate ganglion represents a combination of the inferior cervical and highest, or even the first several, thoracic ganglia. Superficial sympathetic fibers which form a loop around the subclavian artery (ansa subclavia) are also divided. The inferior aspect of the cervicothoracic ganglion lies anterior to the transverse process of the seventh cervical vertebra. The sympathetic chain is followed inferiorly while applying traction to the stellate ganglion. Contributions to the sympathetic ganglia from thoracic nerve roots are divided as they are encountered. The chain passes medially as well as inferiorly in an off-shoot of the pre-vertebral fascia which attaches the inferior rim of the transverse process of C_7 and the inner border of the first rib to the apex of the pleura (Sibson's fascia). At the level of the first rib the sympathetic chain lies laterally, but below this level it passes medial to the heads of the second and third ribs. Sibson's fascia is opened permitting separation of the dome of the pleura from the heads of the ribs and the bodies of the upper thoracic vertebra. This separation is done by finger dissection. As the thoracic sympathetic chain is thus identified, rami will be seen entering and leaving the ganglia. These branches are clipped and divided as they are encountered. These nerves are clipped to avoid bleeding since, with traction on the sympathetic chain, small blood vessels may be mistaken for nerves. The sympathetic chain is clipped and divided below the third thoracic ganglia. Prior to closing, the wound is filled with saline and the anesthetist inflates the lungs. Air bubbles will be seen if a pneumothorax is present. This minor complication is treated by placing an intrapleural catheter to suction and then closing the pleura. The remainder of the wound is carefully reapproximated. Prior to tying the last suture, the anesthetist inflates the lungs and the intrathoracic catheter is removed under continuous suction.

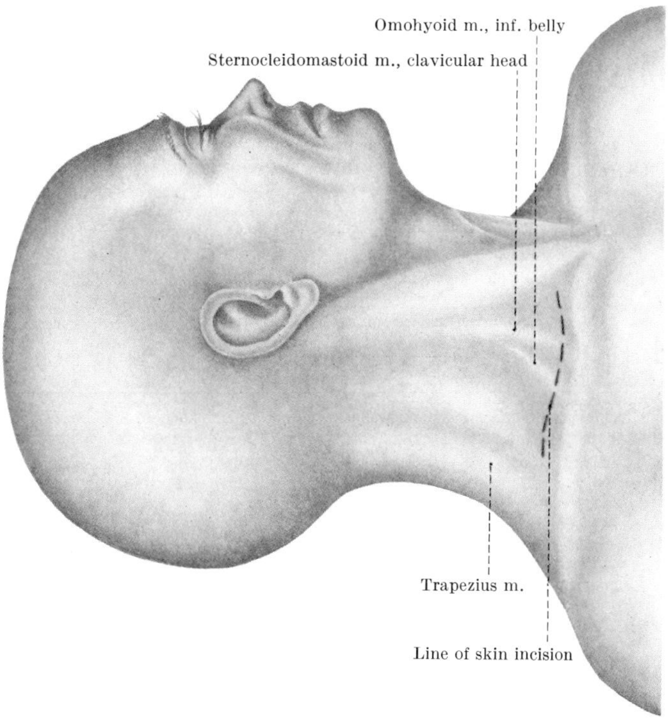

Fig. 252. Sympathectomy, lower cervical-upper dorsal: Skin incision.
Observe: The patient is placed supine on the operating table with the head turned to the side.

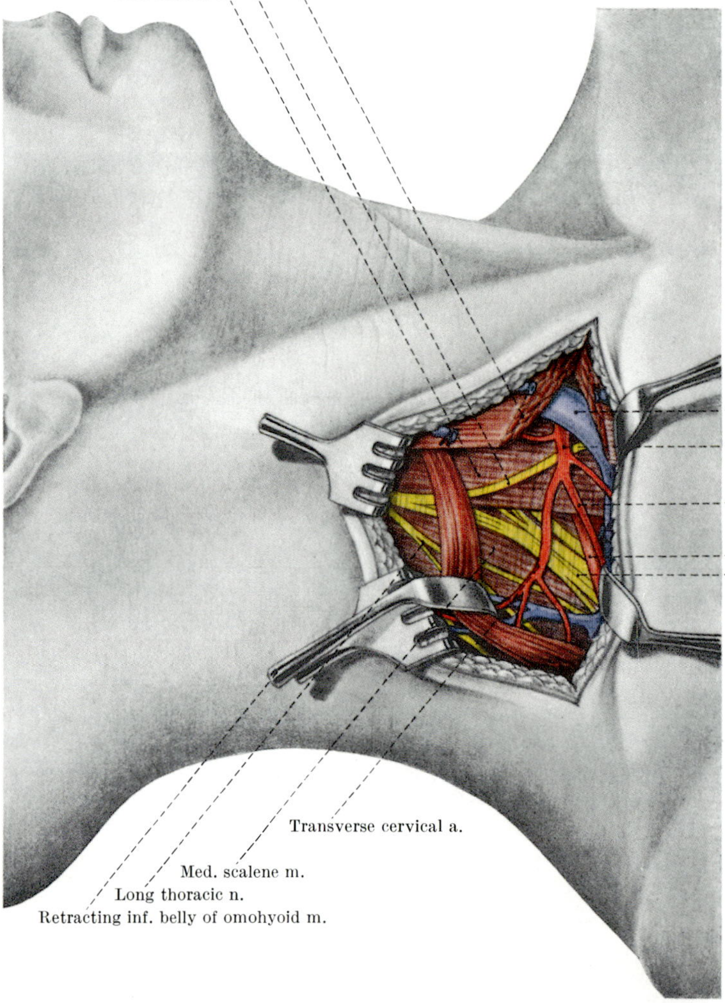

Fig. 253. Sympathectomy, lower cervical-upper thoracic: Exposure of anterior scalene muscle and phrenic nerve.

Observe: 1. The clavicular head of sternocleidomastoid muscle is transected. 2. The venous structures lie in front of the anterior scalene muscle whereas the subclavian artery is behind. 3. The phrenic nerve within the fascial sheat of the anterior scalene muscle passes from posteriosuperiorly to anteroinferiorly.

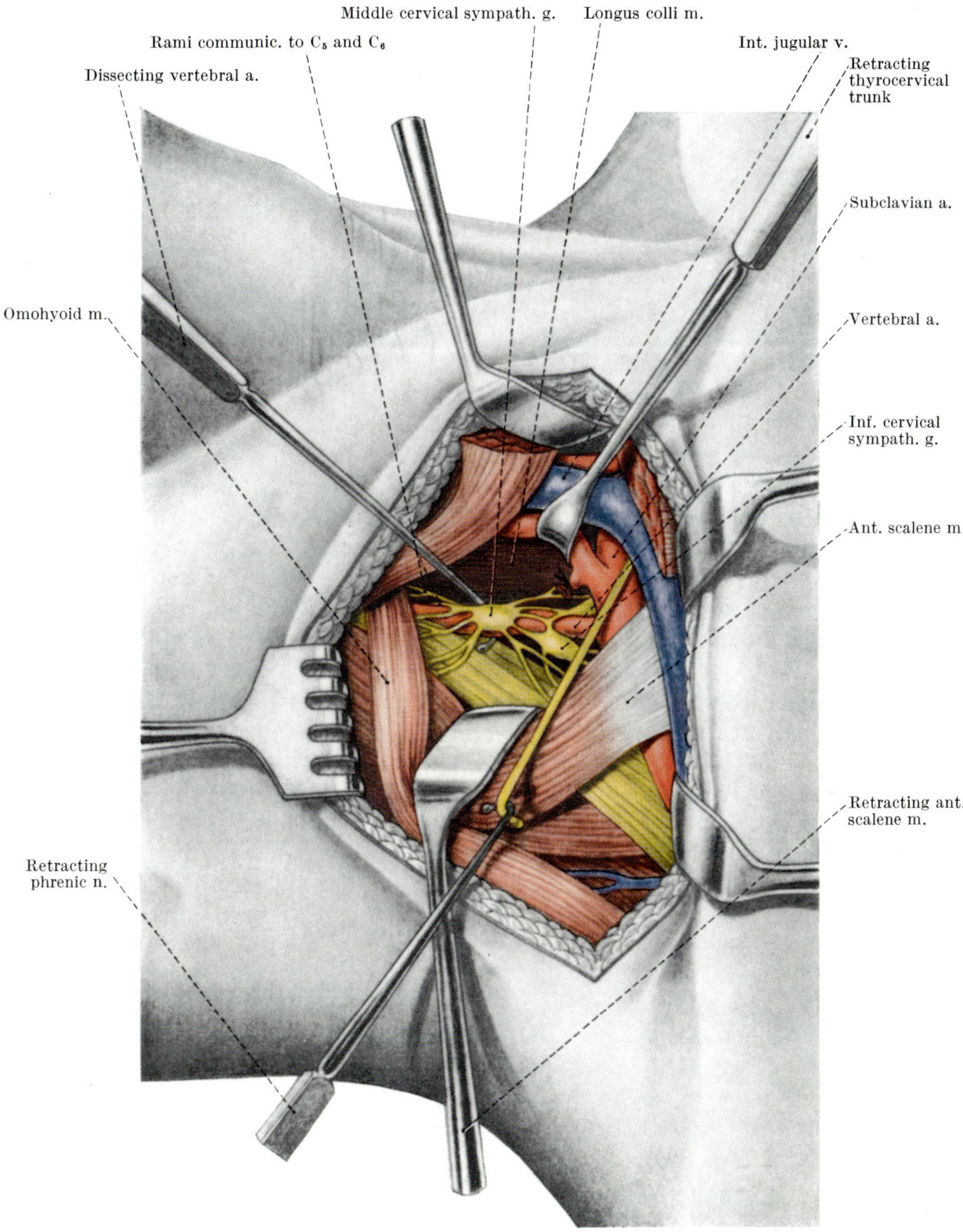

Fig. 254. Sympathectomy, lower cervical-upper dorsal: Exposure of ganglia.

Observe: 1. The phrenic nerve is dissected and retracted laterally. 2. The relationship of the sympathetic ganglia to vertebral artery. 3. The transverse cervical artery is ligated and divided.

B. Lumbar

Indications for lumbar sympathectomy include causalgia and causalgia-like syndromes, hyperhidrosis and vascular disease. The two lumbar sympathetic trunks lie on the vertebral column adjacent to the psoas muscle. Usually there are four or five ganglia but the number is variable. This chain contains preganglionic fibers for pelvic viscera as well as for the lower extremity. For this reason it is well to remember that bilateral removal of the second lumbar ganglia may cause sterility since the emission of semen into the urethra is brought about by sympathetic activity.

The position of the patient for a right lumbar sympathectomy is illustrated in Fig. 255a—c. The hip of the upper leg is flexed slightly to relax the psoas muscle. A kidney bump is used to cause a lumbar scoliosis and, thereby, increase the ilio-costal distance on the upper side. A 10 cm. transverse skin incision is made from the tip of the eleventh rib to just below the umbilicus (Fig. 255). The incision is carried down to the aponeurosis of the external abdominal oblique muscle and the skin and subcutaneous tissues are undermined at this fascial layer. The abdominal muscles are then separated in the direction of their fibers; i.e., the external abdominal oblique muscle obliquely downward, the internal abdominal oblique muscle obliquely upward and the transversus abdominis muscle transversely (Fig. 256). In obese patients it is sometimes wise to extend the muscle incision medially into the lateral border of the rectus sheath. It is important to separate the muscle layers sufficiently so that a funnel does not develop. All retractors are then removed and the surgeon inserts both thumbs as shown in Fig. 257 to separate the peritoneum and renal fascia from the posterolateral abdominal wall. By medial dissection the quadratus lumborum and iliacus muscles are exposed. It is important to remember that the psoas muscle is anterior to and overlaps these muscles. This means that as the lateral border of the psoas muscle is reached dissection must be carried anteriorly onto the belly of this muscle (Fig. 258). The peritoneum is elevated from the psoas muscle and the anterolateral surfaces of the bodies of L_2, L_3 and L_4 are exposed. The sympathetic chain is identified in a groove between the vertebrae and the psoas muscle. The chain is palpated as a fibrous string with periodic enlargements (Fig. 259). A retractor is then placed over the dissecting thumb to retract the peritoneal contents. The posterior abdominal wall must also be carefully protected to avoid injuring the nerves which pass through it (Fig. 260). The genitofemoral nerve emerges through the fibers of the psoas muscle just a centimeter lateral to the sympathetic chain at the level of L_3. The iliohypogastric nerve arising at the L_1 level passes in front of the quadratus lumborum muscle. Injury to these nerves may cause a painful neuritis.

On the right side the vena cava may partially cover the sympathetic chain, and great care must be exercised to avoid tearing small bridging lumbar veins (Fig. 260). These lumbar veins may pass on either side of the sympathetic trunk. Veins passing lateral to the trunk will have to be clipped and divided. The sympathetic chain is elevated with a blunt nerve hook (Fig. 260) or sympathectomy hook, and multiple small rami are clipped and divided. The trunk is then clipped distally at the point where it passes beneath the iliac vessels and proximally at the crus of the diaphragm and removed.

On the left side the sympathetic chain is easier to palpate since the aorta lies medial to it, but it is usually covered by periaortic lumbar lymph nodes. Other than these anatomical differences, the operation is identical on the two sides.

In closing the wound, it will be helpful to remove the kidney bump. This will allow the muscles to fall together as each layer is reapproximated in turn.

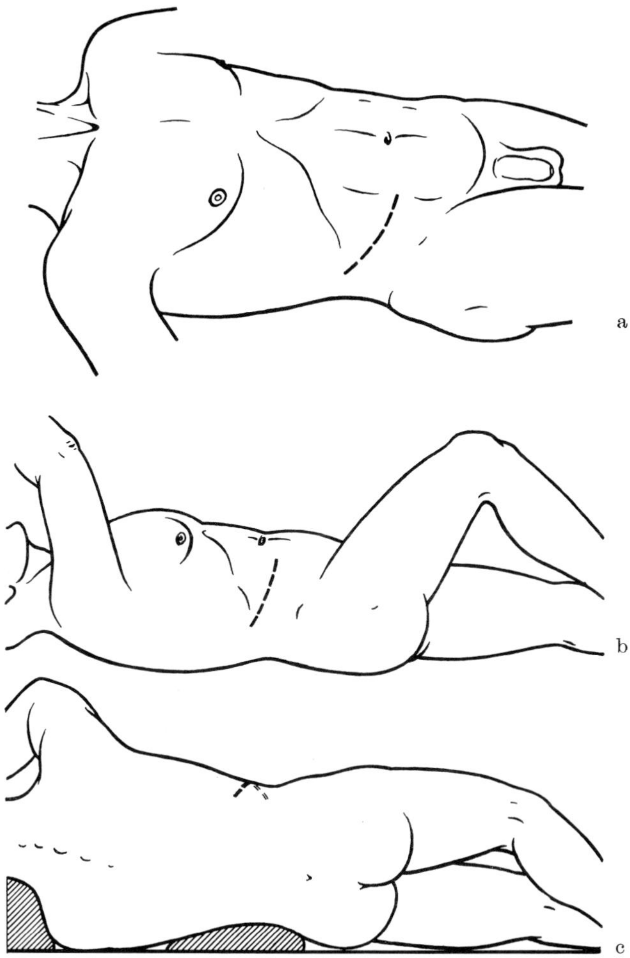

Fig. 255a—c. Sympathectomy, lumbar: Operative position and skin incision.
a Relationship of incision to ribs, iliac crest and abdominal muscles.
b As viewed by surgeon from above.
c Lateral view.

Observe: 1. The thigh is flexed on the side of the incision to relax the psoas muscle.
2. A kidney bump is used to widen the ilio-costal distance.

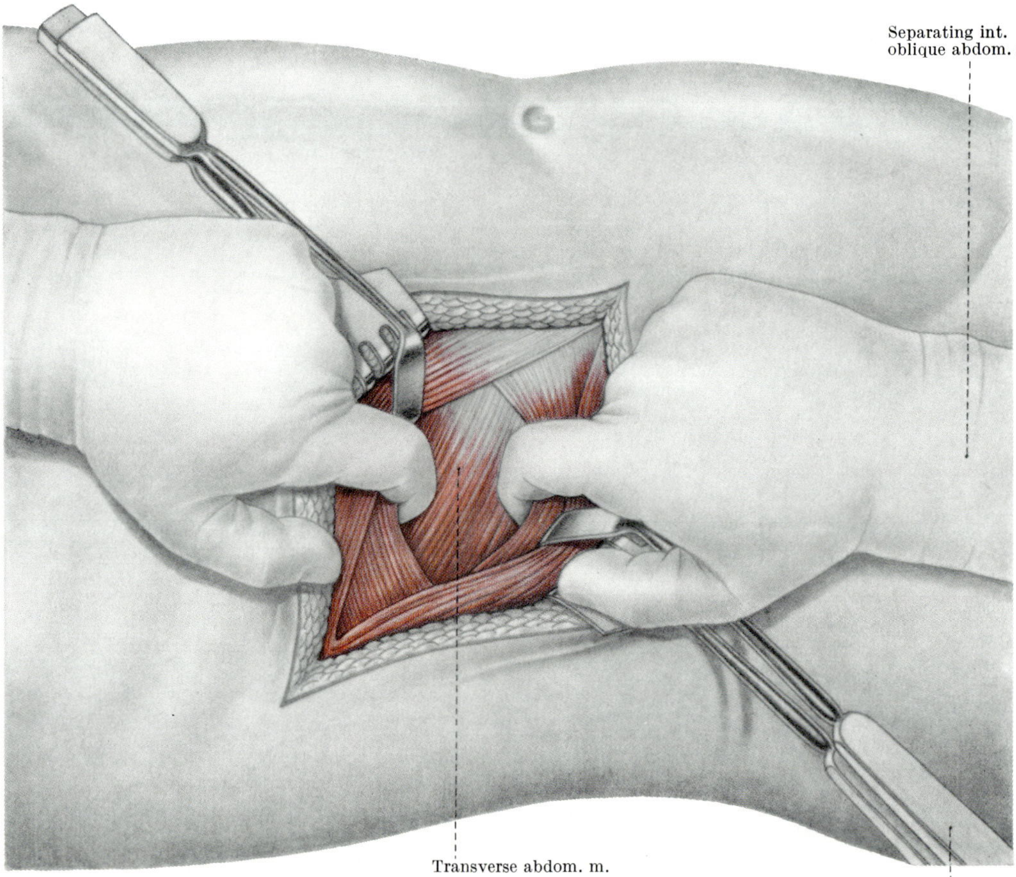

Fig. 256. Sympathectomy, lumbar: Skin and muscle splitting incision.
Observe: Abdominal muscles are separated in the direction of their fibers.

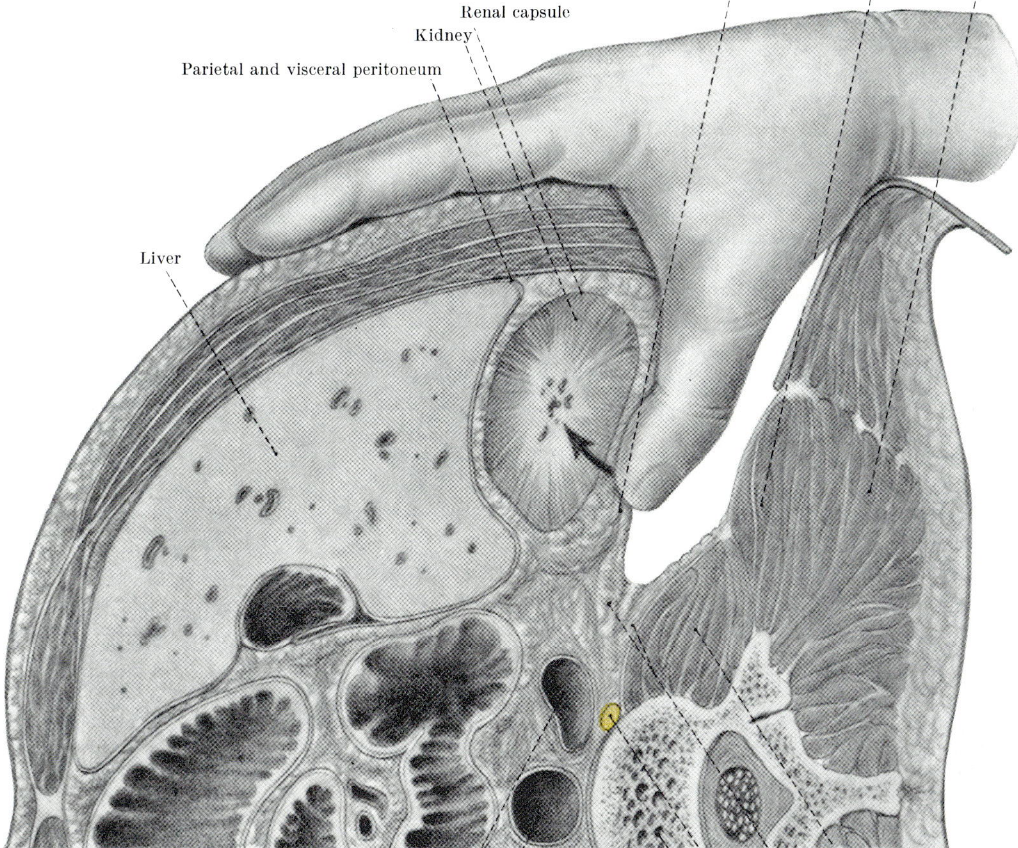

Fig. 257. Sympathectomy, lumbar: Separating renal fascial and peritoneal contents from the lateral and posterior abdominal wall.

Observe: 1. This transverse section is at the level of the third lumbar vertebra. 2. It is important to avoid entering the renal fascia.

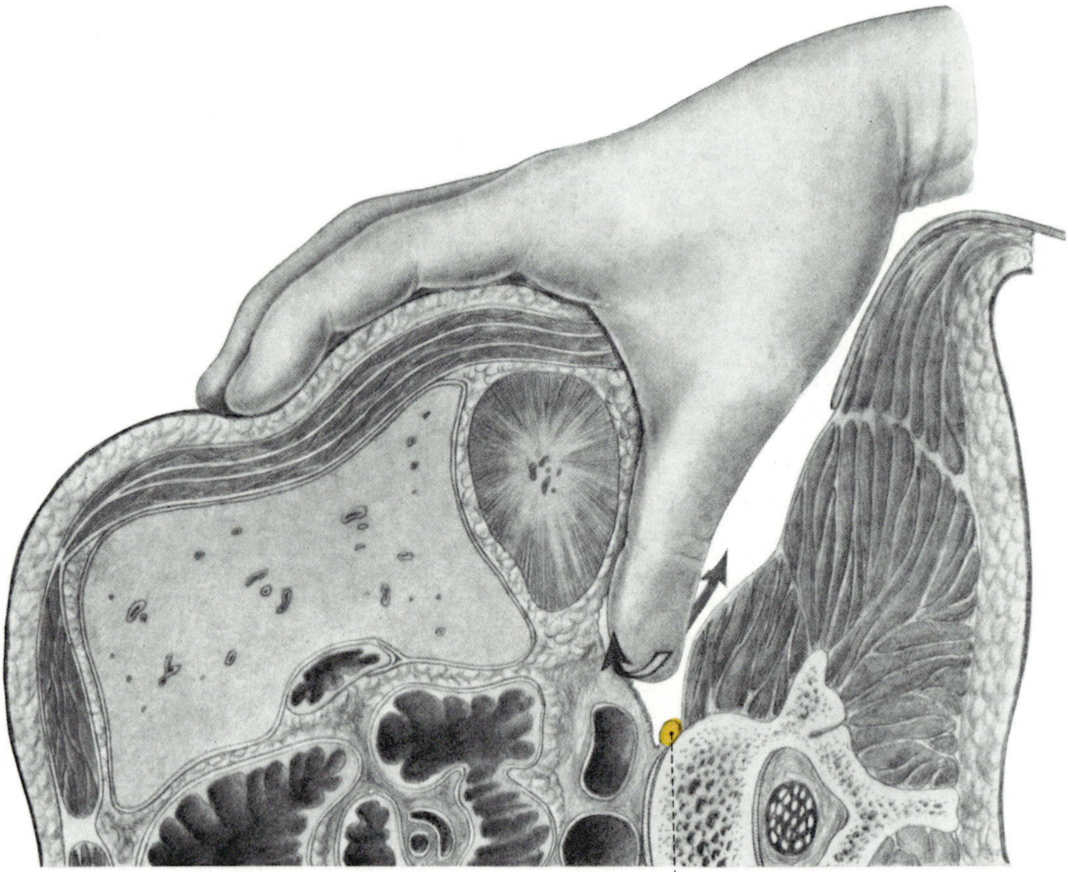

Fig. 258. Sympathectomy, lumbar: Blunt dissection of renal fascia and peritoneum from the posterior abdominal wall.

Observe: The thumb serves as a very sensitive instrument for this maneuver.

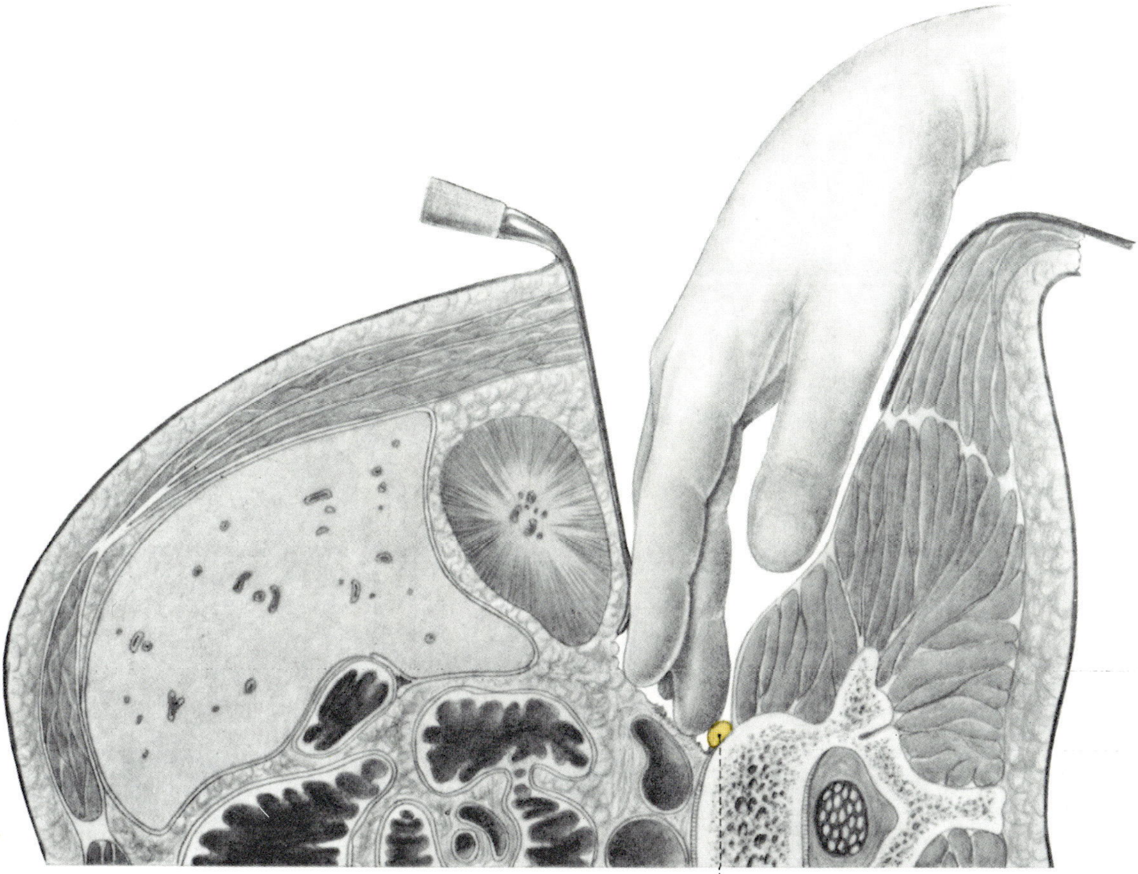

Fig. 259. Sympathectomy, lumbar: Identification of the sympathetic trunk by palpation.
Observe: On the right side the sympathetic trunk may be covered by the inferior vena cava.

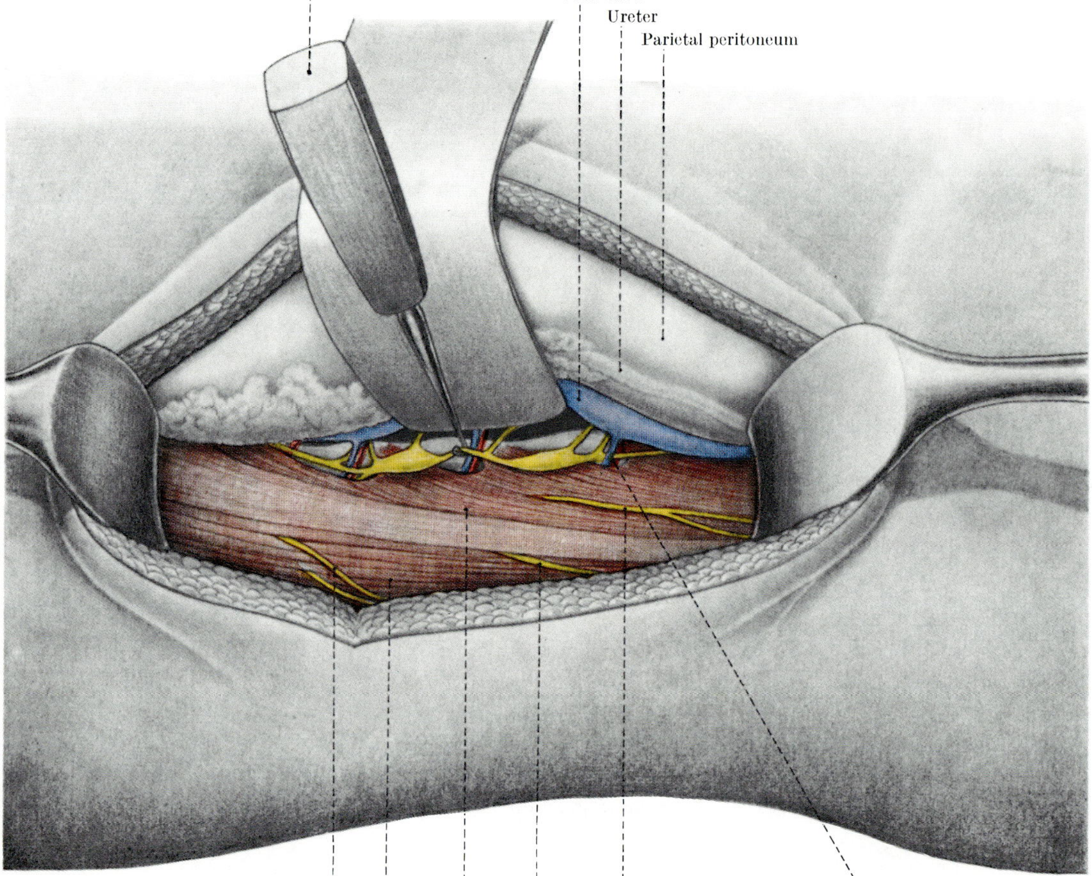

Fig. 260. Sympathectomy, lumbar: Exposure of the third and fourth lumbar ganglia.

Observe: 1. Lumbar veins bridge the sympathetic chain. 2. The position of the genitofemoral nerve about 1 cm. lateral to the sympathetic trunk on the ventral surface of the psoas muscle.

Chapter XXIV

Cervical Radiculoneuropathy

Herniated Intervertebral Disc and Spondylosis

A. Posterior Approach — Laminectomy

Cervical radiculoneuropathy may be due to rupture of an intervertebral disc or spondylosis or a combination of these two processes. The so-called soft disc is caused by rupture of the posterior annulus fibrosis with herniation of the nucleus pulposus. Fig. 261 illustrates a typical laterally extruded disc. The posterior annulus fibrosis is weakest at its lateral extent and the posterior longitudinal ligament is thinnest over the lateral attachment of the annulus. As a result, most degenerated discs present with protrusion or extrusion in this area. Because the nerve root is stretched over this area on its way to the intervertebral foramen, only a minute amount of extruded disc material is necessary to produce symptoms and signs of radiculoneuropathy.

Progressive wear and tear of the mobile connections between cervical vertebrae result in characteristic changes in the intervertebral discs and adjacent structures which are called cervical spondylosis. As the disc degenerates, the intervertebral space narrows. The edges of the vertebral end-plates become elongated, forming osteophytic bars. The uncinate processes bend laterally and spurring occurs along the edges of the uncovertebral joints. All of these changes lead to reduction in the size of the spinal canal and intervertebral foramina. Either myelopathy or radiculopathy may result. Whether these states result from mechanical or vascular causes has not yet been completely elucidated. It is remarkable that this process is often much more severe on one side than the other (Fig. 262). Spondylosis, as well as degenerative disc disease, most often involves the C_{5-6} and C_{6-7} levels.

The author believes that unilateral herniated intervertebral discs can be removed by either the anterior or posterior approach. Cervical spondylosis involving three or less levels is treated with an anterior approach. Cervical spondylosis which is generalized and cervical stenosis should be treated by a total laminectomy which extends well above and below the area of pathology (see Cervical Laminectomy, Chapter XIII).

Preoperative studies should, in our opinion, include myelography. Discography, in our experience, has not proved to be useful. Discography is not reliable enough to warrant the added risk and discomfort to the patient.

A unilateral semi-hemi-laminectomy for a soft disc is illustrated in this chapter.

The patient is placed in the sitting position and all of the precautions necessary with this position (see Chapter I) must be taken. The neck is only slightly flexed (Fig. 263). Venous stasis and tightening of the paravertebral muscles result from marked flexion. In addition to these two good reasons for not flexing the neck, it must be remembered that severe flexion in the anesthetized patient with an already compromised spinal canal may result in an increase in neurological deficit. X-rays, including the myelogram and a lateral view of the cervical spine, must be on the view box in the operating room.

One of the most difficult tasks in this operation is to ascertain the proper vertebral level. The only reliable methop of counting cervical vertebrae at the time of surgery is to identify C_2 and count down. Because this is not always practical (e.g., as in a C_{5-6} and C_{6-7} hemilaminectomy), various methods of x-ray confirmation of the level have been devised. The author prefers to ascertain the appropriate level before making the skin incision.

A spinal needle is introduced, as shown in Fig. 263, in a vertical direction into the spinous process of the vertebra which is thought to be the appropriate level. The direction of insertion of the needle is vertical to prevent penetration of the spinal canal and to afford better visualization on x-ray. A lateral x-ray is taken. If it localizes the needle at the proper vertebral level, two drops of methylene blue are injected to mark the spinous process.

A 6 cm. skin incision is made centering over the marked spinous process. The incision is carried down to the ligamentum nuchae and self-retaining retractors are inserted. The spinous processes and laminae of adjacent vertebrae above and below the level of the lesion are stripped subperiosteally on the symptomatic side. Removal of the bifid process on this side will help in this subperiosteal dissection. The paravertebral muscles are stripped back as far as the facet joints. Using a sharp curette the lower rim of the superior lamina is exposed, and using a fine blunt spatula the ligamentum flavum is dissected free of this lamina. With a thin-lipped Kerrison rongeur the inferior one-half of the lamina is removed as illustrated in Fig. 264. If two lamina overlap to the extent that a rongeur cannot easily be inserted between them, it is sometimes safer to use a Hudson drill with the acorn-shaped burr or a high-speed electric drill to make an opening between the lamina. The upper one-half of the inferior lamina is also removed. Laterally, removal of the bone ends at the facet joint. Sufficient bone must be removed so that the disc can be approached from either above or below the nerve root. The ligamentum flavum, which becomes very thin in the cervical regions, is removed to expose the dura. Using a fine blunt instrument, palpation beneath the nerve root is done from both above and below. This may cause bleeding from epidural veins which can be controlled with tiny cotton pledgets (Fig. 265). These cotton pledgets must not cause pressure on the dural column. The nerve root may be flattened into a ribbon by the protruding disc. Great care is necessary in separating the dural sleeve of the nerve root from the underlying disc and reactive adhesions. The nerve root is either gently elevated or depressed depending on exactly where the disc is presenting. Traction is never placed medially on the dural column. As soon as the disc fragment is visualized, it should be teased out using a pituitary forceps (Fig. 266). Once the extruded fragment is removed the nerve root will be much less tense, and then additional dissection can be carried out looking for other disc material. It may be necessary to widen the opening into the interspace using a small sharp curette. Palpation must be carried out along the nerve root into the intervertebral foramen to make certain that a fragment is not left behind.

If palpation and inspection of the epidural space suggests that the herniation is more medially placed, no attempt should be made to reach this mass extradurally. The dura is opened with a half-moon shaped incision (Fig. 267), and the dura is reflected. Fig. 268 shows the dentate ligament being tightly stretched over the bulging anterior mass. The denticulate ligament is sectioned and the anterior dura is incised over the mass. The herniated disc can then be removed without traction on the nerve root or spinal cord (Fig. 269). The dural opening can be closed with a few fine silk sutures. Epidural bleeding should be readily controlled with a tiny piece of absorbable gelatin soaked in topical thrombin. When epidural bleeding is troublesome, it often indicates that the neck has been flexed too much. A slight adjustment in position may result in a dramatic cessation of bleeding.

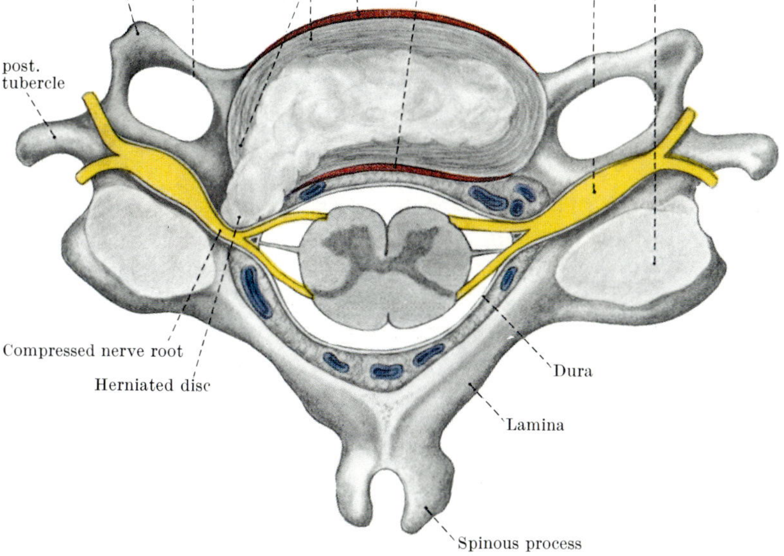

Fig. 261. Cervical radiculoneuropathy: Herniated disc. This transverse section is of the mid cervical region.

Observe: 1. Lateral herniation of the disc. 2. Relationship of herniation to the lateral extent of the posterior longitudinal ligament.

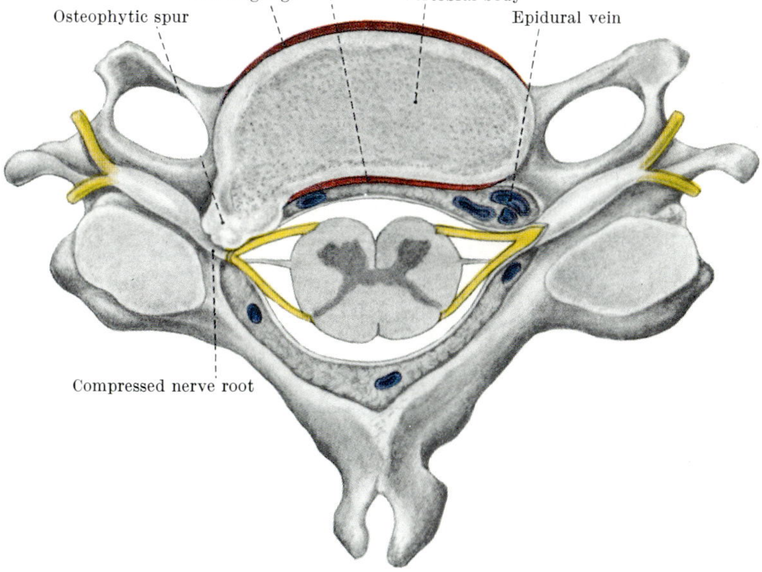

Fig. 262. Cervical radiculoneuropathy: Spondylosis. This transverse section is of the mid cervical region.

Observe: 1. Compression of the nerve root by the bony spur. 2. Extention of the dural sleeve onto the nerve root.

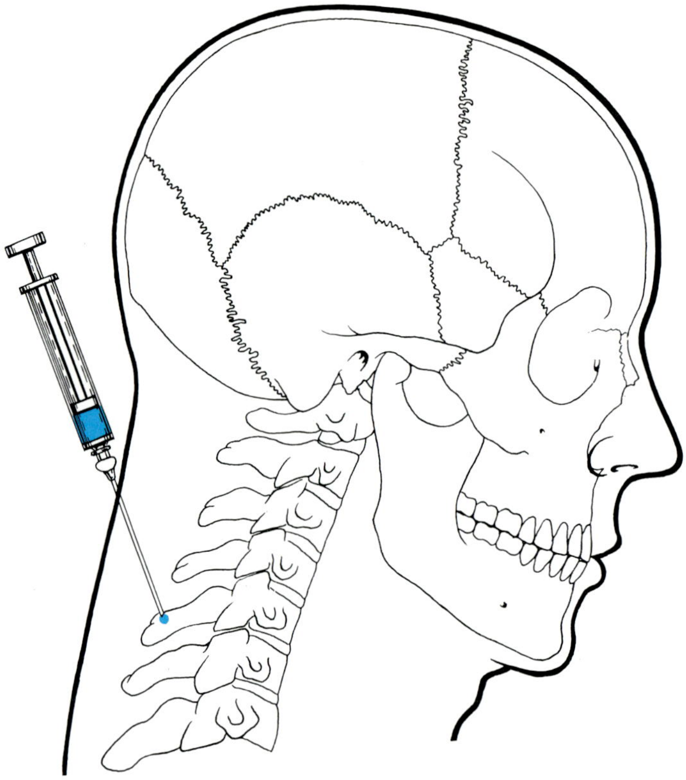

Fig. 263. Cervical hemilaminectomy for herniated disc. The vertebral level may be determined by preoperative x-ray with injection of methylene blue.

Observe: 1. The needle is directed at this angle to avoid entering the theca. 2. The head and neck in this illustration are properly aligned for operation in the sitting position.

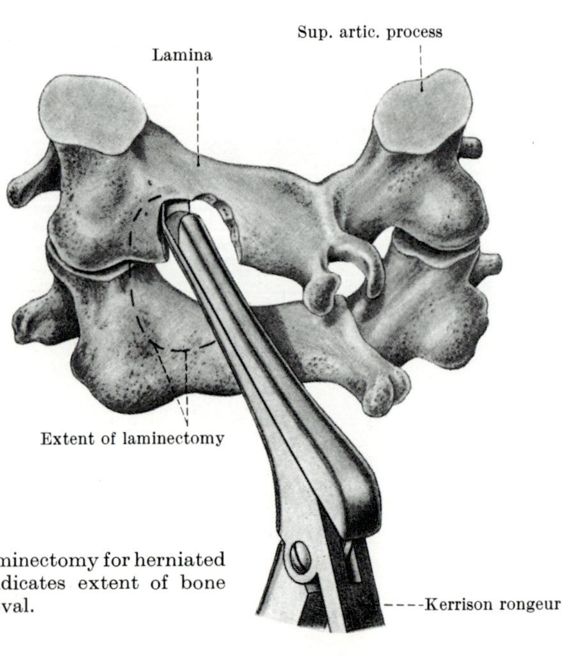

Fig. 264. Cervical hemilaminectomy for herniated disc. The dotted line indicates extent of bone removal.

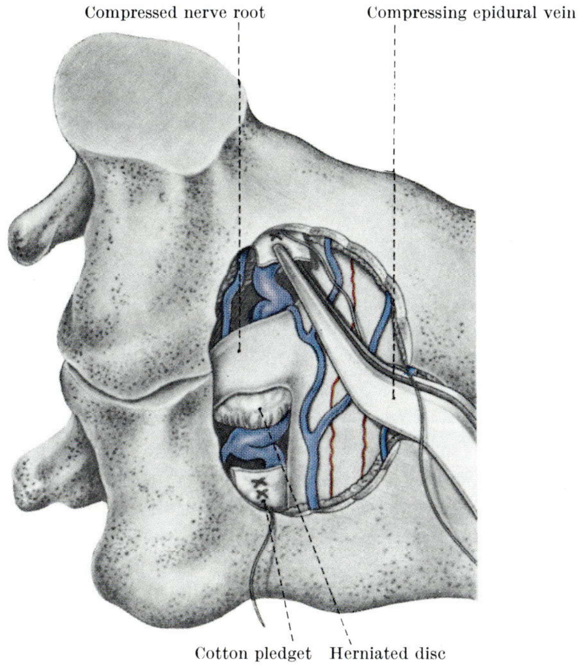

Fig. 265. Cervical hemilaminectomy for a laterally herniated disc. Having exposed the compressed nerve root, tiny cotton pledgets are placed laterally to compress the epidural veins.

Observe: 1. The dura covering the spinal cord does not have to be retracted for this laterally extruded disc. 2. Displacement of nerve root by underlying disc fragment.

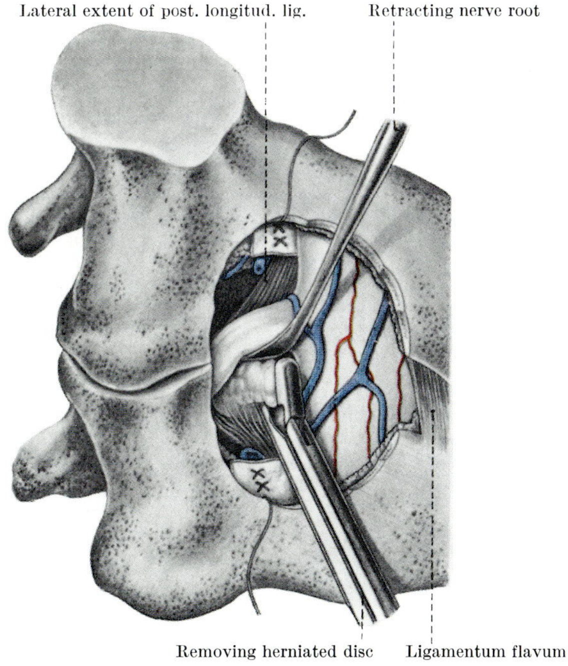

Fig. 266. Cervical hemilaminectomy for a laterally herniated disc. The nerve root is gently retracted and the herniated disc is removed.

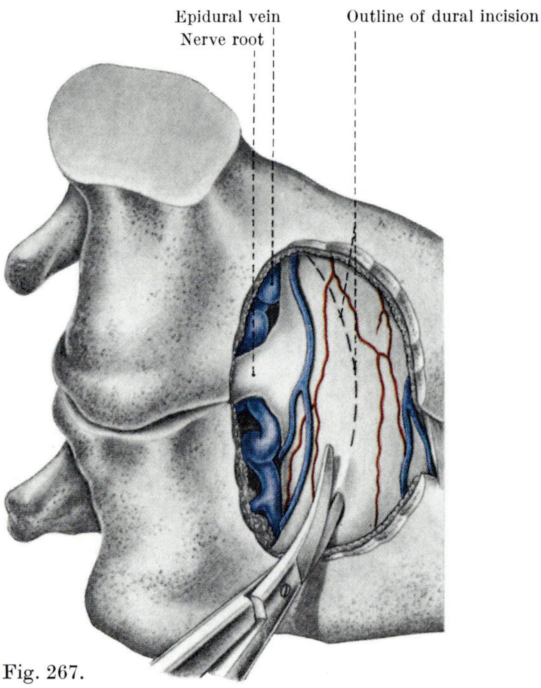

Fig. 267.

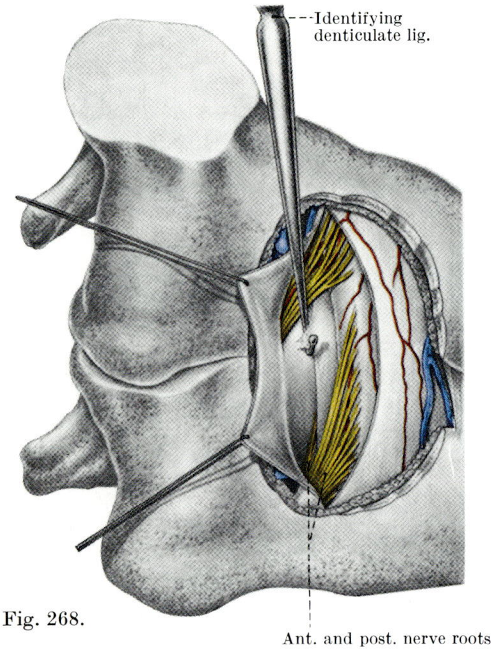

Fig. 268.

Fig. 267. Cervical hemilaminectomy for herniated disc: Transdural approach. This approach is used for a more medially located fragment than depicted in Figs. 265 and 266.

Fig. 268. Cervical hemilaminectomy for herniated disc: Transdural approach.

Observe: 1. Bulging anterior dura over underlying disc. 2. Tense denticulate ligament.

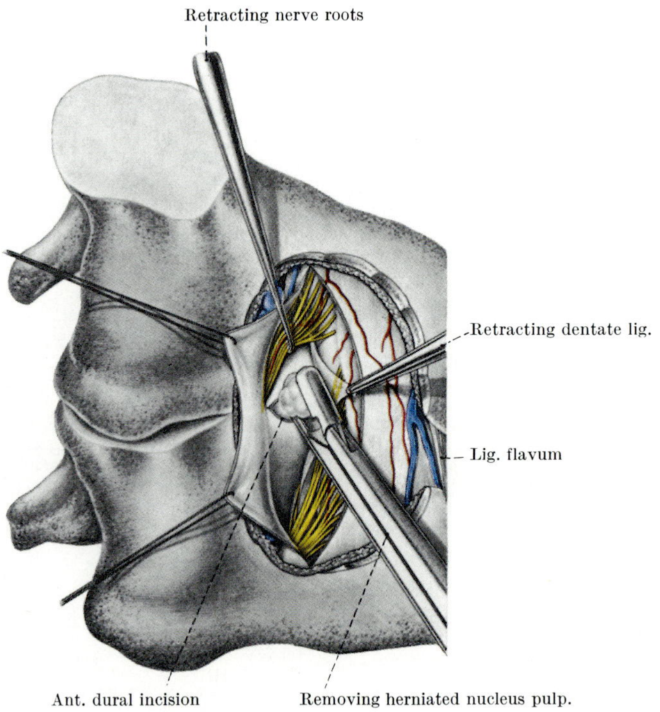

Fig. 269. Cervical hemilaminectomy for herniated disc: Transdural approach.

Observe: 1. The denticulate ligament is transected and retracted.
2. The anterior dura is incised over the ruptured disc.

B. Anterior Approach — Cloward Technique

The anterior approach for the removal of cervical discs and osteophytes has been used almost exclusively since 1960 at Walter Reed General Hospital. A total of over 700 patients with radiculoneuropathy or myelopathy constitute our experience with this procedure. The technique of anterior disc and spur removal with fusion was introduced by CLOWARD[1], and it must be emphasized that the instruments which he has developed are essential to make this operation the safe and elegant procedure which it can be. No attempt will be made to describe the various surgical instruments: only the pertinent steps of the operation will be described.

The patient is placed supine on the operating table with a small sand bag under the nape of the neck (Fig. 271) and a small sand bag under the right hip. The head is kept straight. General endotracheal anesthesia is used. The A-P view of the myelogram is placed on the view box. Using the mind's eye the level of the lesion above the clavicle is measured, and this distance is then transferred to the patient to determine the level of the transverse skin incision (Figs. 270 and 272). The right-handed surgeon will find it easier to work on the patient's right side. The incision is made from the midline to over the anterolateral border of the sternocleidomastoid muscle. The platysma muscle is also incised transversely the entire width of the skin incision. The platysma muscle is elevated at both the inferior and superior margins of the wound and blunt dissection is carried out immediately beneath this muscle. This subplatysmal dissection is imperative if more than one vertebral level is being exposed. The cervical fascia is opened vertically just anterior to the sternocleidomastoid muscle. Using blunt finger dissection the interval between the carotid sheath and midline visceral structures is developed. Using hand retractors the carotid sheath is held laterally and the esophagus and trachea medially. The prevertebral fascia is opened in the midline. Vertebral bodies and intervertebral discs are easily palpable. The level thought to be appropriate is selected and, without further dissection, is labeled by a radio-opaque marker. (A short hypodermic needle serves this purpose well.) A lateral x-ray of the cervical spine is taken.

While waiting for the x-ray to be developed, attention is directed to the region of the right iliac crest. A 6 cm. vertical incision is made 2 cm. behind the anterior superior spine. The incision is carried down to the fascia lata which is then opened using a *T*-shaped incision. The top of the *T* parallels the iliac crest but leaves enough of a rim of fascia for adequate closure. The muscle is stripped back using a sharp periosteal elevator. Using the dowel-cutting instrument perpendicular to the bone (Figs. 278 and 279), as many bone grafts as needed are obtained. The grafts must have cortical layers on each end and should be denuded of any soft tissue attachments. The bone grafts are wrapped in a saline-soaked sponge and saved. Bone wax is used to control bleeding from the ilium. This wound is closed in layers.

Having ascertained the appropriate cervical vertebral level by x-ray, attention must once again be directed to the neck. The hand retractors are inserted as before, and the longus colli muscles are stripped laterally from the anterior surfaces of the two vertebral bodies adjacent to the interspace which will be explored (Fig. 273). Self-retaining retractors are then inserted. The teeth of the laterally retracting blades should be inserted into the longus colli muscles and must not be displaced throughout the remainder of the operation. The anterior longitudinal ligament is scraped off the vertebrae and retracted laterally with the prevertebral muscles. A window is made into the interspace with a No. 11 scalpel blade. The incision should be carried laterally as far as the retractors will permit. Using a pituitary forceps, as much disc material as can be visualized is removed. An interspace spreader may be helpful in enlarging the space so that all disc material can be removed. The interspace spreader is removed, and a burr hole, centered

[1] CLOWARD, R. B.: The anterior approach for removal of ruptured cervical discs. J. Neurosurg. **15**, 602—617 (1958).

on the interspace, is made. The drill must be held perpendicular to the interspace (Figs. 274 and 275). The drill must not deviate to either side but will be pointed slightly superiorly to follow the contour of the disc space. In drilling this hole it is extremely helpful and time saving to wear a head light. The head light makes it possible to look down the drill guard and to see the bottom of the burr hole. This means that the drill guard never has to be moved once it is properly positioned. It is imperative that an assistant hold firmly onto the drill guard throughout the process of drilling the hole. The drilling is stopped at the posterior longitudinal ligament. A cotton pledget soaked in topical thrombin can be used to control bone bleeding. Bone wax should be avoided, if possible, as it will interfere with bony fusion. The lateral margins of the interspace are cleaned out of any remaining soft tissue fragments. A small elevator is used to free the anterior longitudinal ligament from the bone laterally. The region of the nerve root is then palpated bilaterally. Using thin-lipped Kerrison rongeurs and cervical punchs, the bone surrounding the burr hole is removed as illustrated in Figs. 276 and 277. All bone and disc material must be removed from the anterior surface of the nerve root without disturbing the vertebral artery in its position lateral to the vertebral bodies between the foramina transversarium. Beginning laterally where the ligament has already been freed, the posterior longitudinal ligament is removed across the entire width of the interspace. The author firmly believes that the removal of this ligament is an integral part of each anterior cervical fusion. Very commonly extruded fragments of disc material or globular pieces of redundant ligament are removed during this part of the operation. Each neural foramen is then palpated once again to assure the decompression of both nerve roots.

The depth of the space is measured and compared with the height of the graft. The graft should be 2—6 mm. shorter than the hole. The graft is inserted while the interspace spreaders maximally enlarge the vertical diameter of the hole. The graft is inserted so that it lies in the middle of the depth of the burr hole. The graft should always be countersunk slightly from the anterior surfaces of the vertebrae. After removing the interspace retractor, the stability of the cervical spine is examined by having the anesthetist gently flex the neck. Bone chips obtained from drilling the burr hole are placed laterally around the bone plug. The wound is closed in layers after hemostasis has been achieved. Drainage of this wound is not only unnecessary but may lead to infection. The platysma muscle layer is obviously the key layer in this closure. The skin is loosely approximated with fine silk sutures which are removed on the third or fourth post-operative day.

When a fusion is to be accomplished at more than one level, a few additional points are worth remembering. All interspaces involved should be exposed at the same time. When the exposed interspaces are not equally accessible, always do the hardest level first. The burr holes should be placed off-center in both the A-P and lateral dimensions. Each level should be completed in turn before proceeding to the next rather than to drill all the holes at one time.

On the first post-operative day all patients are placed in a Minerva jacket which remains on for six weeks. After comparing 100 consecutive anterior cervical fusions with and without post-operative immobilization, it became our firm conviction that the use of the plaster jacket leads to more prompt fusion with less patient discomfort.

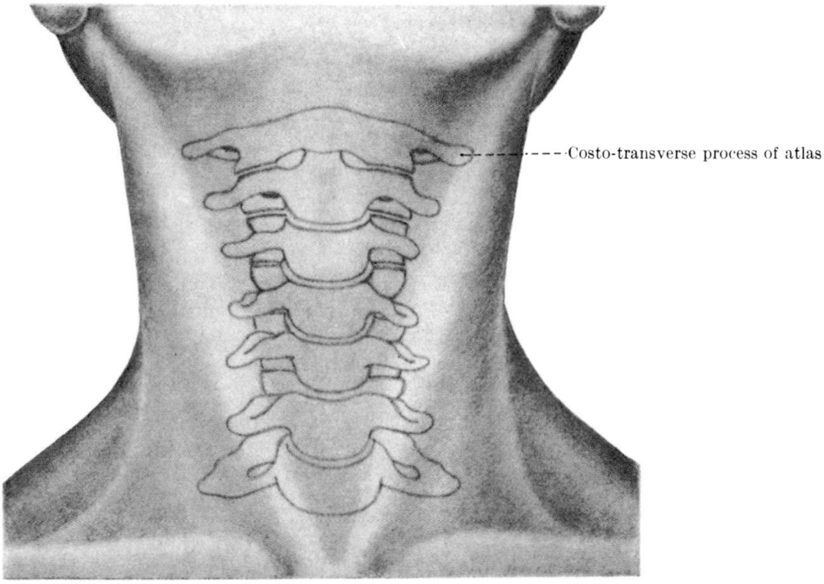

Fig. 270. Anterior cervical fusion (Cloward procedure) for herniated disc or spondylosis. The cervical vertebral column has been superimposed on the skin and soft tissue landmarks of the anterior neck to aid in orientation.

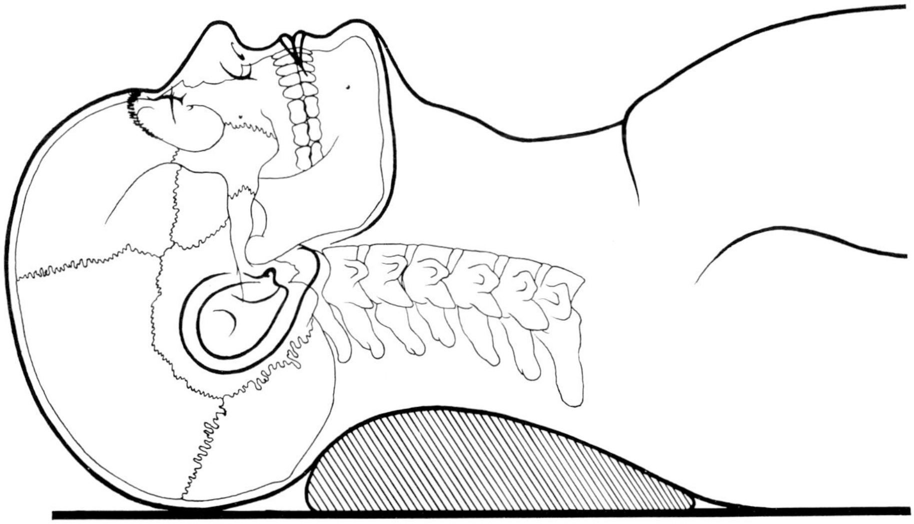

Fig. 271. Anterior cervical fusion (Cloward procedure) for herniated disc or spondylosis: Operative position of the patient.

Observe: 1. Normal cervical lordosis is maintained by a sandbag beneath patient's neck. 2. The face is kept straight.

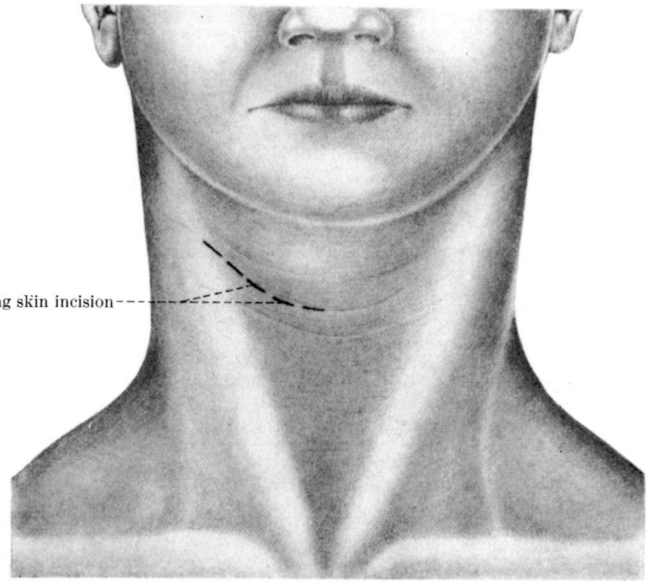

Fig. 272. Anterior cervical fusion (Cloward procedure) for herniated disc or spondylosis: Skin incision.

Observe: The incision begins in the midline and follows a normal skin crease to the anterolateral margin of the sternocleidomastoid muscle.

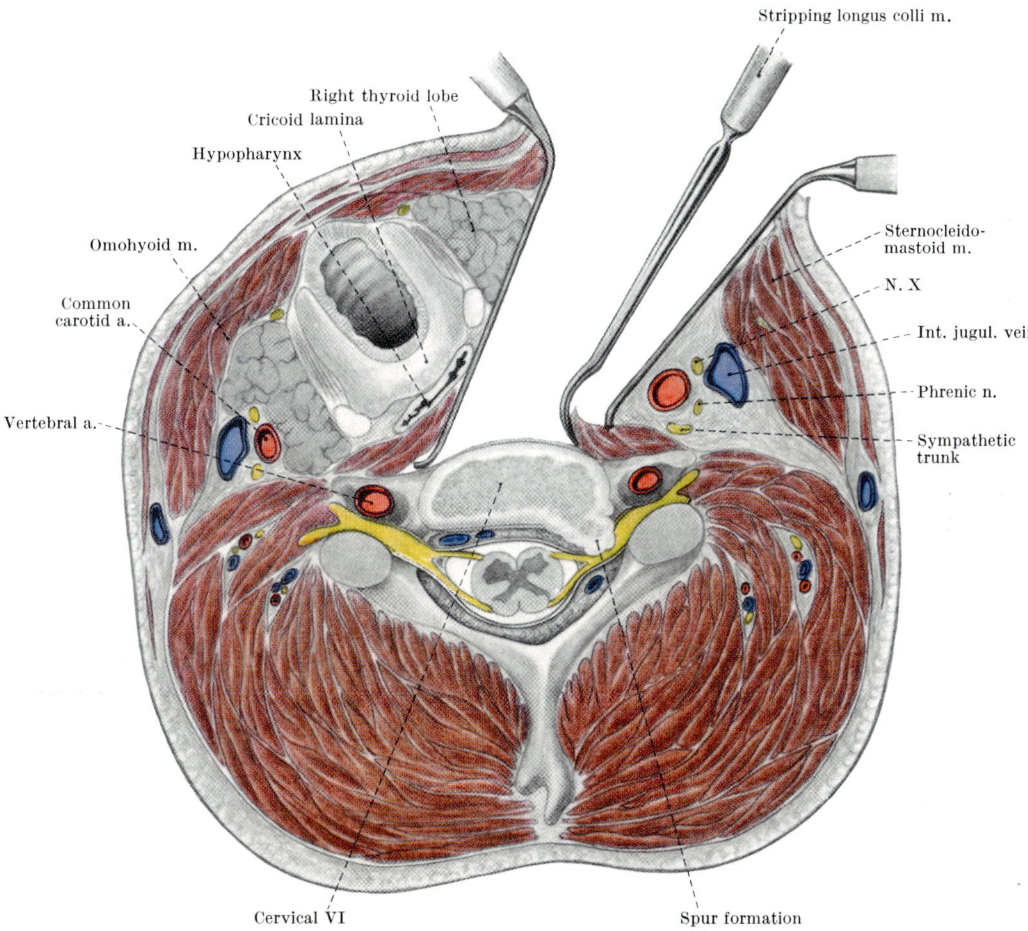

Fig. 273. Anterior cervical fusion (Cloward procedure) for herniated disc or spondylosis: Approach to anterior vertebral surface. This is a transverse section of the neck at the level of C_6.

Observe: 1. The neurovascular structures are retracted laterally and the visceral structures medially. 2. The longus colli muscles are stripped laterally to expose the anterior surface of the vertebrae.

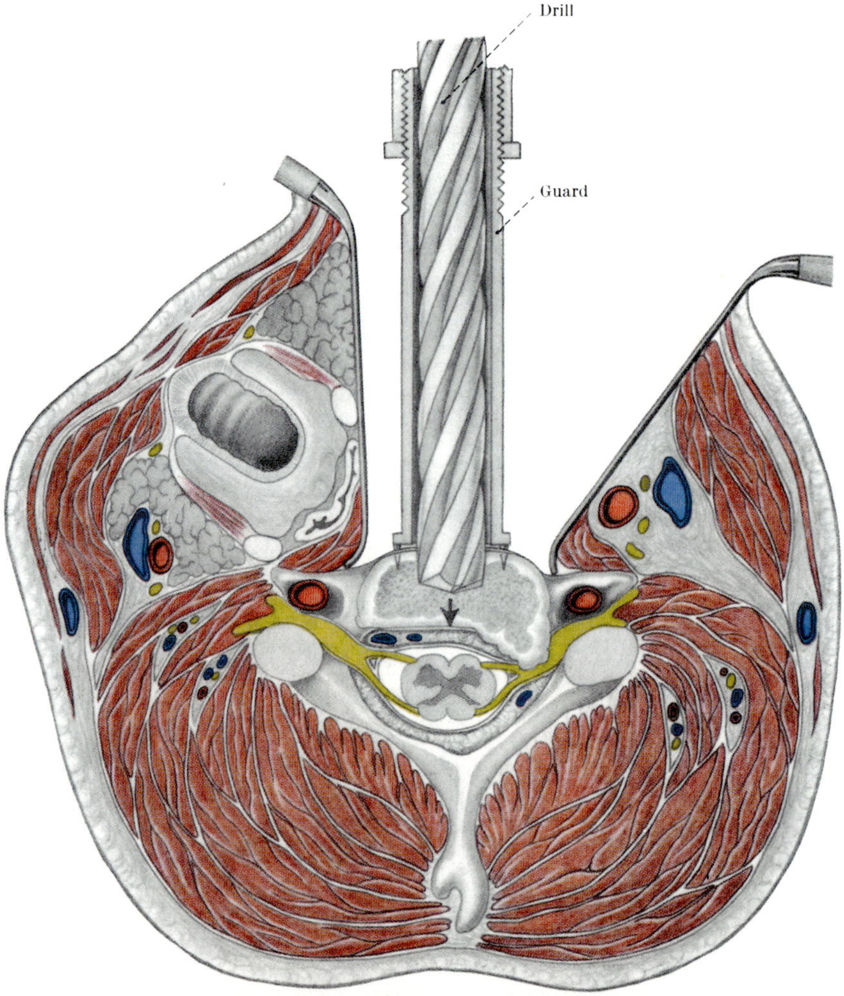

Fig. 274. Anterior cervical fusion (Cloward procedure) for herniated disc or spondylosis: Drilling the hole. This transverse section of the mid cervical region illustrates the proper position of the drill with drill guard.

Observe: The perpendicular position of the drill.

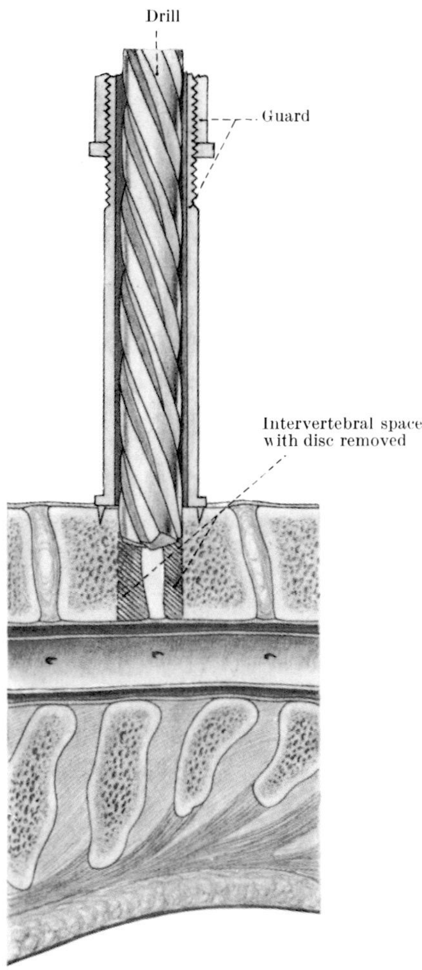

Fig. 275. Anterior cervical fusion (Cloward procedure) for herniated disc or spondylosis: Drilling the hole. This sagittal section of the mid cervical region demonstrates the proper position of the drill with drill guard.

Observe: The disc has been removed prior to drilling the hole.

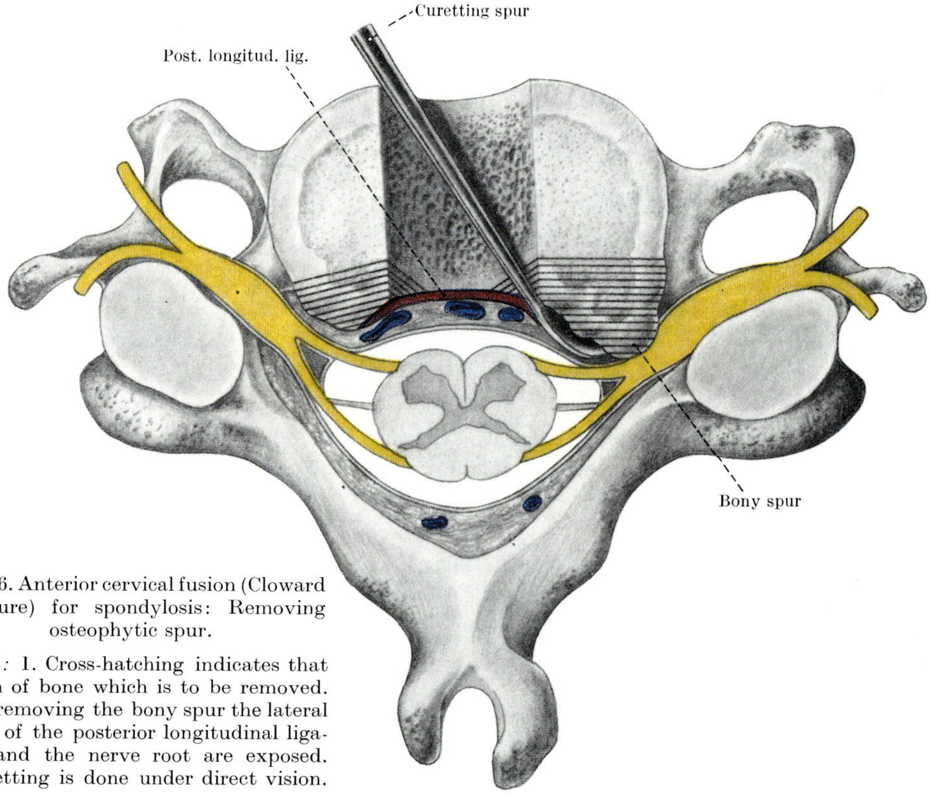

Fig. 276. Anterior cervical fusion (Cloward procedure) for spondylosis: Removing osteophytic spur.

Observe: 1. Cross-hatching indicates that portion of bone which is to be removed. 2. By removing the bony spur the lateral extent of the posterior longitudinal ligament and the nerve root are exposed. 3. Curetting is done under direct vision.

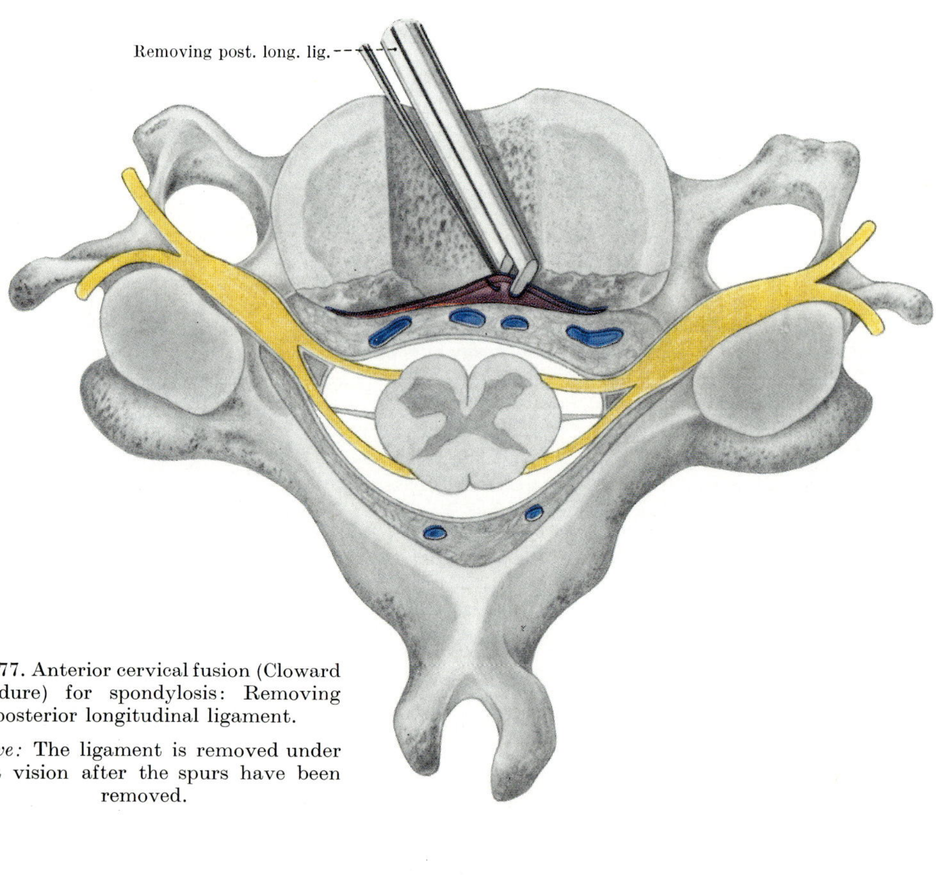

Fig. 277. Anterior cervical fusion (Cloward procedure) for spondylosis: Removing posterior longitudinal ligament.

Observe: The ligament is removed under direct vision after the spurs have been removed.

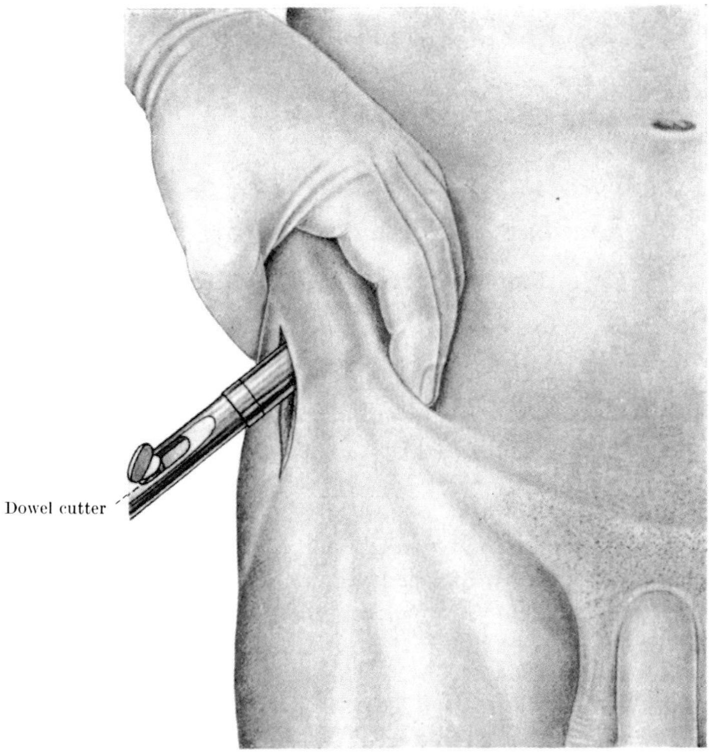

Fig. 278. Anterior cervical fusion (Cloward procedure) for herniated disc or spondylosis: Taking dowel graft from iliac crest.

Observe: 1. Incision starting below iliac crest to prevent irritation of scar by belt clothing, etc. 2. A hand displaces and protects the abdominal viscera.

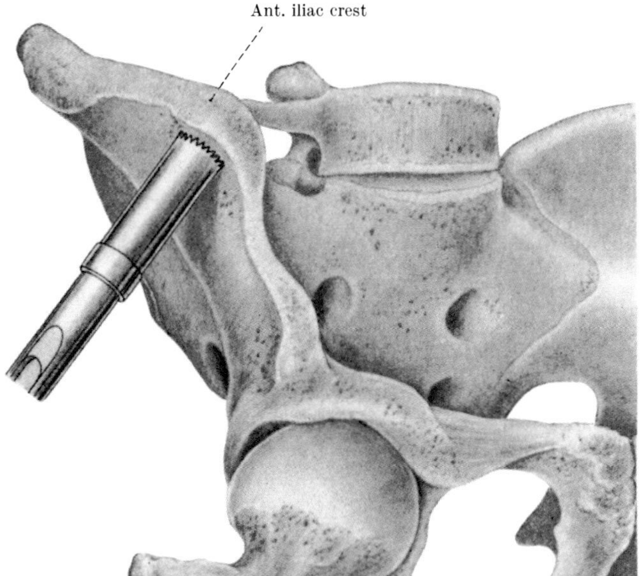

Fig. 279. Anterior cervical fusion (Cloward procedure) for herniated disc or spondylosis: Taking dowel graft from iliac crest.

Observe: The dowel cutter is placed 2—3 mm. below the crest of the ilium to obtain as long a dowel as possible with cortical bone on both ends.

Chapter XXV

Lumbar Radiculoneuropathy

Herniated Intervertebral Disc

The outstanding symptom associated with compression of a nerve root by a herniated lumbar disc is pain radiating down the posterolateral aspect of the lower extremity. The key physical finding in examining such a patient is reproduction of this pain on elevating the leg with the knee extended. In addition to pain, compression of the lumbosacral nerve roots will produce radiculopathy characterized by numbness, weakness and/or loss of deep tendon reflexes.

Lumbar intervertebral discs commonly protrude or extrude posterolaterally (Fig. 280). When this is the case, the disc presses on a specific nerve root with resulting characteristic signs and symptoms of pain and neuropathy in one lower extremity. However, lumbar discs may also herniated in the midline causing symptoms and signs in both lower extremities as well as bowel or bladder dysfunction.

The lowest two lumbar interspaces, i.e. L_{4-5} and L_5—S_1, are the most common sites for herniated intervertebral discs. Characteristically protrusion or extrusion of the L_5—S_1 disc causes compression of the S_1 nerve root with resulting hypalgesia along the lateral surface of the foot, weakness in plantar flexion and depression of the Achilles reflex. However, it is possible for herniations of this disc to impinge on the L_5 nerve. Conversely, although pathology at the L_{4-5} level is most commonly associated with L_5 radiculopathy, i.e. hypalgesia over the dorsum of the foot and weakness of dorsiflexion, herniation at this level may compromise the S_1 nerve root as well. By virtue of a similar anatomical explanation, symptoms suggestive of a L_4 radiculoneuropathy, such as pain in the anterior thigh, hypalgesia on the medial side of the calf and foot, weakness of the knee extensors and depression of the knee jerk, may be associated with either a L_{3-4} or an L_{4-5} herniated disc. Fig. 281 is an anatomical topographic presentation of the common locations for ruptured discs. It illustrates the relationship of the thecal sac and nerve roots to the vertebral bodies and interspaces.

Because of the above mentioned variations, a myelogram is a very helpful preoperative localizing test. In our experience, 15 percent of patients with a herniated lumbar disc will have a normal myelogram. Usually these false negative myelograms are seen in patients with a relatively wide epidural space due to a small thecal sac. A myelogram for lumbar disc disease should always be done with at least nine cc. of contrast material. Films are taken in the A-P, lateral and both oblique views. The patient should be brought to a standing position using the fluoroscopy table. The contrast material must always be carried superiorly as high as T-10 to visualize the conus medullaris.

An electromyogram is not necessary in the routine patient but may be very helpful in cases involving litigation or compensation. Discography, in our opinion, only confuses the situation.

As mentioned previously, the myelogram is not done to decide whether to operate but where to operate. The decision as to when and whether to operate can almost always be made on clinical grounds. Operation without delay is indicated in patients with bladder dysfunction, progressive neurological impairment and intractable pain. Other patients are treated surgically only after conservative treatment has failed.

Most unilateral lumbar discs can be removed by an interlaminar procedure with only very minimal bone removal. This operation is illustrated in this chapter. Quite frequently enough bone of the rostral lamina must be removed to gain adequate exposure so that the operation is termed a semi-hemi-laminectomy. When two adjacent interspaces are explored, some surgeons prefer a hemilaminectomy. Total laminectomy is indicated for midline discs in which the patient has symptoms in both lower extremities and for lumbar stenosis.

As in all neurological surgery, it is essential that the surgeon supervises the positioning of the patient on the operating table. This is crucial in this most common of all neurosurgical operations. After endotracheal anesthesia has been instituted, the patient is placed in the prone position on chest rolls as illustrated in Fig. 282. The operating table is then flexed. Supporting sand bags and pillows must not compress the chest or abdomen over the areas indicated in red on Fig. 283. Respiratory movements must not be impaired, and venous obstruction must be avoided. The very distensible epidural veins will become markedly enlarged if the return of venous blood to the heart is impeded by improper positioning of the patient. This can convert a relatively simple surgical procedure into a nightmare of uncontrollable bleeding with obliteration of normal anatomical structures. Attention to simple details, such as this, is of great importance in all surgical exercises; and this operation is no exception.

In an obese patient whose abdomen cannot be kept uncompressed in the prone position, the lateral decubitus position is preferable. This position presents no added difficulty to the surgeon and is used routinely in all patients by some neurosurgeons.

With the patient properly positioned, x-rays of the lumbosacral spine, as well as the myelogram, are reviewed for the last time. The surgeon must be as familiar with the patient's skeletal structure as he is with the patient's name. The number of lumbar vertebrae must be carefully counted, and the level of the iliac crest should be noted. The possibility of spina bifida should always be kept in mind and looked for on the x-ray. The cauda equina is too often injured by surgeons stripping back the paravertebral muscles without recognizing the presence of a spina bifida.

A midline vertical skin incision is made from over the spinous of L_3 to the sacrum. The fascia is also incised in the midline, and the spinous processes on the side of the lesion are denuded of tendinous attachments by sharp dissection. Using a sharp, broad periosteal elevator, the spinous processes and lamina are stripped of all soft tissue. This subperiosteal elevation should begin at the lowest level and proceed rostrally. Once the lamina is cleared to the facet joint, a gauze sponge is used over the periosteal elevator to aid in hemostasis as well as elevation of the soft tissues. Various types of specially designed retractors are then used to maintain the exposure.

In identifying the vertebral level, the count must always begin at the sacrum. If the level of S_1 is at all in question, the spinous process can be grasped with a towel-clip and movement between adjacent vertebrae evaluated. Obviously, if either lumbarization of S_1 or sacralization of L_5 is present, the surgeon must be aware of it while identifying the level of the lesion.

Having located the appropriate level, any remaining muscle or adipose tissue is removed from between the two lamina to expose the ligamentum flavum. This ligament, which passes from the posterior surface of the lower lamina to the under surface of the lamina above, can be more completely exposed by removing the overhanging rim of the superior lamina. The ligamentum flavum is incised as close to the midline as possible. As soon as the knife blade goes through the ligament, tiny cotton paddies are inserted to protect the dura. The incision of the ligament is then completed along the bone margins (Figs. 284 and 285). After the bulk of the ligament has been sharply excised, the margins of the interlaminar exposure can be enlarged using sharp Kerrison rongeurs (Fig. 286). In removing the ligamentum flavum, it is well to remember that this ligament constitutes the medial wall of the facet joint capsule (Fig. 280). Therefore, as the ligament is removed laterally, the facet joint should not be opened. Opening this joint almost invariably results from using a Kerrison rongeur as a tugging rather than a biting instrument and usually results in a marked increase in post-operative back discomfort for the patient.

The epidural fat should not be removed nor coagulated. It can be displaced very easily, and preserving this tissue reduces postoperative adhesions. Using a fine blunt spatula, palpation is carried out in the lateral gutter beginning as far superiorly as possible. Beginning this dissection rostrally will avoid getting into the axilla of the stretched out nerve root. The nerve root is gradually retracted medially to expose the level of the interspace. At this stage of the operation, the goal is only to locate the epidural mass (Fig. 287). If the nerve root is stretched over the mass so tightly that it cannot be easily displaced, the table should be deflexed slightly. The nerve root is retracted medially and held in this position by a nerve root retractor (Fig. 288). If a fragment of disc material has extruded through the posterior longitudinal ligament, it is removed. Palpation is then carried out into the neural foramen looking for additional free fragments. If none are found then the epidural space may be filled superiorly and inferiorly with small cottonoids to tamponade the epidural veins and to widen the exposure. These cotton pledgets must not exert enough pressure on the dural sac to compress the nerve roots within it. A cruciate incision is made into the posterior longitudinal ligament and the interspace is entered. The interspace is cleaned out of all degenerated disc material using pituitary forceps and various sized curettes. The interspace is curetted in a systematic manner moving the curette about the confines of the disc space in a clockwise manner. A sharp curette can be a dangerous instrument and must always be used with both hands. The cartilaginous plates of both the superior and inferior vertebral surfaces are broken down with the curette and removed with the forceps. An angulated curette will especially be of aid in breaking down medially situated fragments. The forceps should not be inserted into the interspace deeper than the hinge controlling movements of the biting cups. A rim of annulus fibrosis is left anteriorly and laterally to prevent violation of the retroperitoneal vascular and viseral structures. At the L_{4-5} interspace the common iliac artery is especially vulnerable. If a bony spur is associated with the herniated nucleus pulposus, it should also be removed. These spurs can most safely be removed by breaking the spur into the interspace using a sharp dental chisel or an electric drill.

The adequacy of the disc removal from the interspace can be checked by irrigating normal saline into the disc space while holding a sucker in the space. If all disc material has been removed, the sucker will remove the fluid as rapidly as it can be instilled. On the other hand, if fragments of disc material occlude the orifice of the sucker, additional work is indicated. Having completely cleaned out the interspace, attention is once again directed to the epidural space. Using a right-angle dural separator, the epidural space is palpated above and below the nerve root well out into the neural foramen (Figs. 289 and 290). Palpation must also be carried medially beneath the dural sac to make certain that a midline mass is not left behind. Finally, palpation is also done superiorly after all cotton pledgets have been removed. The position of the nerve root leaving at the interspace above must be kept in mind. Review of Fig. 281 will clarify how close this nerve root is to the area from which the disc has just been removed.

If at any point in the procedure the dura has been inadvertantly violated, it should be repaired. Ignoring dural defects may lead to the formation of pseudomeningoceles or cerebrospinal fluid leakage through the wound. Usually a few fine sutures can be used to close the dura. If the dural laceration is in an inaccessible area, the dural opening should be enlarged and covered with an absorbable gelatin strip.

The table is now straightened out. This maneuver is often very helpful in stopping all epidural bleeding and will also make reapproximation of the wound easier. The wound is closed in layers using non-absorbable material such as silk or wire.

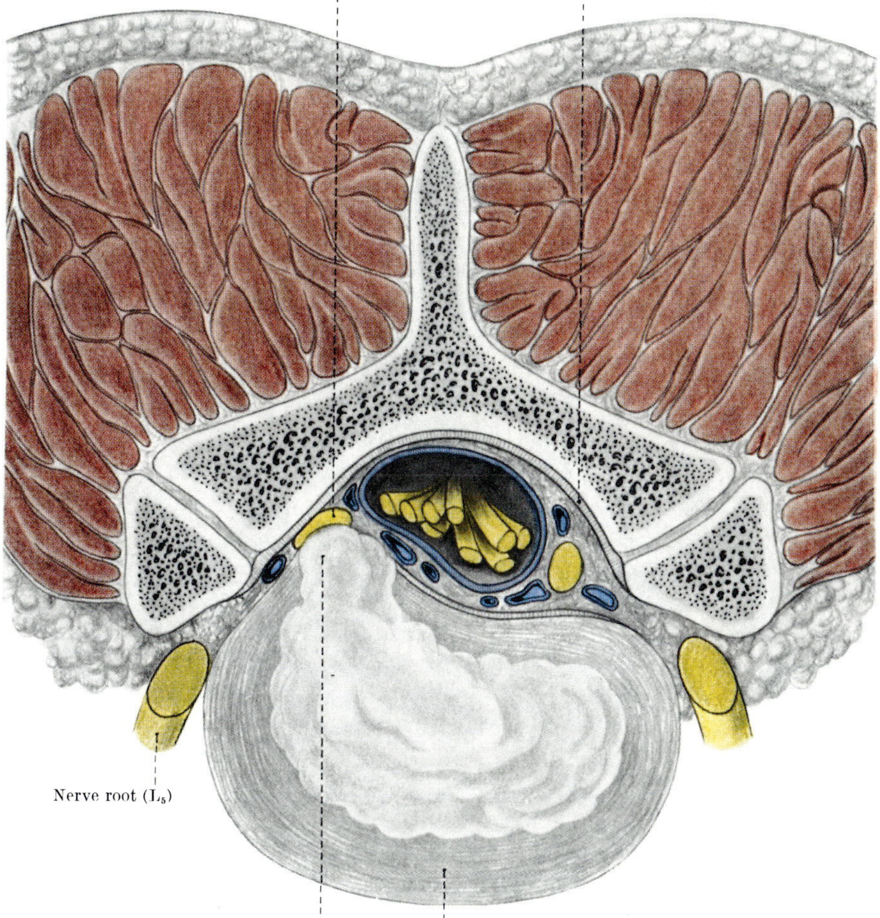

Fig. 280. Lumbar disc: Cross section at level of fifth (L_5—S_1) lumbar intervertebral disc. *Observe:* 1. Ligamentum flavum forms medial wall of articular capsule. 2. Relationship of L_5 nerve root and lateral margin of the disc.

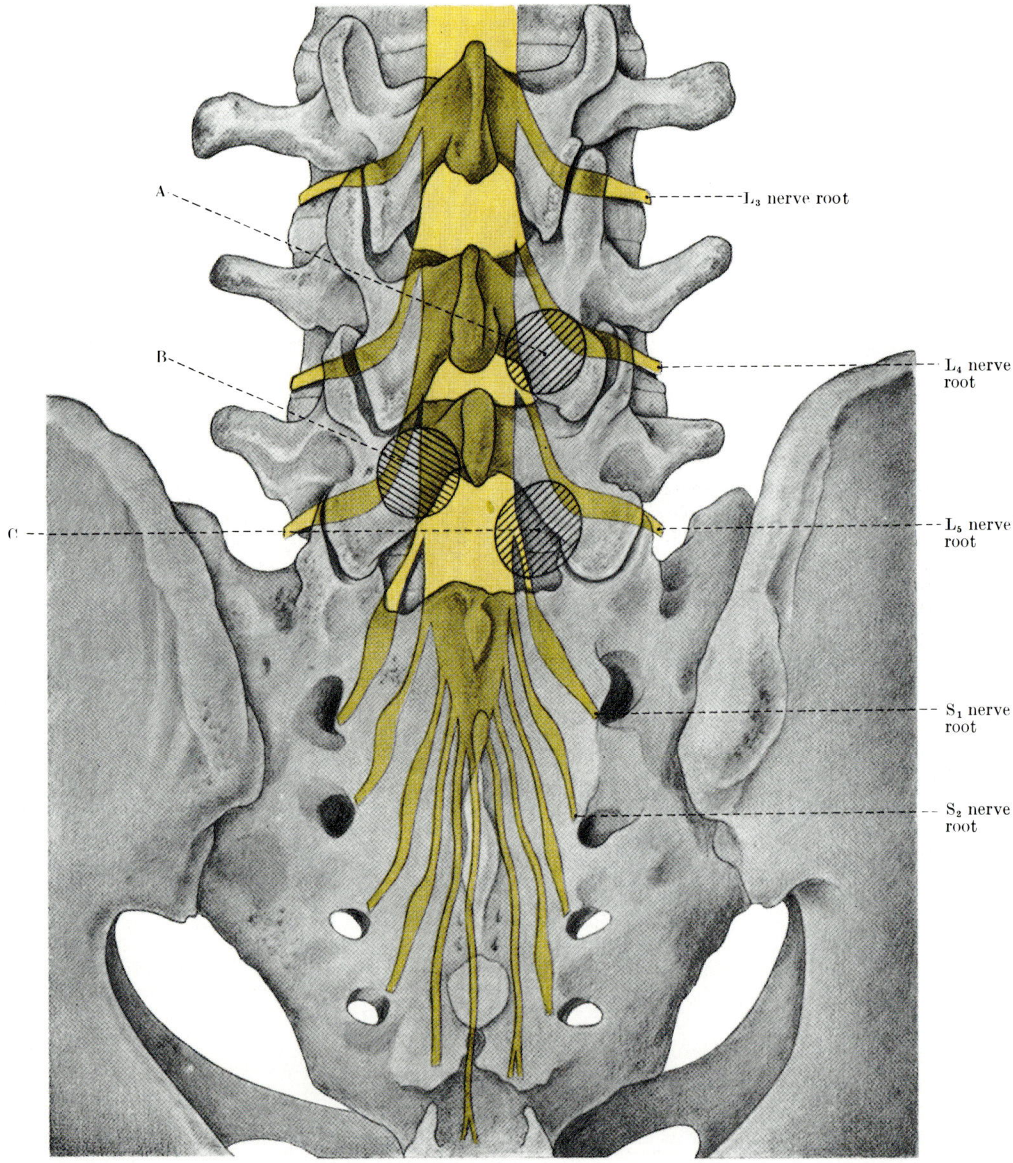

Fig. 281. Lumbar disc: Anatomical-topographical presentation of lumbosacral spine to show the relationship of the thecal sac and nerve roots to the intervertebral disc spaces and foramina.

Observe: 1. At *A* a protruding disc will compress the L_4 nerve root laterally and the L_5 nerve root medially. 2. At *B* a superiorly placed herniated nucleus pulposus of the L_5—S_1 interspace may compress only the L_5 nerve root. 3. At *C* a ruptured nucleus pulposus of the L_5—S_1 interspace may compress the L_5, S_1 and S_2 nerve roots.

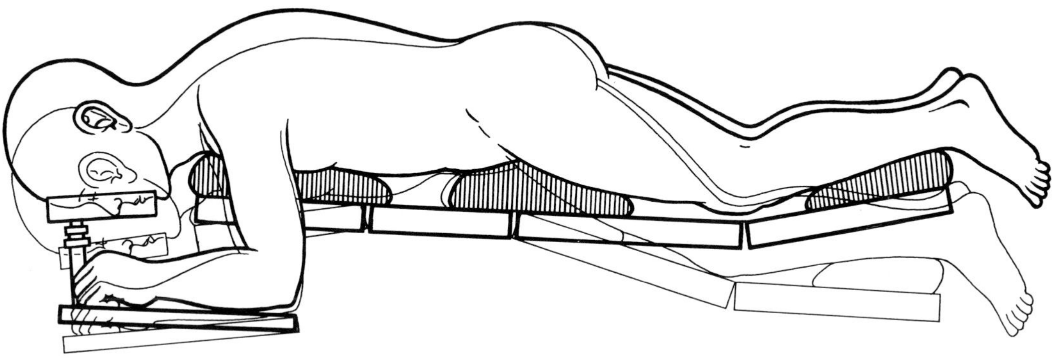

Fig. 282. Lumbar disc: Operative position.

Observe: 1. Prone jacknife position. 2. Placement of pillows beneath patient (compare with Fig. 283).

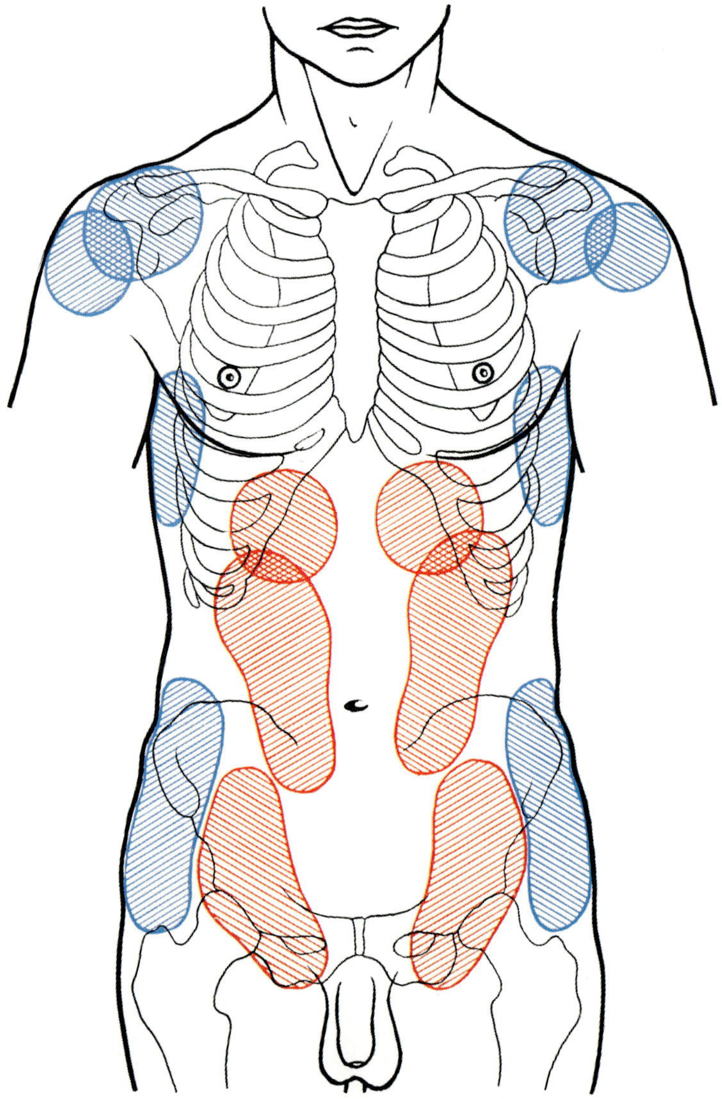

Fig. 283. Lumbar disc. Anterior surface of body showing pressure points to use (blue) and to avoid (red) in the prone position. Compression over red areas will obstruct venous passways and force distension of epidural veins.

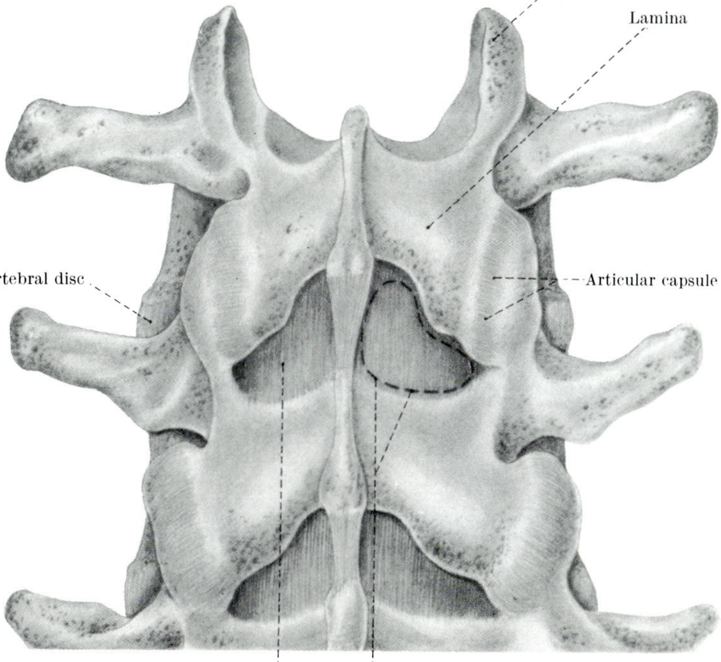

Fig. 284. Lumbar disc: Exposure of lamina and interlaminar space.
Observe: Dotted line indicates extent of the removal of the ligamentum flavum.

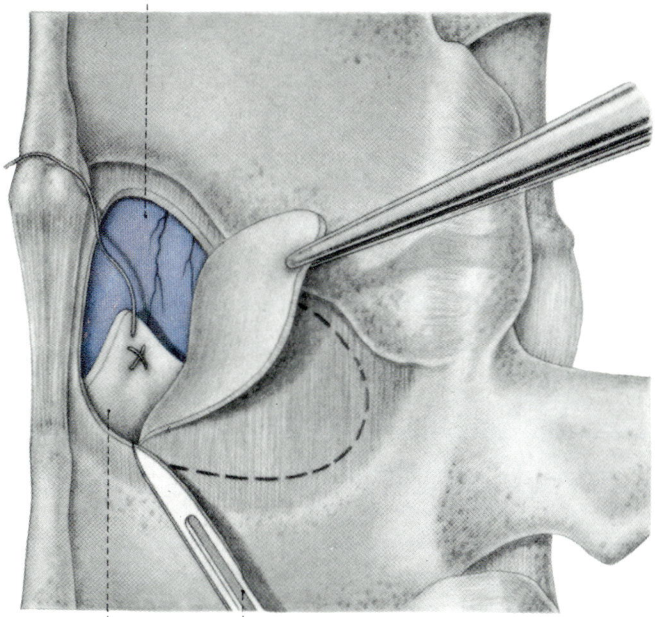

Fig. 285. Lumbar disc: Excision of ligamentum flavum.
Observe: 1. Incision of ligamentum flavum is begun medially.
2. A cotton pledget protects the dura.

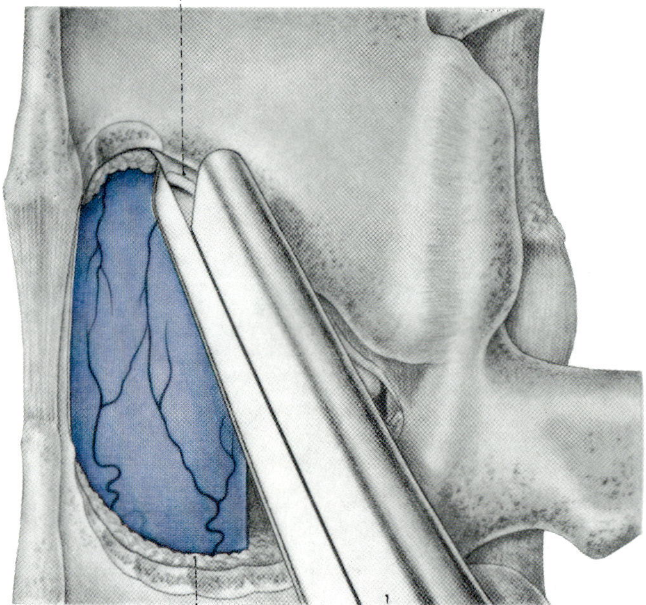

Fig. 286. Lumbar disc: Enlargement of the interlaminar exposure by removing a small portion of both the superior and inferior lamina.

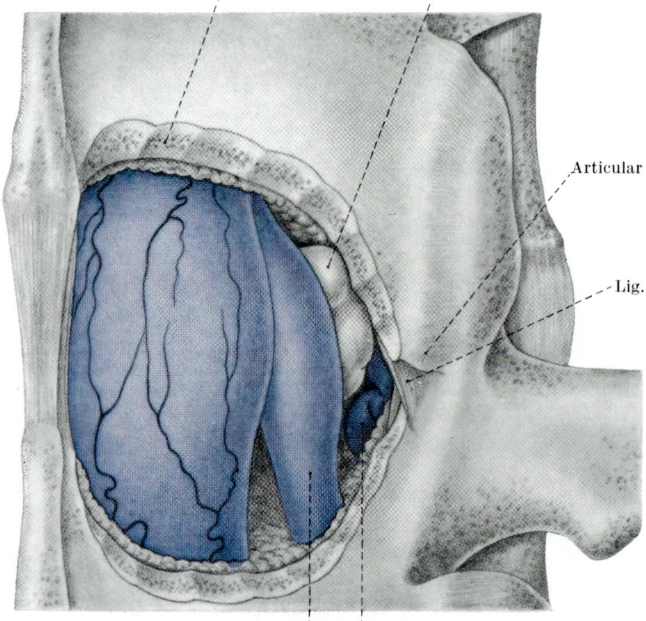

Fig. 287. Lumbar disc: Exposure following removal of bone and ligamentum flavum.

Observe: The ligamentum flavum is left intact close to the articular capsule.

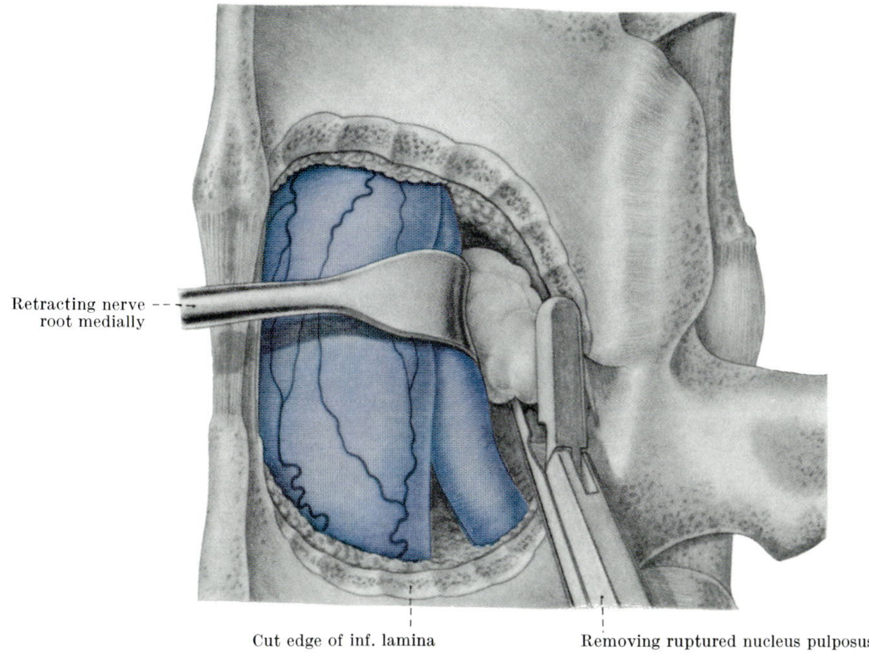

Fig. 288. Lumbar disc: Removal of the disc by pituitary forceps.
Observe: The exiting nerve root is retracted medially.

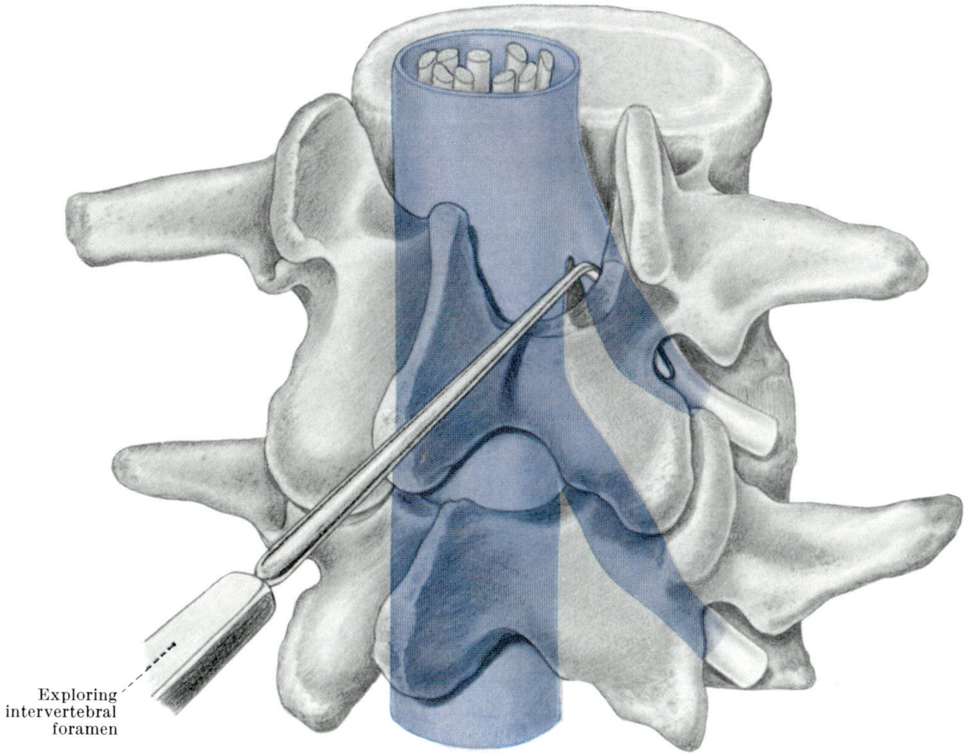

Fig. 289. Lumbar disc: Exploring intervertebral foramen after removal of disc.
Observe: Probe is guided dorsal to the nerve root through the intervertebral foramen.

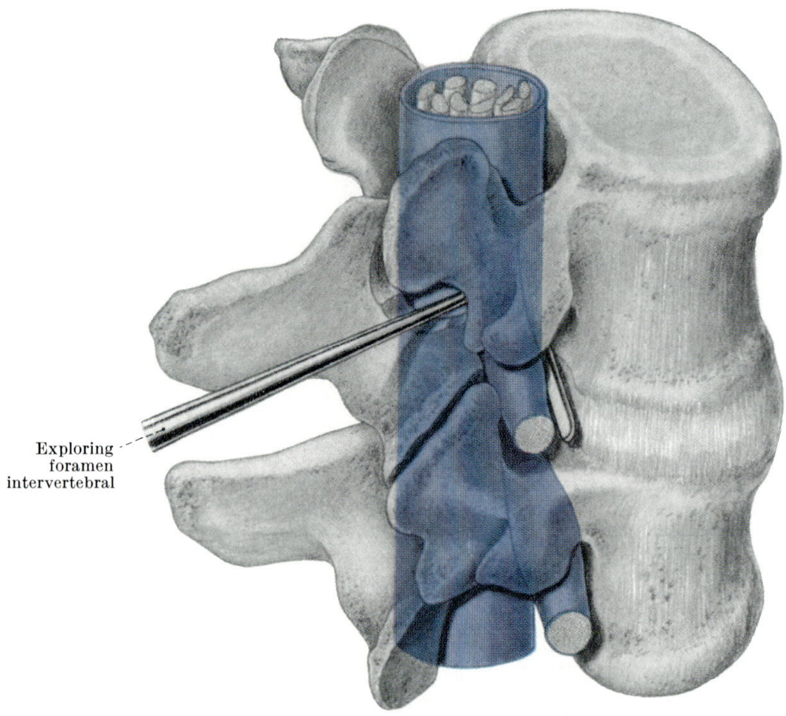

Fig. 290. Lumbar disc: Exploring intervertebral foramen after removal of disc. *Observe:* Probe is guided anterior to the nerve root.

Subject Index

Italics refer to figure numbers. Normal type refers to page numbers.

Universitätsdruckerei H. Stürtz AG Würzburg